Patient-Centered Care Series

Series Editors

Moira Stewart,
Judith Belle Brown
and
Thomas R Freeman

Patient-Centered Medicine

Transforming the clinical method

Second edition

**Moira Stewart,
Judith Belle Brown,
W Wayne Weston,
Ian R McWhinney,
Carol L McWilliam
and
Thomas R Freeman**

Radcliffe Medical Press

Radcliffe Medical Press Ltd
18 Marcham Road
Abingdon
Oxon OX14 1AA
United Kingdom

www.radcliffe-oxford.com
The Radcliffe Medical Press electronic catalogue and online ordering facility.
Direct sales to anywhere in the world.

British Library Cataloguing in Publication Data

A catalogue record for this book is available from The British Library.

ISBN 13: 978 1 85775 981 5

Typeset by Aarontype Ltd, Easton, Bristol
Printed and bound by TJI Digital, Padstow, Cornwall

Contents

Preface

Whereas the essential and interactive components of the patient-centered clinical method remain unchanged, this second edition of the book on patient-centered medicine demonstrates how the clinical method has evolved in both depth and breadth. For example, the centrality of finding common ground with patients, within the framework of patient-centered care, is more fully examined. As well, understanding the whole person now includes ecosystem health. Teaching the patient-centered clinical method has now gained international recognition and with this the learner-centered method of medical education assumes an important role. In addition, the application of a patient-centered curriculum, now a reality, is described. Research on the patient-centered clinical method, both qualitative and quantitative, has made significant strides in the past ten years and is reflected in this book.

This book is divided into four parts. The first section contains an introduction to the patient-centered clinical method including its evolution and relationship to other models of communication. In addition, common misconceptions about the meaning of patient-centeredness are elucidated. The second chapter in this section is a historic perspective written by Ian R McWhinney.

The second section of the book describes the six interactive components of the patient-centered clinical method. Chapters 3 to 9 elaborate in detail components one to six respectively. The clinical reader will notice the cases illustrating each of the six components of the patient-centered approach which are embedded in Chapters 3 to 9. Those most interested in the application of patient-centeredness in everyday practice might enjoy reading the cases first. As McWhinney (2001: 88) has wisely noted, 'an actual case brings things alive for us in a way that aggregated data cannot do'. Taken together the cases represent a typical series of patients in the practice of a busy doctor. All the cases are based on actual clinical encounters; however, the names, dates and places have been altered to ensure the confidentiality of the participants.

The third section, on teaching and learning, contains six chapters. The first chapter examines the context of medical education (Chapter 10). The parallel between the learner-centered method of medical education and patient-centered practice is described in Chapter 11. Practicing, learning and teaching patient-centered medicine has many personal, professional and systemic challenges as Chapter 12 illustrates. Chapter 13 contains details on teaching strategies and practical tips, for teaching the patient-centered clinical method. A particular teaching tool, the patient-centered case presentation is described in Chapter 14.

The final chapter in this section, Chapter 15, describes the development, implementation and evaluation of a patient-centered curriculum. Again, there are cases embedded in these chapters, this time involving patients, learners and teachers, serving to illustrate teaching the patient-centered clinical method.

The fourth section, on research, combines reviews of relevant literature with findings from recent studies. Qualitative and quantitative methodologies are represented. Chapter 16 presents a description of qualitative findings which illuminate the patient-centered clinical method. Chapter 17 is a review of quantitative studies correlating communication with a variety of healthcare outcomes, demonstrating the effectiveness of the patient-centered components. Chapter 18 describes a measure we have developed which uniquely assesses encounters according to the patient-centered clinical method. In Chapter 19 we present measures of patient perceptions of patient-centered care and their use in research and education. Finally, in Chapter 20 we show results of recent studies using the measures described in Chapters 18 and 19.

In the final chapter we conclude with a view on the future and, taking into account the steps already taken, we consider some possible new visions and challenges for patient-centered practice, teaching and research.

Moira Stewart
Judith Belle Brown
W Wayne Weston
Ian R McWhinney
Carol L McWilliam
Thomas R Freeman
February 2003

About the authors

Judith Belle Brown, PhD in Social Work from Smith College, Northampton, Massachusetts is a Professor in the Centre for Studies in Family Medicine, Department of Family Medicine, at The University of Western Ontario (UWO), and in the School of Social Work at King's College, London, Ontario, Canada. She has been conducting research on the patient-centered clinical method for over two decades. Dr Brown has presented papers and conducted workshops both nationally (Canada and the United States) and internationally (UK, Holland, Spain, Hong Kong, Sweden, New Zealand, Denmark, Australia) on the patient-centered method. Dr Brown has coordinated courses on patient-centered communication at UWO at the undergraduate, postgraduate and masters levels. Dr Brown is an Editor of the book *Challenges and Solutions in Patient-Centered Care: a casebook* and is a Series Editor along with Moira Stewart and Thomas R Freeman of *Substance Abuse: a patient-centered approach, Chronic Fatigue Syndrome: a patient-centered approach, Chronic Myofascial Pain: a patient-centered approach* and *Eating Disorders: a patient-centered approach*. She has also published papers dealing with patient–doctor communication in *Social Science and Medicine, Family Practice: An International Journal, Patient Education and Counseling, Canadian Family Physician* and *Journal of Family Practice*. Dr Brown was a recipient of The American Academy on Physician and Patient Award for Outstanding Research in 1996. In the same year, Dr Brown was made an Honorary Member of the College of Family Physicians of Canada.

Thomas R Freeman BSc, MD, MClSc, CCFP, FCFP is a medical graduate of The University of Western Ontario, London, Ontario, Canada and completed his residency training in Family Medicine at Dalhousie University, Halifax, Nova Scotia, Canada. After practicing in a small town in southwestern Ontario for 11 years, during which time he was involved with undergraduate education on a part-time basis, he moved to a full time academic practice at The University of Western Ontario in 1989. He is currently Professor and Chair of the Department of Family Medicine at UWO. Areas of research interest include vaccine adverse effects, risk perception and risk communication and patients' use of metaphor. He has published in *Journal of Family Practice, Family Practice: An International Journal* and the *Canadian Medical Association Journal* and is a Series Editor along with Moira Stewart and Judith Belle Brown of *Substance Abuse: a patient-centred approach, Chronic Fatigue Syndrome: a patient-centered approach,*

Chronic Myofascial Pain: a patient-centered approach and *Eating Disorders: a patient-centered approach*.

Ian R McWhinney, OC, MD, FCFP, FRCP, is Professor Emeritus in the Department of Family Medicine at The University of Western Ontario, London, Ontario, Canada. He was born in Burnley, Lancashire and educated at Cambridge University and St Bartholemew's Hospital Medical School. For 14 years he was a General Practitioner in Stratford-on-Avon. In 1968 he was appointed Foundation Professor of Family Medicine at The University of Western Ontario. He retired in 1992 and now has a post-retirement appointment in the Centre for Studies in Family Medicine. His most recent book, a second edition of *A Textbook of Family Medicine*, was published by Oxford University Press in 1997.

Carol L McWilliam, MScN, EdD, is a Professor in the School of Nursing, Faculty of Health Sciences, at The University of Western Ontario, London, Ontario, Canada, with adjunct appointments in the Department of Family Medicine and School of Occupational Therapy. She conducts research in the areas of health promotion and health services delivery, with a focus on professional–patient and interprofessional communication. She makes a unique contribution to the field as a qualitative research methodologist, with work published in *Social Science and Medicine*, *Family Medicine*, *Patient Education and Counseling*, the *Journal of Advanced Nursing*, the *International Journal of Quality in Health Care* and the *International Journal of Health Promotion*.

Leslie Meredith, MEd from the University of Ottawa, Ottawa, Ontario, Canada is a research associate with the Centre for Studies in Family Medicine, the Department of Family Medicine, at The University of Western Ontario (UWO), London, Ontario, Canada. She has been assisting in primary care research projects for the past five years and has been a co-investigator on two grants related to communication skills and online education. She has also given presentations regarding patient–physician communication and published three papers in the area.

Bridget L Ryan received her MSc in Epidemiology and Biostatistics from The University of Western Ontario, London, Ontario, Canada. She is a project coordinator with the Centre for Studies in Family Medicine, Department of Family Medicine at The University of Western Ontario. She has been involved in primary care research projects including the evaluation of family physician integration into acute home care and the assessment of patient-centered communication. She has also been a co-author on a manual for assessing patient-centered communication.

Moira Stewart PhD. is a Professor in the Department of Family Medicine and Director of the Centre for Studies in Family Medicine at The University of Western Ontario, London, Ontario, Canada. She is an epidemiologist who, for the past 25 years, has conducted research on primary care health services and on communication between patients and doctors. She has published numerous articles in *Social Science and Medicine, Medical Care, Journal of Family Practice, Family Practice: An International Journal, Canadian Medical Association Journal, Journal of the Royal College of General Practitioners* and the *British Medical Journal*. She has been particularly active in fostering an international network of teachers and scientists of communication in medicine, and has published two books on the topic, *Communicating with Medical Patients* and *Patient-Centered Medicine: transforming the clinical method*. Dr Stewart is an Editor of the book *Challenges and Solutions in Patient-Centered Care: a casebook* and is a Series Editor along with Judith Belle Brown and Thomas R Freeman of *Substance Abuse: a patient-centered approach, Chronic Fatigue Syndrome: a patient-centered approach, Chronic Myofascial Pain: a patient-centered approach* and *Eating Disorders: a patient-centered approach*. As a leader in the application of a wide variety of research methodologies in primary care, she was part of a team which sponsored five International Symposia and edited five widely used books in a series called Foundations of Primary Care Research. She is an Honorary Member of the College of Family Physicians of Canada (1991), received a Woman of Distinction Award for London, Ontario (1993), is a recipient of The American Academy on Physician and Patient Award for Outstanding Research (1996) and the Dean's Award of Excellence for Research (2000).

W Wayne Weston MD, CCFP, FCFP, is a Professor of Family Medicine in the Faculty of Medicine and Dentistry, The University of Western Ontario (UWO), London, Ontario, Canada. After graduating from the University of Toronto in 1964, he practiced in Tavistock, Ontario, for ten years before joining the faculty at UWO. He has a special interest in patient–physician communication and faculty development and has been a leader in the development of two large educational projects involving the five Ontario medical schools – the EFPO (Educating Future Physicians for Ontario) Project and Project CREATE (Curriculum Renewal and Evaluation of Addiction Training and Education). He currently serves as a consultant to the Dean on faculty development. He has published over 130 articles and book chapters in such journals as *Canadian Family Physician, Canadian Medical Association Journal* and *Academic Medicine*. Dr Weston is an Editor of the book *Challenges and Solutions in Patient-Centered Care: a casebook*. He has led over 200 workshops for faculty on patient-centered interviewing, problem-based learning, and clinical teaching in Canada, New Zealand, Scotland and the United States. He received the Award for Excellence in Teaching from The University of Western Ontario, the Dean's award of excellence for teaching, the prestigious 3M Award for Excellence in Teaching In Canada and is the first recipient of the McWhinney award for education presented by the College of Family Physicians of Canada and the first family physician to receive the Canadian Association for Medical Education award for distinguished contributions to medical education.

Acknowledgments

We thank the Department of Family Medicine at The University of Western Ontario for providing a supportive environment in which to write this book. In particular we want to express our gratitude to Dr Brian K E Hennen, Chair of the Department of Family Medicine (from 1987 to 1999) for his encouragement of scholarly activities.

We are indebted to our patients and research participants who generously shared their stories of suffering and coping with suffering; our colleagues who shared their stories of caring for patients, exposing both their failures as well as their triumphs; and our students who stimulated our thinking on patient-centered care and encouraged us to clarify the concepts.

Andrea Burt's combination of coordination skills and perpetual aura of calm has been indispensable. Her attention to detail and organizational abilities are extraordinary. Magda Catani has tirelessly worked on many drafts of this manuscript. She has been a steadfast assistant and remained committed to the project throughout the process. We also wish to thank Claire Button, Evelyn Levy and Joanna Asuncion for their help in the final stages of preparing this book.

We would like to extend our sincere thanks to Gillian Nineham and her incredible team at Radcliffe Medical Press Ltd. They have all been fabulous to work with.

Finally, we would like to express our heartfelt appreciation for all the support and encouragement provided by our families, in particular Bonnie and Murray Brown, Kathleen Stewart, Kate and Amy Freeman and Sharon Weston.

The work was conducted in the Thames Valley Family Practice Research Unit, which is supported by the Ministry of Health and Long-Term Care of Ontario as a Health System-Linked Research Unit. The ideas and conclusions contained in this book are those of the authors, and no endorsement by the Ministry is intended or should be inferred.

Dedication

This book is dedicated to Joseph H Levenstein MD, for his inspiration to the authors and his outstanding contribution to the practice of medicine. We are grateful to Dr Levenstein for introducing us to the patient-centered clinical method during his time as a visiting professor in our Department in 1981–1982.

PART ONE

Overview

Introduction

Judith Belle Brown, Moira Stewart, W Wayne Weston and Thomas R Freeman

In the 1980s, when the patient-centered clinical method was first being concep-
tualized and used in research and education, it was at the periphery of medicine
(Brown *et al.*, 1986; Brown *et al.*, 1989; Levenstein *et al.*, 1986; Stewart *et al.*,
1986; Stewart *et al.*, 1989; Weston *et al.*, 1989). Indeed, patient-centered medicine was viewed by many educators and researchers as a 'soft science' – caring
and compassion were acknowledged to be important aspects of humanitarian
care but few people were aware of the pivotal role of patient-centered communication in modern scientific medicine. In the first edition of this book, we
described the full patient-centered clinical method, with the goal of placing it
at the epicenter of clinical practice and medical education (Stewart *et al.*, 1995).

Since that time we have learned much by presenting the patient-centered
clinical method to many groups of medical students, residents, graduate
fellows, community physicians and medical school faculties across North
America, Europe, Australia, New Zealand and South East Asia. The patient-
centered clinical method now forms the basis of many educational curricula
internationally, at both the undergraduate and graduate level. Furthermore,
the patient-centered clinical method serves as the guide for the summative
evaluation of postgraduate training in several countries (Brown *et al.*, 1996;
Tate *et al.*, 1999). Research, focusing on the patient-centered clinical method,
has exploded in the past decade. International studies reinforce not only the
patients' desire for, and satisfaction with, patient-centered care, but also
the positive impact of such care on patient outcomes and healthcare utilization
(Little *et al.*, 2001b; Stewart *et al.*, 2000). These studies support an emerging
international definition of patient-centered care.

Patients want patient-centred care which (a) explores the patients' main
reason for the visit, concerns, and need for information; (b) seeks an integrated understanding of the patients' world – that is, their whole person,
emotional needs, and life issues; (c) finds common ground on what the

problem is and mutually agrees on management; (d) enhances prevention and health promotion; and (e) enhances the continuing relationship between the patient and the doctor. (Stewart, 2001:445)

Given this growing international consensus, the advances in medical education and the accumulating research evidence, the patient-centered model has indeed transformed the clinical method. After 20 years of study and practice, patient-centered care is moving to a central role in healthcare. As biomedical technology proceeds exponentially, what is curious, and indeed compelling, about the interaction between the patient and doctor, is that the fundamental premises remain constant. Indeed, patients continue to expect patient-centered care; it has stood the test of time. As such, so has the theoretical framework of the patient-centered clinical model. In particular, patients notice and resent when biotechnology takes over the agenda of the visit between a doctor and a patient, thus minimizing the importance of the patient's unique personal story. Furthermore, one current area of biomedical research, medical genetics, strongly supports the principle of treating each patient uniquely with a tailored management plan. Patient-centered care and medical genetics go hand in hand in recognising that quality care is as unique as the individual patient.

The patient-centered clinical method

The Department of Family Medicine at The University of Western Ontario began work on the patient–doctor relationship at its inception with the arrival in 1968 of the inaugural Chairperson, Dr Ian R McWhinney. His work elucidating the 'real reason' the patient presented to the doctor (McWhinney, 1972) set the stage for explorations of the breadth of all patient problems, whether physical, social or psychological, and depth, the meaning of the patient's presentation. The research of his PhD student, Moira Stewart, was guided by these interests and began to focus on the patient–physician relationship (Stewart *et al.*, 1975; Stewart *et al.*, 1979; Stewart and Buck, 1977). In 1982, the Department was stimulated by Dr Joseph Levenstein who, as a visiting professor of family medicine from South Africa, shared with us his attempts to develop a model of practice. The patient-centered clinical method evolved further through the work of the Patient–Doctor Communication Group at The University of Western Ontario.

In this book the patient-centered model and method is described and explained. A program of conceptual development, education and research which has been underway for the last two decades provides the material. Although the program took place in the context of family medicine, its messages are relevant to all disciplines of medicine and to other healthcare professions such as nursing, social work and physiotherapy. The overarching framework is the model. The way of implementing the framework reflects the clinical method. This book presents both a framework and its implementation, the patient-centered clinical method.

Patient-centered care presupposes several changes in the mindset of the clinician. First, the hierarchical notion of the professional being in charge and the patient being passive does not hold here. To be patient-centered, the practitioner must be able to empower the patient, share the power in the relationship,

---

Box 1.1 The six interactive components of the patient-centered process

1   Exploring both the disease and the illness experience
  - History, physical, lab
  - Dimensions of illness (feelings, ideas, effects on function and expectations)

2   Understanding the whole person
  - The person (e.g. life history, personal and developmental issues)
  - The proximal context (e.g. family, employment, social support)
  - The distal context (e.g. culture, community, ecosystem)

3   Finding common ground
  - Problems and priorities
  - Goals of treatment and/or management
  - Roles of patient and doctor

4   Incorporating prevention and health promotion
  - Health enhancement
  - Risk avoidance
  - Risk reduction
  - Early identification
  - Complication reduction

5   Enhancing the patient–doctor relationship
  - Compassion
  - Power
  - Healing
  - Self-awareness
  - Transference and countertransference

6   Being realistic
  - Time and timing
  - Teambuilding and teamwork
  - Wise stewardship of resources

and this means renouncing control which traditionally has been in the hands of the professional. This is the moral imperative of patient-centered practice. In making this shift in values, the practitioner will experience the new direction the relationship can take when power is shared. Second, maintaining an objective stance in relation to patients produces an unacceptable insensitivity to human suffering. To be patient-centered requires a balance between the subjective and the objective, a bringing together of the mind and the body.

In this book we describe the six interacting components of the patient-centered clinical method, summarized in Box 1.1 and illustrated in Figure 1.1. The first three interacting components encompass the process between patient and doctor. The second three components focus more on the context within which the patient and clinician interact. Although components are used for ease in teaching and research, patient-centered clinical practice is a holistic concept in which components interact and unite in a unique way in each patient–doctor encounter.

The *first* component of the patient-centered clinical method is to assess the two conceptualizations of ill health – disease and illness. In addition to assessing the disease process by history and physical examination, the physician actively seeks to enter into the patient's world to understand his or her unique experience of illness. Specifically, the doctor explores patients' feelings about being ill, their ideas about the illness, how the illness is impacting on their functioning, and lastly what they expect from the physician.

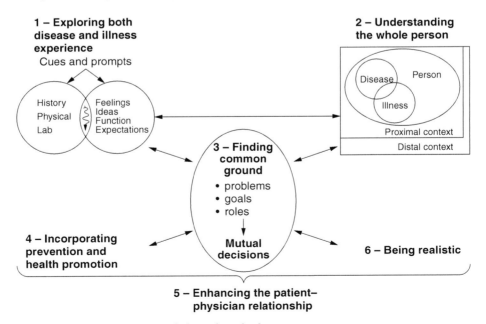

Figure 1.1   The patient-centered clinical method: six interactive components.

The *second* component is the integration of these concepts of disease and ill-ness with an understanding of the whole person. This includes an awareness of the multiple aspects of the patient's life, such as personality, developmental history, life cycle issues and the multiple contexts in which they live, including the ecosystem.

The mutual task of finding common ground between patient and doctor is the *third* component of the method and focuses on three key areas – defining the problem, establishing the goals of treatment and/or management, and identify-ing the roles to be assumed by patient and doctor.

The *fourth* component highlights the importance of using each contact as an opportunity for prevention and health promotion.

The *fifth* component emphasizes that each contact with the patient should be used to build on the patient–physician relationship by including compas-sion, trust, a sharing of power and healing. To enact these skills requires self-awareness as well as an appreciation of unconscious aspects of the relationship such as transference and countertransference.

The *sixth* component requires that, throughout the process, the clinician be realistic about time, participate in teambuilding and teamwork and recognize the importance of wise stewardship in accessing resources.

The patient-centered clinical method in relation to other models of communication

Models of practice are valuable in several ways: first, they guide our perceptions by drawing our attention to specific features of practice; next, they provide a framework for understanding what is going on; third, they guide our actions by defining what is important. A productive model will not only simplify the complexity of reality but will focus our attention on those aspects of a situation that are most important for understanding and effective action. The dominant model in medical practice has been labeled 'the conventional medical model'. No one would question the widespread influence of the conventional medical model; but it has often been challenged for oversimplifying the problems of sick-ness (Odegaard, 1986; White, 1988). Engel (1977: 130) describes the problems with the conventional medical model this way:

It assumes disease to be fully accounted for by deviations from the norm of measurable biological (somatic) variables. It leaves no room within its frame-work for the social, psychological, and behavioral dimensions of illness. The biomedical model not only requires that disease be dealt with as an entity independent of social behavior, it also demands that behavioral aberrations be explained on the basis of disordered somatic (biochemical or neurophysiological) processes.

The term 'patient-centered medicine' was introduced by Balint and colleagues (Balint *et al.*, 1970) who contrasted it with 'illness-centered medicine'. An understanding of the patient's complaints, based on patient-centered thinking, was called 'overall diagnosis', and an understanding based on disease-centered thinking was called 'traditional diagnosis'. The clinical method was elaborated by Stevens (1974) and Tait (1979). Byrne and Long (1984) developed a method for categorizing a consultation as doctor-centered or patient-centered, their concept of a doctor-centered consultation being close to other writers' 'illness' or 'disease'-centered methods. Wright and MacAdam (1979) also described a doctor-centered and patient-centered approach to care.

The patient-centered clinical method we describe joins the work of Rogers (1951) on client-centered counseling, Balint (1957) on person-centered medicine, Newman and Young (1972) on the total person approach to patient problems in nursing, and the 'Two-Body Practice' in occupational therapy (Mattingly and Fleming, 1994). In addition, there are strong similarities between our work and that of Pendleton *et al.* (1984) who defined, independently, a similar model of practice. Their approach of defining their model as a set of tasks for the physician to perform in the consultation appealed to us and we incorporated this idea into our own model. We refer to the elements of our method as components, rather than tasks, to avoid the misconception that the method is a rigid, linear technique. The practice of medicine cannot be reduced to technique but rather is embedded in a way of thinking about the clinical tasks of medicine which need to be explained clearly and pragmatically (White, 1988).

Epstein *et al.* (1993) have described, compared and contrasted a number of approaches to patient–doctor communication including: the biopsychosocial model (Engel, 1977); the three-function model (Bird and Cohen-Cole, 1990); the family systems approach to patient care (Doherty and Baird, 1987; McDaniel *et al.*, 1990); physician self-awareness (Balint, 1957); and the patient-centered clinical method presented in this book. They concluded that 'on a theoretical level, the complementarity of the approaches is more powerful than their difference' (Epstein *et al.*, 1993: 386). In our view, where they are similar is in their attempt to broaden the conventional medical approach to include psychosocial issues, the family, and the physician him- or herself.

Work in the mid-1990s led to a reconceptualization of similar concepts using the term relationship-centered care (Tresolini, 1994). We have chosen not to use the term relationship-centered, concurring with Churchill (1997: 116) that 'the mistake of "relationship-centered medicine" is that it confuses means and ends, stressing the interaction itself, rather than the goal that interaction should serve'. As Churchill (1997: 115) states: 'Doctors can best embark upon therapeutic encounters with patients, it seems to me, not by making the relationship with their patients central, but by making their patients and their patients' needs central'.

More recently a number of conceptual frameworks have been compared and contrasted for research and education purposes (Mead and Bower, 2000; Participants in the Bayer-Fetzer Conference, 2001). The most important distinction to be made between the patient-centered approach described in this book and other frameworks is that it is both a model and a clinical method. It is not a compilation of interviewing skills. Diagrams which depict the interrelations among the components are also unique to the patient-centered descriptions in this book. We have found that these make the concepts, and accompanying skills, much easier to learn and to teach. Where many frameworks differ is the level at which they work. Some are conceptual frameworks or models in the absence of a description of methods or behaviors for implementation. Others focus on practice behaviors within a less well developed framework. Very few have been researched in any systematic way. One strength of the patient-centered model, and the method which we describe, is that it includes both the theoretical framework or grounding, and strategies for implementation in practice and teaching, as well as a body of accompanying research.

Models of patient–doctor communication in general, and the patient-centered clinical method in particular, set out to make the implicit in patient care explicit. While models help clarify the basics in communication, they never completely capture what happens in reality. The tacit knowledge of the doctor and patient are not captured in the models, which are, by definition, oversimplifications. Rudebeck (1992: 67–8) pointed out that a model such as ours 'sets norms for practical medicine by stressing one single aspect (and does) not capture the very essence of practice'. Similarly Stewart (2001: 445) stated that while models do help in teaching and research they 'fail to capture the indivisible whole of a healing relationship'.

Challenges to the patient-centered clinical method in the twenty-first century: the new context of care

There are a remarkable number of changes in our society which challenge the practice of patient-centered care. However, some changes can improve the interaction between patients and doctors, e.g. emphasis on patient autonomy, interest in ethnic diversity and increased attention by the public on prevention and health promotion activities. These changes enhance patients' abilities to become more involved in their own healthcare. Regardless of recent societal changes, research has clearly demonstrated patients' desire for, as well as their expectation of receiving, patient-centered care (Little *et al.*, 2001a; Main *et al.*, 2002; Stewart, 2001).

Some of the changes we are experiencing professionally and as a society may create new difficulties for doctors and patients. For example, many doctors feel uncomfortable with the competing demands placed on them (gatekeeper role); they feel a conflict of interest between their commitment to their patients' welfare and the need to contain costs (Borkan, 1999). This is one key adverse effect of managed care. Another is the loss of continuity of relationship between a patient and a doctor (Emanuel and Dubler, 1995). The use of wise stewardship in accessing resources for patients is discussed in detail in component 6, 'Being realistic' (Chapter 9).

The increasingly litigious environment is fueled by media attention on medical uncertainty and medical errors, resulting in caution and a loss of confidence by doctors. Similarly, patient trust and confidence may be undermined (Green *et al.*, 2002; Kearley *et al.*, 2001; Murphy *et al.*, 2001). The severity of communication problems is reflected in the intensity of patients' reactions of dissatisfaction; complaints to disciplinary bodies are most often due to a communication breakdown between the patient and the physician (Levinson *et al.*, 1997; Moore *et al.*, 2000).

Many doctors, seeking a balance between their professional and personal lives, are no longer prepared to provide care to patients 24 hours a day, seven days a week (Brown *et al.*, 2002a). Juxtaposed to this alteration in the provision of care, are patients' expectations for immediate and convenient care (Brown *et al.*, 2002c). The outcome has been the proliferation of walk-in clinics or after-hours services to fill this niche, yet they threaten some basic premises of patient-centered care, such as continuity and the patient–doctor relationship.

Access to the Internet by the public has added a new dimension to the consultation as patients often arrive with a vast array of information gleaned from various websites – good and bad (Grol, 2001; Kassirer, 2000). The doctor's task is to help the patient sift through what information is reliable and useful. The advent of information technology (IT) has also introduced two other important changes: patient–doctor communication via e-mail; and the electronic medical record. The explosion of IT in the past decade suggests that e-mail communication and the paperless office will be the norm in the not too distant future. To date, however, it has not been widely adopted. As Jerome P Kassirer, editor-in-chief emeritus of the *New England Journal of Medicine*, states: 'To transform care will require new, sophisticated software that permits unconstrained interaction with computers by voice, that incorporates patient information from disparate electronic sources, that unerringly solves clinical problems, and that makes information searching reliable, focused, and fast. With such tools, resistance will vanish' (Kassirer, 2000: 123). This topic is further discussed in Chapter 9.

The sequelae to the human genome era are not yet known, but raise issues of confidentiality, access to testing, and the ripple effect of such testing on the family. These, too, will present specific challenges to physicians in the provision of patient-centered care (Carroll *et al.*, 2003).

Medicine is undergoing a radical transformation which demands fundamental changes in the way we conceptualize the role of physicians. These changes relate to major shifts in the fabric of society just mentioned. Many patients now demand a more egalitarian relationship with their physicians and expect to take a more active part in decisions about their healthcare. But there are still many people, notably the elderly, who value the conventional model of the doctor who 'always knows best'. Details of the patient–doctor relationship are examined in Chapter 8.

The limitations of the conventional medical model have led many patients to seek the help of alternative or complementary practitioners or remedies in order to have all their healthcare needs addressed. Some patients perceive their doctors as skeptical or opposed to these approaches and are reluctant to reveal they are using complementary/alternative medicine even at the risk of adverse effects (Boon *et al.*, 1999). By being patient-centered, doctors may gain an understanding of patients' needs to seek such care.

Doctors are being directed to follow a plethora of clinical practice guidelines (CPGs), with more being produced every day. This can be overwhelming, and particularly daunting when the guidelines are unclear due to insufficient evidence, and at worst conflicting when two or more respected organizations produce differing guidelines. But guidelines are *just* guidelines and their application must be geared to the individual needs and context of each particular patient (Brown *et al.*, 2002e). This is where being patient-centered can be extremely useful (Tudiver *et al.*, 2001). The balance between patient-centered medicine and evidence-based medicine is also explored in Chapter 9 and in the next section.

Evidence-based medicine and the patient-centered clinical method: the confluence of two worldviews

A superficial examination of the current literature of evidence-based medicine and the approach described in this book as the patient-centered clinical method, leads some to conclude that the two are in conflict with one another. This view is sometimes further simplified by saying that evidence-based medicine represents the 'hard science' of medicine and the patient-centered clinical method is the 'soft' side of it. This is to misrepresent both evidence-based medicine and the patient-centered clinical method which, in truth, have significant areas of confluence.

The early writings describing evidence-based medicine make clear that it is not intended to replace clinical judgment. Clinical decision-making is described as consisting of taking into account three elements: the evidence, patient particulars and patient preference (Haynes *et al.*, 2002; Sackett *et al.*, 2000). Evidence-based medicine has made tremendous strides in describing and putting into practice a method for acquiring the best available evidence about an issue in healthcare. The concurrent improvements in electronic databases and retrieval systems make it possible to access this information at the site of care and to integrate with the electronic health record. Evidence-based medicine is, in essence, a robust and extremely useful method for framing questions and evaluating evidence. It is not itself a clinical method, though it does inform the clinician.

Research on the patient-centered clinical method has made clear that finding common ground between both the physician's and the patient's perspective is key to a successful clinical outcome. Evidence-based medicine assists the physician in determining what elements might be appropriate for a part of the physician's perspective. It is not a substitute for clinical judgment or clinical intuition which arises out of a specific interaction between a particular patient and a particular clinician. The patient-centered clinical method describes a method for ensuring that the patient's particulars and preferences are taken into account and an agreed plan arrived at. From this vantage-point, the patient-centered clinical method incorporates or subsumes evidence-based medicine.

One could look at this in another way, however. It is increasingly apparent that the patient-centered clinical method is itself evidence-based. Taking into account the illness experience, the person and the context, and arriving at common ground have together been demonstrated to improve patient health outcomes, patient satisfaction and physician satisfaction. There is a burgeoning literature detailing the evidence to support this clinical method.

In summary, evidence-based medicine and the patient-centered clinical method are not ideas in conflict; rather they are synergistic. The field of action between them is best understood as one of creative tension. Complexity science (Plsek and Greenhalgh, 2001: 627) calls the 'edge of chaos' those circumstances in which there is 'insufficient agreement and certainty to make the next choice obvious, but not so much disagreement and uncertainty that the system is thrown into chaos'. This calls for complex adaptive behavior. Such areas of human interaction are the genesis of humane moral action from which arises true value. The patient-centered clinical method explicitly addresses this domain.

Common misconceptions about the patient-centered clinical method

Over the past 20 years, as the patient-centered clinical method has been disseminated to students, clinicians, educators and researchers, we have observed many misconceptions about the model. These misconceptions have concluded that being patient-centered: takes more time; focuses primarily on the patients' psychosocial issues versus their diseases; requires acquiescing to patients' demands; means seeking out the patient's 'hidden agenda'; expects sharing all information and all decisions with patients; and finally that the patient-centered clinical method is a set of tasks that do not need to be applied during each visit but can be cherry-picked, i.e. some used or some discarded.

In addition, the acronym FIFE (feelings, ideas, function and expectations) can be very useful for students as they are learning to inquire about the patient's illness experience. But it can also be dangerous if it becomes an appendage to the conventional review of systems: 'Any visual problems – blurred vision . . . ?', 'What do you feel about this?', 'How are your bowels – any constipation; diarrhea . . . ?', 'Any ideas about what is causing this?' Thus 'FIFEing' the patient, as we have heard students remark, becomes just another interviewing technique or an additional step in their review of systems and does not reflect a genuine interest in and concern about the patient's unique illness experience.

Having said that, sometimes patients' expectations are very clear and straightforward. They want treatment for their athlete's foot or completion of a medical form for insurance purposes. Thus it is not always essential to explore, in depth, the patient's illness experience. What is essential is that doctors listen to patients' cues and prompts in order to make appropriate and sensitive inquiries. In a similar vein, being patient-centered means taking into account the patients' desire for information and for sharing decision-making and responding appropriately.

Is being patient-centered the same as informed shared decision-making (ISDM)? How does motivational interviewing correspond to the patient-centered clinical method? We contend that ISDM and motivational interviewing are techniques that clinicians can employ in the mutual task of finding common ground with patients and we expand on this in Chapter 6.

The argument that a physician does not need to be patient-centered in all visits, for example when a patient presents a straightforward problem, is supported by the description of visits as falling into types: routines, rituals or dramas (Miller, 1992). Arguing in favor of the view that doctors are not patient-centered all the time, is our own result that doctors with low average scores on patient-centeredness show small standard deviations for these scores. However high-scoring doctors show wide standard deviations. Nonetheless, our contention is that physicians do not know whether the visit ought to be routine, a ritual or a drama, unless they are patient-centered and ask appropriate questions at the beginning of the visit. A brief patient–doctor dialog about a minor sore throat serves as an example:

> Doctor: While I reach over here for the tongue depressor, is there anything unusually worrying about this sore throat?
> Patient: No. (*Pause*)
> Doctor: Do you think this is anything out of the ordinary?
> Patient: No . . . I don't think so.
> Doctor: Anything else going on in your life that you want to tell me about today?
> Patient: No. Things are great!

Only after such a five-second interchange can a doctor be sure that this visit is going to be routine as opposed to a drama.

Adopting a new conceptual framework

Adopting a new conceptual framework and implementing new approaches in practice may sound very threatening to many medical practitioners. Are there risks as well as benefits in changing one's mindset as well as one's methods to a patient-centered approach? Will patients get upset? Will office routine be slowed down? Will the doctor be able to deal with all the feelings expressed? We find that the benefits outweigh the potential risks.

For example, research has shown that patient-centered visits are associated with positive benefits such as: fewer malpractice claims (Hickson *et al.*, 1994); greater physician satisfaction (Roter *et al.*, 1997); greater patient satisfaction (Dietrich and Marton, 1982; Hall and Dornan, 1988a, b; Linn *et al.*, 1982; Stewart *et al.*, 1999); better patient adherence (Golin, 1996; Stewart *et al.*, 1999); reduction of concern (Bass *et al.*, 1986; Headache Study Group, 1986; Henbest and Fehrsen, 1992; Henbest and Stewart, 1990); better self-reported health (Stewart *et al.*, 2000); and improved physiologic status (Greenfield *et al.*, 1988; Kaplan *et al.*, 1989b). A detailed review of studies of a variety of outcomes in relation to patient-centered communication is presented in Chapter 17.

Furthermore, research has indicated that patient-centered consultations do not take longer (Greenfield *et al.*, 1988; Henbest and Fehrsen, 1992; Marvel *et al.*, 1998). Rather they enhance the patient–doctor interaction through a deeper exploration of the patients' illness experience (Arborelius and Bremberg, 1992; Howie *et al.*, 1991; Marvel *et al.*, 1998) and provide opportunities for finding common ground (Greenfield *et al.*, 1988; Marvel *et al.*, 1998;

Williams and Neal, 1998). Nonetheless, longer visits provide an opportunity for more activities relevant to patient-centered clinical practice such as prevention (vaccination) and counseling. A further discussion of time and timing is offered in Chapters 9 and 17.

Another insight from research is that physicians who have learned the patient-centered method are flexible in their approach to individual patients. As mentioned before, physicians who have, on average, high patient-centered scores, show a wide range in scores, implying a flexibility in practice (Stewart *et al.*, 1989).

Finally, research has pointed out the challenges in teaching and learning the patient-centered approach. On the one hand, we have found that many of the methods that we teach can be implemented by residents and practicing physicians over a period of six weeks to three months, e.g. considering patients' ideas and feelings (Stewart *et al.*, 1989). However, students and physicians often have more difficulty with other aspects of the model, e.g. finding common ground. At first they use the method as an add-on to the conventional clinical method and, when they are rushed, tired or feeling threatened, they revert to a focus on disease. It takes considerable experience with the patient-centered clinical method before it becomes second nature. Teachers need to keep in mind this natural history of learning the method and not become impatient or overly critical of students who have trouble integrating the method or who backslide under pressure.

Conclusion

In this introductory chapter we have provided an historical perspective of the evolution of the patient-centered model, and the clinical method which serves as a means for implementation of the theoretical framework. The place of the patient-centered model and clinical method was examined in relation to other models of communication. Challenges in practicing the patient-centered clinical method in the current context were explored with attention given to some common misconceptions about the patient-centered clinical method. The final section in this chapter has provided empirical evidence supporting the adoption of the patient-centered clinical method.

2

The evolution of clinical method

Ian R McWhinney

The clinical method practiced by physicians is always the practical expression of a theory of medicine, even though it is not made explicit. The theory embraces such concepts as the nature of health and disease, the relation of mind and body, the meaning of diagnosis, the role of the physician and the conduct of the patient–doctor relationship. The theory and practice of medicine is strongly influenced in any era by the dominant theory of knowledge and by societal values. Medicine is always a child of its time.

In recent times, medicine has not paid much attention to philosophy. When our efforts have been crowned with such great successes as they have in the past century, why be concerned if someone questions our assumptions? Indeed, we often behave as if they are not assumptions, but simply the way things are. Crookshank (1926) marks the end of the nineteenth century as the time when medicine and philosophy became completely dissociated. Physicians began to see themselves as practitioners of a science solidly based on observed facts, without a need for inquiry into how the facts are obtained and, indeed, what a fact is (Fleck, 1979). We believe ourselves to be at last freed from metaphysics, while at the same time maintaining a belief in the theory of knowledge known as physical realism.

Although continuous with the Hippocratic tradition of Greek medicine, the clinical method which has dominated Western medicine for nearly 200 years had its main origins in the European Enlightenment of the seventeenth century. AN Whitehead called this the century of genius, on whose capital of ideas we have lived ever since. It was the century of Galileo and Newton, of Descartes, Locke and Bacon. Bacon urged mankind to dominate and control nature, thus lightening the miseries of existence. In his *Advancement of Learning*, he provided, as his agenda for medical science, a revival of the Hippocratic method of recording case descriptions, with their course towards recovery or death; and the study of the pathological changes in organs – the 'footsteps of disease' – with a comparison between these and the manifestations of illness during life. Clinical medicine at this time was dominated by untested theory ungrounded in bedside observation. The new scientific ideas had recently been applied to medicine by men such as Vesalius and Harvey, but their discoveries had been in anatomy and physiology, not in pathology and clinical science. Medicine was still practiced in ignorance of these discoveries. If Bacon set the agenda for science, it was Descartes who provided the method: the separation of mind and matter, with value residing only in mind; the separation of subject and object; and the reduction of complex phenomena to their simplest components.

Of all seventeenth century figures, none has had more influence on science and medicine than René Descartes. In his *Traité de l'homme*, published in 1634, he wrote: 'The body is a machine, so built up and composed of nerves, muscles, veins, blood and skin, that even though there were no mind in it at all, would not cease to have the same functions' (Foss, 2002: 37). Descartes' concept of the body as machine had enormous consequences for medicine. It replaced the vitalist concept of pre-modern medicine and made possible the basic sciences of medicine and all the benefits they have conferred on us. Descartes' reductionist approach to inquiry, and his separation of *res extensa* from *res cogitans* enabled biology to make great progress. But the problems left unresolved by Descartes have been gnawing away at the conceptual foundations of medicine and science. The questions include: how can a non-material mind act on a material substance, and what is the relationship between the mind of the observer and the world of phenomena. The philosopher EA Burtt (1954: 324) wrote: 'An adequate cosmology will only begin to be written when an adequate philosophy of mind has appeared'.

It was in the century of genius that reason was enthroned and modern science was born. But it was a reason defined as formal logic, divorced from human experience and seeking for universal laws to explain natural phenomena. Mathematics was the model and Newton's *Principia* was the great exemplar. The idea of nature as a vast machine – including the human body – seemed eminently plausible. The aim was to attain knowledge that was universal and certain. Toulmin (1992) describes this as a radical shift in the paradigm of knowledge: 'From 1630 on, the focus of philosophical inquiries has ignored the particular, concrete, timely and local details of everyday human affairs: instead it has shifted to a higher, stratospheric place on which nature and ethics conform to abstract, timeless, general and universal theories' (Toulmin, 1992: 34–5). In his book *Return to Reason* (1991), Toulmin reminds us that a 'universal' was for the Greeks a concept which was true 'on the whole' or 'generally', but not invariably applicable in every case. 'In real-life situations, many universals hold generally rather than invariably' (1991: 11). This applies especially in biology and the human sciences.

Since the seventeenth century, physics has been the model for all sciences. But physics, writes the biologist FE Yates (1993: 189), is 'characterized by uniformity and generality':

Biology, in contrast, presents diversity and specialness of form and function and sometimes a striking localness of distribution of its objects. Biological systems are *complex*. Physics is a strongly reductionist science and has prospered in that style; [the metaphor of organisms as machines] is false and destructive of conceptual advances in the understanding of complex living systems that self-organize, grow, develop, adapt, reproduce, repair and maintain form and function, age and die. (emphasis in original)

Our patients do all these things. They are complex systems – organisms – and our clinical method should enable us to deal with complexity.

Thomas Sydenham

It was in the intellectual climate of the 1600s that there arose the first modern physician to use systematic bedside observation: Thomas Sydenham. Sydenham described the symptoms and course of disease, setting aside all speculative hypotheses based on unsupported theories. He classified diseases into categories – a novel idea at the time – believing that they could be classified by description in the same way as botanical specimens. Finally, he sought a remedy for each 'species' of disease, exemplified by the newly introduced Peruvian bark (quinine). His great innovation, however, was to correlate his disease categories with their course and outcome, thus giving them predictive value. His method bore fruit in the distinction, for the first time, of syndromes like acute gout and chorea. Sydenham was a close friend of John Locke, who took a great interest in his observations, sometimes accompanying him on his visits to patients.

From Sydenham to Laennec

After Sydenham, the work of classifying diseases was taken up by others, notably Sauvages of Montpellier, a physician and botanist, who sought to group diseases into classes, orders, and genera in the same way that biologists were classifying plants and animals. Biology and medicine were at this time predominantly descriptive sciences. Sauvages was a strong influence on Carl von Linné, the Swedish physician and botanist who was responsible for the Linnaean system of botanical classification – another instance of the connection between medicine and the ideas of the Enlightenment. The groupings of Sydenham's successors, however, were of little practical value because they were not correlated with the course and outcome of disease and represented only random combinations of symptoms with no basis in the natural order.

Sydenham died in 1689 and for the next hundred years no system for classifying diseases proved to be of lasting value. The next great step, and the one which laid the foundations for the modern clinical method, was taken by the French clinician-pathologists in the years after the French revolution. The political turmoil engendered by Enlightenment ideas was associated with a further application of these ideas to medicine. The method was described by Laennec, the greatest genius of the French school:

> The constant goal of my studies and research has been the solution of the following three problems:
>
> 1   To describe disease in the cadaver according to the altered states of the organs.
> 2   To recognize in the living body definite physical signs, as much as possible independent of the symptoms . . .
> 3   To fight the disease by means which experience has shown to be effective: . . . to place, through the process of diagnosis, internal organic lesions on the same basis as surgical disease. (Faber, 1923: 35)

For the first time, clinicians examined their patients, using new instruments like the Laennec stethoscope. Then they linked together two sets of data: signs and symptoms from the clinical inquiry, and the descriptive data of morbid anatomy. At last medicine had a classification system based on the natural order of things: the correlation between symptoms, signs, and the appearance of the organs and tissues after death. The system proved to have great predictive value, and it was further vindicated when Pasteur and Koch showed that some of these entities had specific causal agents. The clinical method based on this system developed gradually during the nineteenth century, until by the 1870s it had taken the form familiar to us today.

As is always the case, this development in clinical method was associated with a change in the perception of disease. Since classical times, Western medicine has used two different explanatory models of illness (Crookshank, 1926; Dubos, 1980). According to the ontological model, a disease is an entity located in the body and conceptually separable from the sick person. According to the physiological or ecological model, disease results from an imbalance within the organism, and between organism and environment: individual diseases have no real existence, the names being simply clusters of observations used by physicians as a guide to prognosis and therapy. According to the latter view, it becomes difficult to separate the disease from the person and the person from the environment.

Each model is identified with a clinical method, the ontological with a conventional or academic, and the physiological with a natural or descriptive method. The natural, concerned with the organism and disease, attempts to describe the illness in all its dimensions, including its individual and personal features. The conventional, concerned with organs and diseases, attempts to classify and name the disease as an entity independent of the patient. Crookshank (1926), who introduced these terms, also observed that the best physicians in all ages have used a balance of the two methods. The patient-centered clinical method can be seen as the restoration of balance to a clinical method that has gone too far in the ontological direction.

The success of the new clinical method in the late 1800s soon resulted in a dominance of the ontological model, a dominance it has retained ever since. Whereas in former times the word diagnosis often meant the diagnosis of a patient, the aim of diagnosis was now to identify the disease. Disease was located in the body. As in all taxonomies, the disease categories were abstractions which, in the interest of generalization, left out many features of illness, including the subjective experience of the patient.

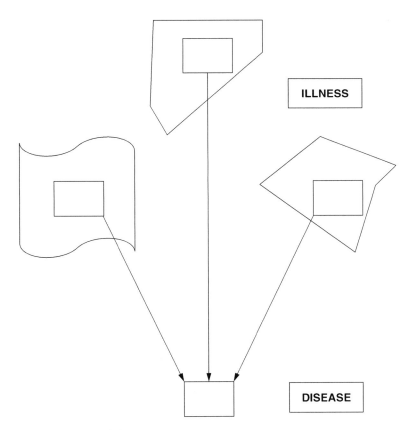

Figure 2.1   The process of abstraction.

Figure 2.1 illustrates the process of abstraction. The three irregular shapes represent patients with similar illnesses. They are all different because no two illnesses are exactly the same. The three squares represent what the patients have in common. In the process of abstraction we take the common factors and form a disease category: multiple sclerosis, carcinoma of the lung, and so on. Abstraction gives us great predictive power and provides us with our taxonomic language. It enables us to apply our therapeutic technologies with precision: but it comes at a price. The power of generalization is gained by distancing ourselves from individual patients and all the particulars of their illness. 'A large acquaintance with particulars', said William James (1958: *ix*), 'often makes us wiser than the possession of abstract formulas, however deep.' If we look closely, every patient is different in some way. It is in the care of patients that the particulars become crucial. If we are to be healers, we need to know our patients as individuals: they may have their diseases in common, but in their responses to disease, they are unique.

With its predictive and inferential power, the new clinical method was highly successful. Indeed, the application of new technologies to medicine depended on it. It had other strengths: it gave the clinician a clear injunction: 'identify the patient's disease or rule out organic pathology'; it broke down a complex process into a series of easily remembered steps; and it provided canons of verification: the pathologist was able to tell the clinician whether he was right or wrong.

So successful was the method that its weaknesses only became apparent much later, as its abstractions became further and further removed from the experience of the patient. No abstraction is ever a complete picture of what it represents: it becomes less and less complete as levels of abstraction and power of generalization increase. Table 2.1 illustrates degrees of abstraction in a

Table 2.1   Levels of abstraction in a patient with multiple, fluctuating, neurological symptoms and signs

Level 1	Level 2	Level 3	Level 4
Patient's sensations and emotions	Patient's expressed complaints, feelings, interpretations	Doctor's analysis of illness: clinical assessment	MRI scan
Preverbal	Second-order abstraction	Third-order abstraction	Fourth-order abstraction
Illness	'Illness' (doctor's understanding)	'Disease' (clinical diagnosis: multiple sclerosis)	'Disease' (definitive diagnosis: MS)

Source: McWhinney IR (1997: 77). Reprinted with permission of Oxford University Press, New York.

patient with multiple, fluctuating neurological symptoms. The first and lowest level is the patient's experience before it has been verbalized: his raw experience that something is not right. Level 2 is the patient's expressed sensations, feelings and interpretations, and their understanding by the doctor. Level 3 is the doctor's clinical assessment and analysis of the illness: the clinical diagnosis of multiple sclerosis (MS). Level 4 is the definitive diagnosis after an MRI scan. As we increase the levels of abstraction, individual differences are ironed out in the interest of generalization. The lower levels of abstraction are closest to the patient's lifeworld. As we increase the level of abstraction, the danger is that we forget that our abstraction is not synonymous with the real world. The diagnosis of MS and the MRI scan are not the patient's experience. To forget this is, in Alfred Korzybski's aphorism, mistaking the map for the territory (Korzybski, 1958). Many of the recently published illness narratives have drawn our attention to this weakness.

Illness narratives

In the past three decades there has been a remarkable increase in the number of books and articles describing personal experiences of illness. These writings, by patients themselves or by their relatives, are often bitterly critical of clinicians and, by implication, of the modern clinical method. Hawkins (1993) sees this literature as a possible reaction to a medicine 'so dominated by a biophysical understanding of illness that its experiential aspects are virtually ignored'. Two themes recur in these stories: 'the tendency in contemporary medical practice to focus primarily not on the needs of the individual who is sick but on the nomothetic condition we call the disease, and the sense that our medical technology has advanced beyond our capacity to use it wisely' (Hawkins, 1993).

Some illness narratives are written by patients who have a professional perspective as physicians, philosophers, sociologists or poets. Sacks (1984) viewed his experience of a body image disorder from the perspective of an existential neurologist and medical theorist. Stetten (1981) found that his fellow physicians were interested in his vision, but not in his blindness. Toombs (1992), a phenomenologist who has multiple sclerosis, noted that physicians' attention is directed to their patients' bodies rather than to their problems of living. The patient feels 'reduced to a malfunctioning biological organism' (1992: 106). Toombs writes: 'no physician has ever inquired of me what it is like to live with multiple sclerosis or to experience one of the disabilities that have accrued . . . no neurologist has ever asked me if I am afraid, or . . . even whether I am concerned about the future' (1992: 106). Writing of his experience with testicular cancer, A Frank (1991), a sociologist, observed that the more critical his illness became, the more his physicians withdrew.

True to its origins in the age of reason, this clinical method was analytical and impersonal. Feelings and the life experience of the patient did not figure in the process. The meaning of the illness was established on one level only – that of physical pathology. The focus was on diagnosis, with much less attention to the detailed care of the patient. In keeping also with its Cartesian origins, it divided mental from physical disorder, bringing the two together in dubious terms like 'functional illness', 'psychosomatic disease' and 'somatization' (McWhinney *et al.*, 1997).

The central idea on which the modern clinical method was based came into being at a time when Enlightenment ideas had become the dominant worldview of the West. Man had become the measure of all things, metaphysics devalued, tradition weakened, progress proclaimed and knowledge put to practical use for the benefit of mankind. The fruits borne by these ideas in our own time include this clinical method and all the benefits and problems of modern medicine.

Modern medicine continues to make great advances, many of them based on the mechanical metaphor. Training these technologies on their target has required diagnostic precision and the modern clinical method has rightly attached great importance to the linear logic of differential diagnosis. But the promise of new technologies often falls short of expectations when they are applied in the real world of practice. It is here that linear logic meets the logic of complexity. Whether they are preventative, therapeutic or rehabilitative, the technologies require acceptance by the patient, motivation, cooperation and often determination. They may require a different way of life and the giving up of lifelong habits or cherished pleasures. The changes must be timely, and consistent with life time goals and priorities. The patient must be convinced that their efforts are justified.

Many illnesses are themselves complex and multifactorial, requiring an approach different from the linear logic and targeted technology which can work so well in diseases with a specific etiology. Illnesses such as chronic pain, eating disorders, depression and addiction have an existential dimension which must be addressed if they are to be understood. Attention must be paid to patients' sufferings, to their emotions, beliefs and relationships, not only for humanitarian reasons, but because they have an important bearing on the origins of illness (Foss, 2002).

The patient-centered clinical method is designed to deal with complexity. While using linear logic where appropriate, its essence is the understanding of the patient as a whole, a knowledge of his/her illness experience and an attempt to attain common ground. Common ground is the key to therapeutic success, but it is often difficult to obtain. It tests the doctor's ability to motivate the patient by resolving objections, laying doubts to rest, allaying fears and clearing up misconceptions (Botelho, 2002). The art of persuasion has ancient roots in medicine. The Greeks spoke of a 'therapy of the word' (Entralgo, 1961). Before the Enlightenment, rhetoric – the art of persuasion – was a respected field of study. Its purpose was to take general fundamental principles and apply them in practical situations such as clinical medicine, taking into account all the local circumstances of time and place. The fact that rhetoric is now a derogatory term is a reflection on the limits of our knowledge. The search for common ground should be an exchange and synthesis of meanings. The physician interprets the patient's illness in terms of physical pathology, the name of the disease, causal inferences and therapeutic choices. The patient interprets it in terms of experience: what it is *like* for him or her to suffer from the illness, beliefs about its nature, and expectations of therapy. Ideally, the exchange results in a synthesis of perspectives: they are, after all, different perspectives – concrete or abstract – of the same reality. But there are some reasons why synthesis may not be achieved – at least initially. For the patient, the encounter with the physician is often emotionally charged. The physician's interpretation or management of the illness may be rejected. The physician may not believe the patient – a disbelief not necessarily conveyed in words. There are a hundred ways of saying: 'I don't believe you.'

Attaining empathetic understanding requires attention to the patient's emotions. This is something which the modern clinical method does not do in any systematic way. True to Descartes' supposed separation of mind from body,* the method of most clinical disciplines does not include attention to the emotions. Internal medicine attends to the body; psychiatry attends to the emotions. Family practice is one of the few clinical fields that transcend this deep fault line. As long ago as 1926, FG Crookshank, writing on the theory of diagnosis, noted that the handbooks of clinical diagnosis, which appeared in the early 1900s, 'give excellent schemes for the physical examination of the patient while strangely ignoring, almost completely, the psychical [*sic*]' (1926: 941). The price we have paid for the benefits of abstraction is a distancing of doctor from patient. We have justified this to ourselves as objectivity, but to our patients it is often seen as indifference to their suffering.

The teaching with regard to the patient–doctor relationship was 'don't get involved'. In one respect, fear of the emotions was well founded. To be involved at the level of one's unexamined emotions is potentially harmful. But what the teaching did not say was that involvement is necessary if one is going to be a healer as well as a competent technician. There are right and wrong ways of being involved and the teaching gave no guidance about finding the right way. The teaching was also profoundly mistaken in suggesting that one can encounter suffering and not in some way be affected. Our emotional response may be repressed, but this exacts a heavy price, for repressed emotion may be acted out in ways that are destructive of relationships. There is no such thing as non-involvement and only self-knowledge can protect us from the pitfalls of

---

* Contrary to modern assumptions, Descartes did not deny mind–body interactions but maintained that most aspects of affective states are primarily somatic.

involvement at the level of our egocentric emotions. Without self-knowledge, moral growth is likely to have shallow roots. This is why the patient-centered clinical method includes attention to the patient–doctor relationship, and, by implication, to the physician's self-awareness. The daily encounter with suffering can evoke strong emotions: helplessness in the face of incurable illness, fear of discussing questions that frighten us, guilt at our failures, anger at our patient's demands, and sadness at the suffering of someone who has become a friend. If we fail to acknowledge and deal with our disturbing emotions, they may be acted out in avoidance of the patient, emotional distancing, exclusive concentration on the technical aspects of care, and even cruelty. Lack of emotional insight can disturb or destroy the relationship between patient and doctor, adding to the patient's sufferings and often leaving the doctor with a sense of failure. It is not easy to look suffering in the face without flinching.

All this implies that we see ourselves no longer as detached observers and dispassionate dispensers of therapy. To be patient-centered means to be open to a patient's feelings. It means becoming involved in a way that was made difficult by the old method. This has the potential for making medicine a much richer experience for us, as well as more effective for our patients. But there are pitfalls. There are right and wrong ways of becoming involved. There are ways of dealing with some of the disturbing things our new openness will expose us to. Hence the importance of the knowledge and insight I have referred to. It is through such experiences that students can develop emotionally as well as intellectually.

If we are to recapture our capacity to heal, we will have to transcend the literal-mindedness that seems to follow when we become prisoners of our abstractions. A new clinical method should find room for the exercise of imagination and for restoring the balance between thinking and feeling.

A different way of thinking about health and disease

Most difficult of all perhaps, will be the transition from linear, causal thinking to cybernetic thinking. Linear thinking is deeply ingrained in our culture. The notion of a cause is based on the Newtonian model of a force acting on a passive object, as when a moving billiard ball impacts on a stationary one. The action is in one direction only. In medicine, this notion is exemplified by the doctrine of specific etiology – of an environmental agent acting on a person to produce a diseased state.

The notion of cybernetic causation is based on the model of self-organizing systems. The human organism can be viewed as a self-organizing system, maintaining itself by interaction with its environment and by a system of feed-back loops from the environment and from its own output. Self-organizing systems have the ability both to renew and to transcend themselves. Healing is an example of self-renewal in which constituent parts are renewed while the integrity of the organization is maintained. Organisms transcend themselves by learning, developing, and growing. Self-organizing systems require energy, but as organizations they are maintained and changed by information. The notion of cause in self-organizing systems is based on the model of information which triggers a process that is already a potential of the system. The response is not the direct result of the original stimulus but the result of rule-governed behavior that is a property of the system. If the process is long term, destabilizing, and self-perpetuating, then the question of cause becomes much more complex than that of identifying the trigger. The trigger which initiated the process may be quite different from the processes perpetuating it. We have to consider the processes in the organism that are perpetuating the disturbance. The key to enhancing healing may be in strengthening the organism's defenses, changing the information flow or encouraging self-transcendence, rather than neutralizing an agent.

Non-linear logic is 'both-and' rather than 'either-or'. Perspectives that we regard as opposites can be seen as complementary polarities: different aspects of the same reality. The pitfalls of either-or thinking are exemplified by a leading neurologist's perspective on migraine: 'Practitioners should realize that migraine is a neurobiologic, not a psychogenic disorder' (Olesen, 1994: 1714). Non-linear logic would say: 'Why can it not be both?'

It is self-knowledge that enables us to know where we are on the scale of these complementary polarities: between involvement and detachment, between concrete and abstract, between the particular and the general, or between uncertainty and precision.

The reform of clinical method

It is not surprising that criticism of the modern clinical method from within the profession has come mainly from fields of medicine that most experience the ambiguities of abstraction and the importance of the patient's life story, notably general practice and psychiatry. In the 1950s, Michael Balint (1964), a medical psychoanalyst, began to work with a group of general practitioners, exploring difficult cases and the doctors' affective responses to them. Balint distinguished between 'overall' diagnosis and traditional diagnosis; he emphasized the importance of listening and of the personal change required in the doctor; and he introduced new terms such as: 'patient-centered medicine', 'the patient's offers' and the doctor's 'responses', the doctor's belief in his 'apostolic function' and the 'drug doctor' – the powerful influence for good or harm of the patient–doctor relationship. The idea that physicians should attend to their own emotional development as well as the emotions of the patient was revolutionary in its day. In other ways, Balint's method conformed to the dualistic approach of the period. The method was intended to apply only to certain patients with 'neurotic illnesses', not to those with straightforward clinical problems.

In the 1970s, Engel (1977, 1980), an internist and psychiatrist with a psychoanalytic orientation, used systems theory as a model for integrating biologic, psychologic and social data in the clinical process. Engel's critique of the modern clinical method focused on the unscientific nature of the physician's judgments on interpersonal and social aspects of patients' lives, based on 'tradition, custom, prescribed rules, compassion, intuition, common sense, and sometimes highly personal self-reference' (1980: 543).

Any successor to the modern clinical method must propose another method with the same strengths: a theoretical foundation, a clear set of injunctions about what the clinician must do, and canons of verification by which it may be judged. Lain Entralgo (1956) attributes the failure of Western medicine to integrate the patient's inner life with the disease to the lack, among other things, of a method – 'a technique [for] laying bare, to clinical investigation and to subsequent pathological consideration the inner life of the patient . . . an exploration method – the dialogue with the patient . . .'. Balint and Engel both provided a theory, but were less clear about what the clinician must do and how the process is to be validated. Although Engel emphasized that the verification must be scientific, validation of both models was bound to depend on qualitative methods which were barely accepted as scientific. A model is an abstraction; a method is its practical application; and medicine had to wait longer for the transition to occur. The patient-centered clinical method is an answer to Lain Entralgo's challenge.

Clinical medicine, it seems, took a long time to fall under the domination of the Enlightenment paradigm of knowledge. Although the modern clinical method was concerned with abstractions, until our own time the individual case or series of cases remained the focus of attention for study and for teaching. Our abstractions have been low-level, not far removed from experiences of patients. In more recent times, however, the development of clinical method can be seen as moving towards increasing levels of abstraction, and an increasing distance from the experience of illness. The fact that a ward round can now be done round the charts rather than round the beds, is an indication of how far we have gone.

The difficulties of change

It is important not to underestimate the magnitude of the changes implied by the transformation of our clinical method. It is not simply a matter of learning some new techniques, though that is part of it. Nor is it only a question of adding courses in interviewing and behavioral science to the curriculum. The change goes much deeper than that. It requires nothing less than a change in what it means to be a physician, a different way of thinking about health and disease, and a redefinition of medical knowledge.

A glance at any medical school curriculum is usually sufficient to show that it is dominated by the modern paradigm of knowledge. Of course, this kind of knowledge is important, but restoring the balance in medicine requires that it be balanced by other kinds of knowledge: an understanding of human experience and human relationships, moral insight, and that most difficult of accomplishments, self-knowledge. Whitehead (1975) criticized professional education for being too full of abstractions, a condition he described as 'the celibacy of the intellect' (1975: 223), the modern equivalent of the celibacy of the medieval learned class. Wisdom, he believed, is the fruit of a balanced development. What we need is not more abstractions, but an education in which the necessary abstractions are balanced by concrete experiences, an education which feeds both the intellect and the imagination. Much of this is not the kind of knowledge that can be learned in the classroom or from books, though some of it can. There is now, for example, a rich literature describing personal experiences of illness. If we are to give as much attention to care as we give to diagnosis we will need to feed our imagination with accounts of what it is like to go blind, have multiple sclerosis, suffer bereavement, bring up a handicapped child, and the many other experiences our patients live with. We will need also to know the many practical ways in which life for them can be enriched or made more tolerable.

Human relationships and moral insight, again, are not principally classroom subjects, except insofar as students learn moral lessons from the way they are treated by their teachers. However, once its importance is acknowledged, and time allowed for it, understanding of relationships can be deepened with the help of teachers who are sensitive, reflective, and prepared to expose their own vulnerability. Self-knowledge, by definition, cannot be taught. But its growth can be fostered by teachers who are themselves embarked on this difficult journey – a journey that is never complete. The patient-centered clinical method is the most recent version of the historic struggle to reconcile two often competing notions of the nature of disease and the role of the physician. The past century has seen the increasing dominance of abstraction and the devaluation of experience. The patient-centered clinical method can be viewed as a move to bring medical practice and teaching back to the center, to reconcile clinical with existential medicine (Sacks, 1982). It may seem paradoxical that the modern clinical method does not have a name. It is simply the way clinical medicine has been taught in the medical schools in modern times. Giving the successor method a name has its dangers, notably that of conveying different meanings to different people. In this transition period, however, it does seem necessary to have a name for the new method. But when the transition is complete, perhaps it can simply become 'clinical method'.

The new method should not only restore the Hippocratic ideal of friendship between doctor and patient, but also make possible a medicine which can see illness as an expression of a person with a moral nature, an inner life and a unique life story: a medicine that can heal by a therapy of the word and a therapy of the body.

PART TWO

The six components of the patient-centered clinical method

Introduction

*Judith Belle Brown, Moira Stewart
and W Wayne Weston*

In this section of the book, the six interactive components of the patient-centered clinical method are described in detail with each component being illustrated by several case examples. Of note, the 'Whole person' component, because of its magnitude, is examined in two separate but interconnected chapters. While each component is, for the most part, described as a discrete entity, the expert clinician weaves among the components throughout the process in response to the patient's expressed needs and concerns. There is both an art and a science to this process that comes together with time, training and experience.

3

The first component: exploring both the disease and the illness experience

Judith Belle Brown, W Wayne Weston and Moira Stewart

Disease and illness

There is a long history documenting the failure of conventional medical practice in meeting patients' perceived needs and expectations. Component 1 of the patient-centered clinical method addresses this failure by proposing that clinicians explore both the disease and the illness experience.

To practice patient-centered medicine, clinicians must make a distinction between two conceptualizations of ill health: disease and illness. Effective patient care requires attending as much to patients' personal experiences of illness as to their disease. Disease is diagnosed by using the conventional medical model, but understanding illness requires a different approach. Disease is diagnosed by objective observation; it is a category; the 'thing' that is wrong with the body-as-machine or the mind-as-computer. Disease is a theoretical construct, or abstraction, by which physicians attempt to explain patients' problems in terms of abnormalities of structure and/or function of body organs and systems and includes both physical and mental disorders. Illness, on the other hand, is the patient's personal and subjective experience of sickness; the feelings, thoughts, and altered behavior of someone who feels sick.

To be patient-centered requires a balance between the objective and the subjective, a bringing together of the body and mind. The connection between biology and emotions, between body and mind, has been described recently and convincingly in psychoneuroimmunology studies. Haunting literary examples are contained in the stories of Alistair MacLeod about the depth of caring of his male characters, Scottish immigrants living on the unforgiving soil of Cape Breton, whose lives are inexorably bound to the physical. 'You know', says the narrator in *Vision*, 'the future scar will be forever on the outside while the memory will remain, forever, deep within.' By associating memory with blood and body, MacLeod suggests that emotion is biological and genetic and can never, therefore, be connected to that which is ephemeral or casual (Urquhart, 2001: 41).

In the biomedical model, sickness is explained in terms of pathophysiology: abnormal structure and function of tissues and organs. This model is a conceptual framework for understanding the biological dimensions of sickness by reducing sickness to disease. The focus is on the body, not the person. A particular disease is what everyone with that disease has in common, but the illness experiences of each person are unique. Disease and illness do not always coexist. Patients with undiagnosed asymptomatic disease do not feel ill; people who are grieving or worried may feel ill but have no disease. Patients and doctors who recognize this distinction and who realize how common it is to feel ill and have no disease, are less likely to search needlessly for pathology. However, even when disease is present, it may not adequately explain the patient's suffering, since the amount of distress a patient experiences refers not only to the amount of tissue damage but to the personal meaning of the illness.

Several authors have described this same distinction between disease and illness from different perspectives. In analyzing medical interviews, Mishler (1984) identifies two contrasting voices: the voice of medicine and the voice of the lifeworld. The voice of medicine promotes a scientific, detached attitude and uses questions such as: 'Where does it hurt? When did it start? How long does it last? What makes it better or worse?' The voice of the lifeworld, on the other hand, reflects a 'common sense' view of the world. It centers on the individual's particular social context, the meaning of illness events, and how they may affect the achievement of personal goals. Typical questions to explore the lifeworld include: 'What are you most concerned about? How does it disrupt your life? What do you think it is? How do you think I can help you?'

Mishler (1984) argues that typical interactions between doctors and patients are doctor-centered; they are dominated by a technocratic perspective. The physician's primary task is to make a diagnosis; thus, in the interview, the doctor selectively attends to the voice of medicine, often not even hearing patients' own attempts to make sense of their suffering. What is needed, he maintains, is a different approach, in which doctors give priority to 'patients' lifeworld contexts of meaning as the basis for understanding, diagnosing and treating their problems' (Mishler, 1984: 192).

In a recent qualitative study, Barry *et al.* (2001) applied Mishler's concepts in the analysis of 35 case studies of patient–doctor interactions. Their findings revealed an expansion of Mishler's ideas, adding two communication patterns 'lifeworld ignored', where patients' use of the voice of the lifeworld was ignored, and 'lifeworld blocked', where doctors' use of the voice of medicine blocked patients' expressions of the lifeworld. These two communication patterns were found to have the poorest outcomes. When both the patient and the doctor used the voice of medicine exclusively Barry *et al.* (2001) called this 'strictly medicine' as the emphasis was on simple, acute physical complaints. 'Mutual lifeworld' was the term applied to interactions where both the patient and doctor used the voice of the lifeworld, thus highlighting the uniqueness of the patient's life and experience. Of note, Barry *et al.* (2001) found that the best outcomes were in patient–doctor encounters categorized as either 'mutual lifeworld' or 'strictly medicine'. They interpret the latter finding in four different ways: patients have come to view their problems from the perspective of the voice of medicine; patients have learned from experience that the voice of the lifeworld has no value in medical encounters; patients are goal-oriented in these encounters and want a quick, efficient encounter; and finally the structure of these encounters is such that the patient has no opportunity to use the voice of the lifeworld. Because the encounters incorporating 'mutual lifeworld' reflected excellent outcomes, too, Barry *et al.* (2001) conclude that doctors need to be sensitized to the importance of attending to patients' concerns of the lifeworld.

Eric Cassell (1985a) has a corresponding message:

> The story of an illness – the patient's history – has two protagonists: the body and the person. By careful questioning, it is possible to separate out the facts that speak of disturbed bodily functioning, the pathophysiology that gives you the diagnosis. To do this, the facts about the body's dysfunction must be separated from the meanings that the patient has attached to them. Skillful physicians have been doing this for ages. All too often, however, the personal meanings are then discarded. With them goes the doctor's opportunity to know who the patient is. (1985a: 108)

The patients' 'explanatory model' is their own personal conceptualization of the etiology, course, and sequela of their problem (Green *et al.*, 2002). Medical anthropologists such as Kleinman have described ways to elicit the patients' 'explanatory models' of their illness and offer a series of questions to ask patients which they call a 'cultural status exam'. The physician might ask, for example: 'How would you describe the problem that has brought you to me? Does anyone else that you know have these problems? What do you think is causing the problem? Why do you think this problem has happened to you and why now? What do you think will clear up this problem? Apart from me, who else do you think can help you get better?' (Galazka and Eckert, 1986; Good and Good, 1981; Katon and Kleinman, 1981; Kleinman *et al.*, 1978).

Research has long supported the contention that disease and illness do not always present simultaneously. For some illnesses patients do not even seek medical advice (Freer, 1980). When they do, fewer than half result in a known etiology or diagnosis after six months (Blacklock, 1977; Jerritt, 1981; Wasson *et al.*, 1981). There is a variety of reasons for this: the problem may be transient; it may be treated so early that it never reaches a diagnosis, e.g. pneumonia; it may be a borderline condition which is difficult to classify; the problem may remain undifferentiated; and/or the problem may have its source in factors such as an unhappy marriage, job dissatisfaction, guilt, or lack of purpose in life (McWhinney, 1997).

The following two views on the importance of distinguishing between disease and illness are offered from the perspective of the patient and the doctor. The patient is Anatole Broyard who taught fiction writing at Columbia University, New York University and Fairfield University. An editor, literary critic, and essayist for the *New York Times*, he died from prostate cancer in October, 1990.

> I wouldn't demand a lot of my doctor's time. I just wish he would brood on my situation for perhaps five minutes, that he would give me his whole mind just once, be bonded with me for a brief space, survey my soul as well as my flesh to get at my illness, for each man is ill in his own way ... Just as he orders blood tests and bone scans for my body, I'd like my doctor to scan me, to grope for my spirit as well as my prostate. Without some such recognition, I am nothing but my illness. (Broyard, 1992: 44–5)

The doctor is Loreen A Herwaldt, an internist and epidemiologist in Iowa.

> The big lesson for me was learning the difference between treating the disease and treating the human being. It's not always the same thing. There are times you can kill the person – in a sense, killing their spirit – by insisting that something be done a certain way. (Herwaldt, 2001: 21)

The latter quote illustrates the dilemma from the doctor's perspective. The doctor seeing the person, in addition to attending to classification of disease, is an ongoing challenge. This is similar to the challenge of artists who contend that a major barrier to creating the unique vision in the painting is the classification or labeling that results from familiarity. 'It was Monet, the painter, who said that in order to see, we must forget the name of the thing we are looking at' (Patterson, 1979: 10). Finally, Broom (2000) observes:

> ... physicians generally take their first responsibility to be a diagnosis, especially the diagnosis of physical disease. And what is a diagnosis but essentially a process based on the physician's recognition of a typical pattern of symptoms and signs, combined with the results of important technical investigations? This is the focus of the observer within the biomedical model. In this approach, then, the patient is essentially an object. In our alternative view, the patient must also be seen as a subject with a meaningful story relevant to the appearance of illness. (2000: 164)

The stages of illness

The reasons patients present themselves to their doctors when they do are often more important than the diagnosis. Frequently the diagnosis is obvious or is already known from previous contacts; often there is no biomedical label to explain the patient's problem. Thus, it is often more helpful to answer the question, 'Why now?' than the question, 'What's the diagnosis?' In chronic illness, for example, a change in a social situation is a more common reason for presenting than a change in the disease or the symptoms.

The illness experience has several stages. Illness is often a painful crisis that will overwhelm the coping abilities of some patients and challenge others to increased personal growth. It is helpful to understand these reactions as part of a developmental process that has three stages: awareness, disorganization, and reorganization (Reiser and Schroder, 1980). The first stage, awareness, is characterized by ambivalence about knowing: on the one hand, wanting to know the truth and to understand the illness and on the other, not wanting to admit that anything could be wrong. At the same time patients are often struggling with conflicting wishes to remain independent and longing to be taken care of. Eventually, if the symptoms do not go away, the fact of the illness hits home and their sense of being in control of their own lives is shattered.

This disrupts the universal defense – the magical belief that somehow we are immune from disease, injury and death. The patient who has struggled to forestall his awareness of serious illness and then has finally recognized the truth is one of the most fragile, defenseless and exquisitely vulnerable people one can ever find. This is a time of terror and depression and reflects the second stage-disorganization (Reiser and Schroder, 1980).

At this stage patients typically become emotional and may react to their caretakers as parents rather than as equals. They often become self-centered and demanding, and, although they may be aware of this reaction and embarrassed by it, they cannot seem to stop it. They may withdraw from the external world and become preoccupied with each little change in their bodies. Their sense of time becomes constricted and the future seems uncertain; they may lose a sense of continuity of self. They can no longer trust their bodies, and they feel diminished and out of control. Their whole sense of their personal identity may be severely threatened. One reaction to this state of mind in some patients is rebellion, a desperate attempt to have at least some small measure of control over their lives even if it is self-destructive in the end.

The third stage is reorganization. In this stage patients call upon all of their inner strengths to find new meaning in the face of illness and, if possible, to transcend their plight. Their degree of mastery will be affected, of course, by the nature and severity of the illness. But in addition, the outcome is profoundly influenced by the patients' social supports, especially loving relationships within their families, and by the type of support their physician can provide.

These stages of illness are part of a normal human response to disaster and not another set of disease categories or psychopathology. This description emphasizes how the humanity of the ill person is compromised and points to an added obligation of physicians to their wounded patients.

> So great is the assault of illness upon our being that 'it is almost as if our natures themselves were ill, as if the strands or parts of us were being forced apart and we verged on the loss of our own humanness'. A phenomenon so great in its effects that it can threaten us with the loss of our fundamental humanness clearly requires more than technical competence from those who would 'treat' illness. (Kestenbaum, 1982: *viii–ix*)

Patients' cues and prompts

Patients often provide physicians with cues and prompts about the reason they are coming to the physician that day. These may be verbal or non-verbal signals. The patients may look tearful, sigh deeply, or be breathless. They may say directly, 'I feel awful, Doctor. I think this flu is going to kill me.' Or, indirectly, they may present a variety of vague symptoms that are masking a more serious problem such as depression. Other authors have described patients' cues and prompts using different terminology, such as clues (Lang *et al.*, 2000; Levinson *et al.*, 2000) or offers (Balint, 1964) but regardless of the name assigned, the patient behaviors are the same. Lang *et al.* (2000) describe a useful taxonomy of clues revealed in patients' utterances and behaviors reflecting their underlying ideas, concerns and/or expectations:

1 expression of feelings (especially concern, fear or worry)
2 attempts to understand or explain symptoms
3 speech clues that underscore particular concerns of the patient
4 personal stories that link the patient with medical conditions or risks
5 behaviors suggestive of unresolved concerns or expectations (i.e. reluctance to accept recommendations, seeking a second opinion, early return visit).

Levinson *et al.* (2000) define a clue 'as a direct or indirect comment that provides information about any aspect of a patient's life circumstances or feelings. These clues offer a glimpse into the inner world of patients and create an opportunity for empathy and personal connection ... [Thus] physicians can deepen the therapeutic relationship' (2000: 1021). In order to assess how primary care physicians and surgeons respond to patient clues, they assessed 116 patient–doctor encounters (54 of primary care physicians and 62 of surgeons). Through their qualitative analysis, Levinson and colleagues found that patients initiated the majority of clues and most were emotional in nature. The physicians frequently missed opportunities to acknowledge patients' feelings adequately and as a result some patients repeatedly brought up the clue only to have it ignored again and again.

Thus as doctors sit down with patients and ask them, 'What brings you in today?' they must ask themselves, 'What has precipitated this visit?' They need to listen attentively to patients' cues of not only their disease but their experience of illness. Of equal importance to hearing patients' cues and prompts are empathic responses which help patients feel understood and recognized.

Four dimensions of the illness experience

We propose four dimensions of illness experience that physicians should explore: patients' feelings, especially their fears, about their problems; their ideas about what is wrong; the effect of the illness on their functioning; and their expectations of the doctor (*see* Figure 3.1).

What are the patients' *feelings*? Do they fear that the symptoms they present may be the precursor of a more serious problem such as cancer? Some patients

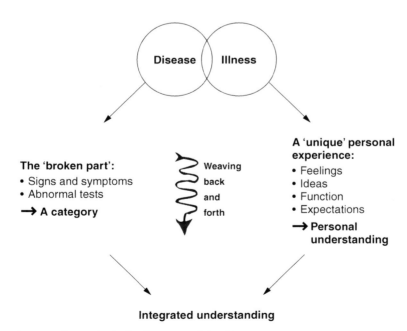

Figure 3.1 Exploring both the disease and the illness experience.

may feel a sense of relief and view the illness as an opportunity for relief from demands or responsibilities. Patients often feel irritated or culpable about being ill.

What are the patient's *ideas* about their illness? On one level the patient's ideas may be straightforward, e.g. 'I wonder if these headaches could be migraine headaches.' But at a deeper level patients may struggle to find the meaning of their illness experience. Many persons face illness as an irreparable loss; others may view it as an opportunity to gain valuable insight into their life experience. Is the illness seen as a form of punishment or, perhaps, as an opportunity for dependency? Whatever the illness, knowing its meaning is significant for understanding the patient.

What are the effects of the illness on *function*? Does it limit a patient's daily activities? Does it impair their family relationships? Does it require a change in lifestyle? Does it compromise their quality of life? Does the patient see any connection between his headaches and the guilty feelings he has been struggling with?

What are their *expectations* of the doctor? Does the presentation of a sore throat carry with it an expectation of an antibiotic? Do they want the doctor to do something or just listen? In a recent review and synthesis of the literature on patient expectations of the consultation, Thorsen *et al.* (2001) provide a further conceptualization of patients' expectations of the visit. They suggest that patients may come to a visit with their doctor with '*a priori* wishes and hopes for specific process and outcome' (2001: 638). At times these expectations may not be explicit and, in fact, patients may modify or change their expectations during the course of the consultation.

The following examples of patient–doctor dialog contain specific questions that physicians might ask to elicit the four dimensions of the patient's illness experience.

To the doctor's question, 'What brings you in today?' a patient responds, 'I've had these severe headaches for the past few weeks. I'm wondering if there is something that I can do about them.'

The patient's feelings about the headaches can be elicited by questions such as: 'What concerns you most about the headache? You seem anxious about these headaches, do you think that something sinister is causing them? Is there something particularly worrisome for you about the headaches?'

To explore the patient's ideas about the headaches, the physician might ask questions such as: 'What do you think is causing the headaches? Have you any ideas or theories about why you might be having them? Do you think there is any relationship between the headaches and current events in your life? Do you see any connection between your headaches and the guilty feelings you have been struggling with?'

To determine how the headaches may be impeding the patient's function, the doctor might ask: 'How are your headaches affecting your day-to-day living?

Are they stopping you from participating in any activities? Is there any connection between the headaches and the way your life is going?'

Finally, to identify the patient's expectations of the physician at this visit, the doctor might inquire: 'What do you think would help you to deal with these headaches? Is there some specific management that you want for your headaches? In what way may I help you? Have you a particular test in mind? What do you think would reassure you about these headaches?'

As the following case illustrates, listening to the patient's story – exploring both the disease and illness experience are essential aspects of patient-centered care.

Case example

At 3 a.m. Jenna Jameison was awakened by a sharp pain in her right lower quadrant. She dismissed it as bothersome menstrual pain and tried to get back to sleep. But sleep was not an option as the pain became unremitting.

Jenna was a 31-year-old single woman who lived alone. A committed teacher of special needs children, she had just begun working at a new school. She was also an accomplished rower who had led her team to several national victories. At 3.30 a.m. Jenna, feeling feverish and nauseated, staggered to the bathroom. In her stupor of pain she was thankful on two counts. It was Saturday – at least she would have a couple of days to recover from whatever this was before returning to school – and being winter there was no rowing practice.

By 6 a.m. the pain had reached the point that Jenna could hardly get her breath. She felt weak, sweaty and nauseated. In desperation Jenna called a close friend to take her to the hospital.

Three hours later, after undergoing numerous tests and examinations, the surgeon on call diagnosed acute appendicitis. Jenna was promptly taken to the OR for surgery. While medication had alleviated Jenna's pain, her anxiety and fear had intensified. In a few brief hours she had gone from feeling healthy and vital to someone who was very ill.

In the recovery room Jenna felt groggy and disoriented. She sighed and then blinked to see her surgeon standing over her. 'Well Jenna,' he said. 'It was not your appendix after all. In fact it was a bit more serious.' Jenna had had a Meckel's diverticulitis requiring a partial bowel resection. She would be in hospital for ten days with an open wound and significant pain. Her recovery would require at least four to six weeks. The diagnosis was a shock and the surgery had been intrusive. Jenna found it hard to comprehend how all this had transpired and to some extent denied her current reality.

Daily, her surgeon came to see her and offer support. On one occasion, sensing her irritability, he asked Jenna if she was angry. While initially surprised by his question, upon reflection Jenna realized that she *was* angry and also felt as if her once-healthy body had betrayed her. She was struggling to make sense of why this had happened. Her life had been turned upside down and the things that were important to her were now even more precious. She missed her students and her work and wondered if she would have the physical stamina to return to work. She was also fearful that her other passion, rowing, would have to be forsaken – at the pinnacle of her career. Her team was so close to an international victory – an event she might now miss.

Jenna's surgeon listened and understood her anger and fears. He did not dismiss them or render them superfluous. Rather, he validated Jenna's concerns and reassured her that she would be able to enjoy all her activities and zest for living. These actions on the part of the doctor were central to Jenna's recovery. The doctor's acknowledgment of her present anger and future fears assisted in Jenna's own self-knowledge and belief in becoming well again. Had the surgeon only focused on her disease, her emotional recovery could have been delayed. Exploring Jenna's unique illness experience and supporting her through the recovery period was as important as the surgical intervention.

Certain illnesses or events in the lives of individuals may cause them embarrassment or emotional discomfort. As a result, patients may not always feel at ease with themselves or their physician, and may cloak their primary concerns in multiple symptoms. The doctor must, on occasion, respond to each of these symptoms to create an environment in which patients may feel more trusting and comfortable about exposing their concerns. Often, the doctor will provide them with an avenue to express their feelings by commenting: 'I sense that there is something troubling you or something more going on. How can I help you with that?'

Identifying the key questions to be asked ought not to be taken lightly. Malterud (1994) has described a method for clinicians to formulate and evaluate the wording of key questions. The wording of questions should be comfortable for the doctor and suited to each individual patient's context. It is important for physicians to explore patients' understanding of their problems and their expectations of the physician with enough depth that the doctor will know what words to use with each patient.

Metaphors and narratives of illness

Metaphors and narratives provide important ways of understanding patients' experiences of illness. Skelton *et al.* (2002) observe that patients and doctors may use very different metaphors, hence limiting the physician's ability 'to enter the patient's conceptual world' (2002:114). Doctors tend to see disease as 'a puzzle' and something to solve and hence 'control' (2002:116). In contrast, patient metaphors reflect the perspective of the body as 'a container of the self' and the experience of illness as often inexplicable, a sense of being out of touch, for example, is described as 'I'm the cotton wool man' (2002:116). Stensland and Malterud (2001) reveal, in their report of a case study, that eliciting and engaging in the patient's metaphor gives 'colour back to the patient's symptom experience' (2001:428) and empowers not only the patient but the clinician as well.

Recent publications (Borkan *et al.*, 1999; Brown *et al.*, 2002a; Greenhalgh and Hurwitz, 1998) also illustrate the importance of patients' narratives – their recounting of their story of illness. As Arthur Kleinman (1999) observes, narratives of illness, the patients' stories of being unwell, open up untold vistas of experience and knowing.

> Stories open up new paths, sometimes send us back to old ones, and close off still others. Telling (and listening to) stories we too imaginatively walk down those paths – paths of longing, paths of hope, paths of desperation. We are, actually, all of us, physicians and patients and family members too, storied folk: stories are what we are; telling and listening to stories is what we do. (Kleinman, 1999: *x*)

Hunter's (1991) vision of the narrative expands this view, in that the story is not one-sided but involves two (and we suggest multiple) protagonists or storytellers.

> Understanding medicine as a narrative activity enables us – both physicians and patients – to shift the focus of medicine to the care of what ails the patient and away from the relatively simpler matter of the diagnosis of disease. (Hunter, 1991: *xxi*)

Expanding the focus of inquiry from simply the disease to include the patient's illness experience can provide a richer, more meaningful and more productive outcome for all participants.

Yet research spanning almost 25 years (Beckman and Frankel, 1984; Marvel *et al.*, 1999; Rhoades *et al.*, 2001) indicates that physicians interrupt patients' accounts of their symptoms early in the consultation and hence their stories of illness are often untold. This reflects a failure on the physicians' part to weave back and forth between exploring the disease and illness experience, following the patients' cues. The patients' story of a troublesome sore throat may be cloaked in their fear that this is a precursor to cancer or patients may minimize their severe shortness of breath, explaining it as allergies, which from the doctor's perspective may indicate a more severe medical problem such as COPD.

However, when the clinician assists patients in telling their story of illness, they are helped in gaining meaning, and ultimately mastery, of the illness experience (Stensland and Malterud, 1999). When patients do not have a voice in the consultation, important dimensions of the illness experience such as their feelings and ideas will not be expressed (Barry *et al.*, 2000). Of equal concern is the potential for problematic outcomes, such as non-use of prescriptions and non-adherence to treatment (Barry *et al.*, 2000). Thus patient-centered practice defines attending to the patient's unique experience of illness as an important part of practicing good medical care.

The following case provides another illustration of the patient-centered method.

Case example

Rex Kelly was a 58-year-old man who had been a patient of the practice for ten years. Until eight months ago, when he had a massive myocardial infarction and required triple coronary artery bypass surgery, he had been a healthy man with few problems. He was married, with grown children and worked as a plumber. He had come to the office for diet counseling about his elevated cholesterol.

The following excerpt from the visit demonstrates the doctor's use of the patient-centered approach. The interaction began with Dr Wason stating, 'So, Rex, you're in about your diet. Looks like your cholesterol levels are dropping nicely.'

'Yes,' responded Rex. 'That's good news and I'm feeling pretty good about my weight. I'm down five more pounds and almost at my goal.' The doctor proceeded to explore Rex's diet in some detail.

The interview then shifted to Rex's exercise program, and he stated that he had been dutifully following his exercise regimen throughout the summer months and was walking up to four miles a day. Dr Wason asked, 'Will you be able to continue your walking during the winter?'

'Oh, yes,' indicated Rex. 'I don't mind walking in the winter. I quite enjoy it. I just have to be careful on those very cold days.'

'Yes, you do need to be cautious during the severe weather,' replied Dr Wason. Rex looked away and appeared sad. The doctor paused and asked, 'Is there something concerning you, Rex?'

'Oh well . . . no,' stated Rex quickly. 'No, not really.'

'Not really?' reflected Dr Wason.

'Well', replied Rex, 'I was just thinking about the winter and . . . well . . . no, I guess I'll be able to snowmobile if I just keep warm.'

'Why are you concerned that you won't be able to do that, Rex?' asked the doctor.

'Well, I don't know. I'd just miss it if I couldn't participate.'

'It sounds as if that activity is important to you,' responded Dr Wason.

'Well, yes, it has been a very important family activity. We have some land and a little cabin up north of here, and it's really how we spend our winter weekends the whole family together.'

'It sounds as if not being able to participate in something that's been an important family activity would be very difficult for you,' reflected the doctor.

'Oh, yes it would be. I just feel that so many things have been taken away from me that I really would miss not being able to do that.'

The doctor responded, 'Rex, it seems that in the past several months, you have experienced a lot of changes and a lot of losses. I sense it has been very difficult for you.'

Rex replied: 'Yes, Doc, it has. It's been tough. I've gone from being a man who is really healthy and has no problems to having a bad heart attack and a big operation and being a real weight watcher. It has been a big change, and it has had its tough moments, but I'm alive and I guess that is what matters.'

'It seems that you still have a lot of feelings surrounding your heart attack and the surgery and the changes that have occurred,' observed Dr Wason.

'Yes, I have', Rex replied soberly, '. . . I have.'

'Would it be helpful at some time for us to talk about that more, to set aside some time just to look at that?' inquired Dr Wason.

'Yes, it would. It's hard to talk about, but it would be helpful,' Rex emphatically replied.

'Are you encountering any problems with sleep or appetite, Rex?' asked the doctor.

'No, none at all,' stated Rex.

The doctor asked a few more questions exploring possible symptoms of depression. Finding none, he again offered to talk further with Rex at their next visit. The patient answered affirmatively.

In this example the patient's situation can be summarized by using the disease and illness framework which is part of the patient-centered method illustrated in Figure 3.2.

The doctor already knew the patient's disorders before the interview began. He picked up on the patient's sadness and his hesitancy in exploring how he was experiencing his illness. At the same time, the doctor ruled out serious depression by asking a few diagnostic questions and offered the patient an opportunity to explore further his feelings about his illness. The reader will notice that the interview effortlessly weaved back and forth between the disease issues and the illness experience.

By considering the patient's illness experience as a legitimate focus of inquiry and management, the physician has avoided two potential errors. First, if the

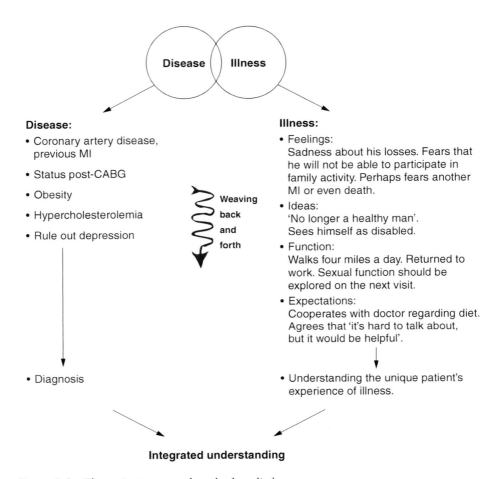

Figure 3.2   The patient-centered method applied.

conventional biomedical model only had been used, by seeking a disease to explain the patient's distress, the doctor might have labeled the patient depressed and given him unnecessary and potentially hazardous medication. A second error would have been to conclude that the patient was not depressed. Had the physician decided that the patient's distress was not worthy of attention, he may have delayed the patient's emotional and physical recovery and his adjustment to living with a chronic disease.

This case also illustrates that doctors are often very limited in what they can do about a patient's disease. However, dealing with this patient's experience of illness may be helpful in alleviating fears, correcting misconceptions, encouraging him to discuss his discouragement, or simply 'being there' and caring about what happens to him. At the very least this compassionate concern is a testimony to the fundamental worth and dignity of the patient; it might help prevent him from becoming truly depressed; it might even help him to live more fully.

Conclusion

In this chapter we have articulated the first component of the patient-centered clinical method, exploring both the disease and the patient's illness experience. Prior research has demonstrated how physicians have failed to acknowledge the patient's personal and unique experience of illness. The importance of exploring the illness experience, particularly the four dimensions of the patient's illness experience – feelings, ideas, function and expectations (FIFE) – has been described and demonstrated through case examples. The inextricable link between the patient's disease and illness experience with their position in the life cycle, context and environment is addressed in the next chapters.

Case example: 'I don't want to die!'

Judith Belle Brown, W Wayne Weston and Moira Stewart

With shock and disbelief Hanna felt the lump in her breast. She felt it again and with mounting fear realized her cancer may have returned. Hanna had been diagnosed with localized cancer in her left breast four years earlier. Treatment included lumpectomy and adjuvant radiotherapy. Axillary dissection showed no cancer in the axillary lymph nodes. She was given tamoxifen at that time, which she had taken faithfully. Since her surgery and treatments Hanna had been healthy with no symptoms. With vigor and determination she had resumed her active and busy life as a wife, mother, daughter and worker.

Now, recognizing the need to seek medical advice immediately, Hanna contacted Dr Maskova, her surgeon, who performed a biopsy. A few days later, Hanna was called into the doctor's office, at which time Dr Maskova broke the news that the biopsy results indicated a new cancer in the right breast. During the appointment, Hanna, a normally strong and independent woman, became distraught and wanted to leave immediately after her physical examination. Dr Maskova, surprised by Hanna's response, suggested they meet again in a week to discuss the next steps. Hanna agreed.

Up until that fateful appointment with her surgeon Hanna had kept her fear of recurrence a secret. Hanna, age 48, had not wanted to alarm her 50-year-old husband, Arnold, who had been recently diagnosed with hypertension. A manager at a local food store, Arnold had been under extreme stress due to a possible strike action by the cashiers at the store. The last thing Hanna wanted to do was to add more stress to her already overburdened partner. Nor did Hanna wish to frighten her two children, Rachel, aged 14, and Jonah, aged 16. They had been very anxious and afraid of losing their mother when she was first diagnosed four years ago. Their worries had subsided and they were both currently excelling in their individual academic and social circles. Finally, Hanna wished to protect her 70-year-old mother from the fear and angst it would evoke to learn that her daughter might have cancer again. Her mother had endured enough losses in life: the loss of an infant son from SIDS and then the death of her husband six years ago of a myocardial infarction at age 64, just as he was about to retire. And now to possibly lose her daughter would be too much to bear. Hanna resolved to keep the diagnosis a secret – just a little longer.

Hence, in the intervening week until her next visit to her surgeon, Hanna searched the Internet. She also spoke with several friends regarding breast cancer recurrence and treatment. Since Hanna worked as a copywriter for a medical journal, she was comfortable with medical terminology and tests. She was also the type of patient who needed as much information as possible in order to make any decisions about her health. In addition, she had talked at length to her friend, Adelle.

Hanna's friend Adelle was also a breast cancer survivor. Unlike Hanna, Adelle had tried several different kinds of alternative therapy. Her cancer had not recurred in over seven years and Hanna began to question if she should have also tried these alternative treatments. She had begun to question her faith in conventional treatments and although normally quite decisive she now felt confused and uncertain about how to proceed.

A week later Hanna returned to Dr Maskova's office.

Dr Maskova: Hello Hanna – I am glad to see you back today. How are you doing?

Hanna: Hi, Dr Maskova. It has been a hard week since I last saw you.

Dr Maskova: How so?

Hanna: Oh, Doctor, I'm really scared, I wasn't expecting anything like this. I haven't slept in a week. I can't eat, and my stomach is in knots . . .

Dr Maskova: It does sound like it's been an awful week for you.

Hanna: Yes, it has been awful, I have so many questions, and I am so confused. Will I have to stop working? I'm already finding it hard to work.
I DON'T WANT TO DIE. I'm not ready to die; my children are just teen-
agers – they still need me.

Dr Maskova: There is a lot going on Hanna – a lot to consider. Tell me more
about what is happening.

Hanna: Yes, and I have been on the Internet and I've been talking to
friends. I need to know if I should have done things differently.
Should I have restricted fat from my diet? Should I have taken shark's
cartilage or Essiac? My friend has done these things and her breast
cancer has not come back in over seven years. Could it be that they
prevented a recurrence for Adelle? Why did I get a new cancer? Isn't
that very rare? What am I doing wrong?

Dr Maskova: (*Feeling overwhelmed by the multitude and rapidity of his patient's
concerns the doctor decided to try to gain a better understanding of Hanna's
life and context.*) You're asking a lot of important questions Hanna.
I feel I need more information before I can answer them properly.
Can you tell me Hanna, what's happening at home – with you and
the family?

Hanna explained that she had not told her family because her husband was
under tremendous strain at work and had high blood pressure. She
described her children's fear that they would lose their mother. Most
importantly, Hanna did not want to upset her mother; she had already
had enough losses in one lifetime. Hanna perceived that the well-being
of all these people was basically on her shoulders and she clearly felt
overwhelmed.

Hanna's confusion and anxiety dissipated as Dr Maskova took time to
listen to her story. He was honest, caring, and understanding. Dr Maskova
validated her concerns and worries about the effect of her diagnosis on her
family and explored ways to address how best to involve them. He listened
to her growing doubts about conventional treatments and allayed her fears
that she could have, or should have, done more to stop her cancer from
recurring. With respect, he explored her inquiries about alternative therapies and discussed how they could examine the efficacy of such treatments
together. The doctor also provided Hanna with sufficient information at
the appropriate moments and provided guidance in making informed decisions. Dr Maskova gave Hanna permission to seek help or information
about support groups and alternative medicine. Dr Maskova made it clear
to Hanna that she would be given opportunities to choose between treatment options and be involved as much as she wanted in all the decisions
throughout the course of her treatment.

At the conclusion of the consultation, Hanna felt more informed, more certain, more in control and less overwhelmed. The doctor had achieved this by exploring Hanna's feelings and expectations by resisting his desire to take over and provide all the answers and by building on his relationship with Hanna. Dr Maskova indicated that he would be there for her through her treatment and recovery.

Hanna's interactions with her surgeon consequently became pivotal in regaining control. She needed information from him that would assist her in the multiple treatment decisions before her. She needed a surgeon who would listen to and respect her concerns and wishes. For Hanna, a relationship with her surgeon, built on honesty and reciprocity, was paramount. Hanna also needed a surgeon who expressed an interest in both her and her family – taking into consideration their needs and anxieties. By developing a trusting and respectful relationship with her surgeon, Hanna was able to regain some semblance of control over the chaos she was experiencing. Dr Maskova did not dismiss Hanna's questions or negate her worries; rather he took the time necessary to explore her fears and that in itself helped to alleviate her concerns.

As Hanna progressed from the shattering realization of the recurrence of cancer to the treatment phase, she and her physician engaged in a process of establishing a mutual understanding of what should and would transpire. At each point in her treatment they discussed the current situation, her various options and what would be the most appropriate plan. Hanna, by choice, became an active and informed partner in her care, thereby regaining the courage to live with cancer.

4

The second component: understanding the whole person, Section 1: individual and family

Judith Belle Brown and W Wayne Weston

Cassell (1991) has observed that patients' diseases are only one dimension of their personhood: hence they are a narrow means of understanding the patients' illness and suffering. Many of the dimensions of personhood proposed by Cassell (1991) are examined in this chapter and in Chapter 5. For example, in this chapter, we will examine the influence of personality in the context of human development; the relationship between past events and current behaviors and responses to illness and care; the role of spirituality in patients' lives; and the strong and potent effect of how family history and current dynamics influence patients' responses to health and illness. In Chapter 5 broader contextual issues that influence patients' health and well-being are addressed.

The person: individual development

There are multiple theoretical frameworks that can help clinicians understand patients' individual development and provide both explanation and prediction about patient behavior and responses to illness. For example, they include: psychoanalytic theory, i.e. ego psychology, object relations, and self psychology; feminist theory; and cognitive theory. A comprehensive overview of these various theoretical frameworks has been provided by numerous authors (e.g. Berzoff *et al.*, 1996; Eagle, 1984; Erikson, 1950, 1982; Gilligan, 1982; Jordan *et al.*, 1991; Kohut, 1971, 1977; Mishne, 1993; Piaget, 1950).

The intent of this section of the chapter is to highlight understanding individual development and to demonstrate how this can be achieved in the practice of patient-centered care.

Healthy individual development is reflected by a solid sense of self, positive self-esteem, a position of independence and autonomy, coupled with the capacity for connectedness and intimacy. The motives, attachments, ideals and expectations that shape each individual's personality evolve as they negotiate each developmental phase. Each person's life is profoundly influenced by each developmental phase which may be isolated and lonely for an elderly widow or vast and complex for a middle-aged woman with the multiple responsibilities as wife, mother, daughter, worker. Thus their position in the life cycle, the tasks they assume and the roles they ascribe to will influence the care patients seek. As an illustration of the impact of illness on human development, consider the teenager, grappling with the demands of peer acceptance, who is ostracized because of his or her acne, or the middle-aged woman, coping with the 'empty-nest syndrome', who is reminded of her loss of fertility by the symptoms of menopause.

Understanding the patient's current stage of development and the relevant developmental tasks which need to be accomplished assists doctors in several ways. First, knowledge of expected life cycle crises that occur in individual development helps the doctor recognize the patient's problems as more than isolated, episodic phenomena. Second, it can increase the doctor's sensitivity to the multiple factors that influence the patient's problems and broaden awareness of the impact of the patient's life history. For example, the onset of a chronic illness at an early age may interfere with negotiation of age-specific tasks. Such is the case of juvenile onset diabetes, which may create difficulty for an adolescent attempting to negotiate the turbulent process of becoming independent. Third, understanding the whole person may also expand the doctor's level of comfort with caring as well as curing.

In the following case example we observe how an accumulation of life events had a powerful influence on a patient's response to coping with a fatal illness.

Case example

Marianna engaged her cancer as she engaged her life – with determination, ingenuity and humor. But not all her healthcare providers had appreciated these qualities. In fact, on occasion they had been rather threatened by them. In one instance, when a collection of Marianna's friends had gathered at her bedside to form a healing circle, involving the burning of sweetgrass, the hospital was adamantly opposed. Marianna, with her consummate ability to invoke humor commented: 'Going to sue a dying woman for setting fire to some old weeds?!?'

For ten years Marianna endured her cancer as it ravaged her body and as the treatments to stop it did even more damage. She lost her hair, her bones became weak and fragile and her teeth disintegrated as a result of her cancer treatments. Yet, she continued to paint, to assert her expressions of life, both beautiful and poignant. When she was able to, she reveled in the small things – the sweet taste of a mango dripping off her lips; the exquisite details of a monarch butterfly in flight; the lingering smell of a gardenia; the multitude of colors cast by a prism caught in a ray of sunshine; the soft touch of her infant granddaughter's cheek and – best of all – the delightful sounds of her family chatting all around her.

It took considerable time for Marianna's healthcare professionals to understand and appreciate the uniqueness of this woman, and how her approach to battling cancer was embedded in her own personal health beliefs and experiences. Marianna had been the last child in a sibline of six – the three before her had died, all of stillbirth. Hence, she had been designated as the 'precious child' – a miracle. She had borne this mantle for many years. It was not until her marriage to Ned, and her parents' deaths shortly thereafter, that she broke free and began to stake out her own independence.

But this was short-lived as Ned's aging parents demanded more attention, initially to their business needs, and ultimately for their personal care. For many years Marianna set aside her own needs and interests to provide her ailing in-laws with the care they needed. Despite her devotion and attention to their needs they never acknowledged her care and concern. Marianna's primary regret during this time was not devoting sufficient energy and care to her only daughter Nadine who was, in Marianna's view, 'growing up on her own'. It had only been in the past few years, when Nadine had married and become a mother, that they established a 'special bond'. The linchpin of this connection was Marianna's granddaughter, Angela.

All these events in Marianna's life – her early years, her place in the sibline, her assigned role, her expectations of herself and others, her ambitions and lost opportunities, all affected her as a person – well or dying. In Marianna's final days the healthcare professionals attending to her care developed an appreciation of these many factors that culminated in Marianna's peaceful death.

Understanding the patient's personality structure, in particular the defense mechanisms they use to ward off anxiety, both internal and external, can enhance clinicians' understanding of patients' varied responses to disease and illness. Defense mechanisms which are automatic and unconscious serve an important function in protecting the self or the ego from real or perceived danger (Schamess, 1996). Patients use a variety of defense mechanisms, including more primitive or immature defenses, such as denial and projection. Higher level or more mature defenses, such as repression, rationalization, displacement and sublimation are used to ward off toxic threats to the ego and thus help patients cope. The defenses are used to prevent ego disintegration and as such need to be respected. As Broom (1997: 66–7) observes:

> The patient defends himself against the 'intolerable' by setting in place structures that are not ideal but are actually adaptive within the patient's total economy, and we should expect resistance to any change in this. I may be imprisoned and long for freedom, but also be terrified of venturing out into a wider world. There may also be some comforts in the prison cell that those of us outside may scorn as objects to be clung to, but this may be very understandable within the patient's perspective.

The following case serves as an example of a patient's use of defense mechanisms and takes place in the context of what is normally a happy event, the birth of a child.

Case example

> When the delivery room nurse announced to 28-year-old Roseanne that her baby was a healthy eight-pound boy, the patient loudly exclaimed: 'I didn't want a boy!' She refused to hold the baby and the shocked nurse handed the baby over to his father.
>
> A few days later when the visiting nurse made a home visit she found Roseanne stiffly holding her infant. She denied that there were any problems and rationalized her outburst in the delivery room as a result of exhaustion from a long labor. Over the next several weeks as the nurse continued to visit Roseanne she observed that mother and child were bonding well. Roseanne's initial displeasure about the baby's sex seemed to have disappeared. Her anger was now being displaced onto her husband, Gregory, whom she described as never being around or helping out with young Timothy. The source of the marital discord was apparently Gregory's 'obsession with work'. Her husband was, from Roseanne's perspective, just like her father who had never been physically or emotionally available during her childhood. 'All men are the same', concluded Roseanne, 'never there when you need them most.'
>
> The nurse's attempts to further explore Roseanne's feelings during subsequent visits were met with denial and rationalization. Because mother and child were doing well the nurse's role had been fulfilled, yet as she closed the case she had a nagging feeling that Roseanne's defenses were protecting the patient from some deeper distress. We will return later in this chapter to Roseanne's story.

An understanding of the whole person enhances the clinician's interaction with the patient and may be particularly helpful when signs or symptoms do not point to a clearly defined disease process, or when the patient's response to an illness appears exaggerated or out of character. On these occasions, it is often helpful to explore how the patient is dealing with the common issues related to his or her stage in the life cycle. Knowing that a patient has minimal family interaction or limited social supports alerts the physician to an individual at risk. Also, being aware of prior losses or developmental crises assists the doctor to identify vulnerable junctures in the patient's life.

Case example

Dr Grant was perplexed. This was the sixth time he had seen his 23-year-old patient, Suzy, and her daughter, Michelle, in the past two months. At each visit Suzy had expressed concern about her 5-year-old daughter's health. But from the doctor's perspective Michelle's, or rather her mother's, complaints were minor, such as a sore throat or a stomach ache. On each occasion, Dr Grant reassured Suzy that her daughter's problem was self-limiting and would resolve quickly. Yet Suzy continued to bring her daughter to see the doctor.

Suzy and her daughter had joined the practice a year ago and upon reflection Dr Grant realized he knew little of Suzy's life and experiences. At the end of the next visit he asked Suzy if she would be interested in coming back alone to talk to him regarding her concerns about Michelle. She agreed and when she returned the following story was revealed.

Suzy, a single parent on welfare, was finding it more difficult to cope with the demands of her active daughter. She had become increasingly more physical with Michelle in her attempts to control her behavior and was concerned that she might unintentionally harm her when her anger got 'out of control'. In order to cope with the pressure and calm herself down, she had started to drink 'the odd shot of vodka', which at times had led to consuming the whole bottle.

Suzy described her feelings of guilt after having struck Michelle and how these feelings added to her sense of helplessness and growing reliance on alcohol. She often ruminated about 'what could have been' if her boyfriend had not 'got her pregnant and taken off'. Her goal had been to go to university and train as a physiotherapist: her above-average high school grades would have ensured admission into the program. Suzy was angry at herself for 'wasting' her life. She felt extremely lonely and confused. Finally, she questioned her ability to be a 'good' mother and in turn demanded near-perfection in her mothering skills (e.g. with regard to hygiene and child nutrition).

The doctor then asked about her early years and learned important information about Suzy's past that illuminated her current problems and concerns. Suzy, the eldest of three daughters, was raised in a rural community. Her father had held an executive position with a nearby food processing and distributing company for 30 years. He was an alcoholic who controlled his binge-drinking in such a way that it did not interfere with the demands of his job. However, when intoxicated, he would emotionally and physically abuse his wife. Often, Suzy and her younger sisters 'got in the way' and would also suffer physical and emotional abuse from their father.

Her pregnancy had been a shameful experience for the family and became a well-kept family secret. Forced to leave the family home, and small close-knit community where she had been raised, all Suzy's supports and connections had been severed. Furthermore, her father had forbidden her to have contact with her mother and sisters. Consequently, Suzy was raising Michelle on her own with no family support and limited social supports.

In listening to Suzy's story the doctor gained a greater understanding and deeper appreciation of the influence of the patient's past on her current behavior. Her frequent visits to the doctor and her 'over-concern' about her daughter's health were being fueled by multiple factors, both present and historical. A pattern of multigenerational behaviors and responses was now evident. Dr Grant was no longer perplexed by his patient's actions but informed by her difficult and tragic history of abuse and alcoholism. The patient's disclosure of this important information would assist the patient and doctor in their work together – helping Suzy be the best mom she could be.

An individual's past can haunt them, immobilizing their ability to act in the present and preventing their movement towards future goals and aspirations. As Fraiberg *et al.* (1975) so aptly wrote there are 'ghosts in the nursery'; demons of the past that can be dissipated by the clinician's careful and attentive listening to the patient's life story, not just their disease.

Finally, the normal achievement of developmental milestones by a child can often serve as triggers for the parent of their unresolved issues of the past. Returning to the case of Roseanne serves as an illustration.

Case example

When Roseanne's son Timothy was aged $2\frac{1}{2}$, she began presenting to her family doctor with a variety of complaints including headaches, dizziness, leg weakness and buzzing in her ears. Each round of investigations failed to uncover a cause for her symptoms. Reassurance from her doctor that 'nothing was wrong' did not alleviate her distress, rather her symptoms intensified and the frequency of her visits to the doctor increased. Finally, during a visit Roseanne burst out crying and said, 'I think I'm dying.' The doctor was initially baffled by the extreme nature of his patient's response, as none of her symptoms were life-threatening. She appeared to have a happy home life, with a healthy and active toddler and a loving husband. But clearly her ongoing presentation of multiple and unexplained physical symptoms was a signal of some deeper distress in Roseanne's life.

What unfolded was a complex, multigenerational story, activated by the normal developmental progression of a toddler. As Roseanne's son Timothy began to assert his autonomy and independence, she felt anxious and abandoned. The root of these powerful emotions rested in the patient's own childhood and her family of origin.

Roseanne was the eldest in a sibline of five, all of whom had been born in rapid succession, hence propelling her out of the maternal nest. The patient described how, by the age of four, she had become her mother's 'little helper' assisting in the care of her younger siblings. She had assumed this role in an attempt to have her unmet needs addressed. When this failed, Roseanne turned in desperation to her father. But he was self-absorbed with his failing business and own physical problems, including chronic leg weakness as a result of having polio in his youth. Roseanne's father frequently complained how the burden of providing for his family was 'killing him'.

Roseanne's early years had been fraught with abandonment and uncertainty. Now in her late twenties these feelings had re-surfaced as her son, in whom she had invested all her love and attention, was asserting his own agency. Unable to articulate her profound sense of loss she had voiced her feelings through bodily symptoms.

This is a difficult and multi-faceted case and the patient's story was uncovered over many visits with the family doctor and assisted by the expert skills of a therapist. It highlights the intricate relationship between the mind and body; the past and present (Broom, 1997, 2000). While not all patients' stories are this complex, this case demonstrates how clinicians can use their understanding of the whole person to enhance patient-centered care. Learning about the patient's developmental journey helps clinicians realize that patients are more than just their diseases. As Broom (1997) observes:

> The patient's story is, amongst many other things, a woven tapestry – of events, of perceptions of events, and of highly idiosyncratic responses to events. Many of the very significant events have to do with the vicissitudes of the patient's relationships with the world, and with other significant persons. Therefore, when a patient and a doctor collaborate together to look for the meaning of an illness, they are usually looking for the story of a person in relationship. (1997: 1–2)

The final segment of this section examines the role of spirituality in patients' lives and responses to illness. Until recently physicians have abdicated issues of patient spirituality to the clergy (King and Bushwick, 1994). Physicians are hesitant to discuss religious or spiritual issues with their patients, perhaps because they feel such inquiry is outside their area of expertise or from fear of offending patients (Post *et al.*, 2000). But research has revealed patients' desire for their physicians' involvement in the spiritual aspects of their personhood (Ehman *et al.*, 1999). A survey in an inpatient rehabilitation unit indicated that 74% of patients considered their religious and spiritual beliefs to be important and 54% desired pastoral counseling. Yet only 16% of physicians in this study ever inquired about these matters (Anderson *et al.*, 1993). In another study of 203 adult family practice patients in Kentucky and eastern North Carolina, 77% of patients wanted physicians to consider their spiritual needs, 37% wanted doctors to discuss these needs more often, and 48% wanted their physicians to pray with them (King and Bushwick, 1994). Furthermore, physicians have expressed an interest in engaging their patients in discussions about spirituality, recognizing that this must be approached with 'sensitivity and integrity' (Craigie and Hobbs, 1999; Ellis *et al.*, 2002: 249). While physicians recognize the relationship between spirituality and patient's overall well-being, barriers to assessing patients' spiritual resources include lack of time and inadequate training (Ellis *et al.*, 1999; Matthews *et al.*, 1998; McBride *et al.*, 1998). Broom (1997) views the person's mind, body and spirituality as an integrated whole: to separate off one piece for examination is to minimize, or at worst deny, the importance of the other.

Serious illness raises questions about meaning – why has this happened, why me, what did I do to deserve this, what will become of me? These are spiritual questions that may have no easy answer and which are unique to each person. These questions may lead to a deepening of patients' spiritual lives or, conversely, to a loss of faith based on a feeling that God has abandoned them. Thus, these questions are intensely important. And yet, because they are so personal, they may not be discussed with anyone, not even family or close friends. This may leave the patient alone with these fundamental doubts and concerns at a time when they most need to share them – a challenge to all members of the healthcare team to be open to discuss these issues.

May (1991) observes that there are two kinds of ethical question in medicine: 'On the whole, medical ethics has tended to explore those moral issues that cluster around the admittedly important question "What are we going to do about it?" but at the expense of those deep, troubling issues which patients and families often face: How can they manage – whatever the decision or whatever the event – to rise to the occasion?' (May, 1991: 14). He comments further: '... the latter type of problem resembles a mystery more than a puzzle; it demands a response that resembles a ritual repeated more than a technique' (1991: 4). The following example illustrates the dilemma faced by patients struck down by illness: '... suddenly a blood clot stalls in his coronary artery; the rescue unit pulls him out of his car and wheels him into an intensive care unit. Suddenly he finds his time even more limited than he thought. The catastrophe confronts him with problems to solve; but these problems pale before the deeper question: who and what is he now that he has suffered this explosion from within? Accustomed to commanding his world, the patient suddenly finds himself helpless in the hands of nurses down the hospital corridor; used to total obedience from his subordinates, he discovers that the very humblest of his subordinates, his own body, has rebelled against him' (May, 1991: 5). How does such a man come to terms with the loss of a job that gave his life excitement and meaning? Adopting a less demanding role, perhaps as a mentor to junior colleagues, and learning to pace himself may help, but these technical solutions do not address the fundamental crisis involved in losing his former identity. Such questions are at the heart of religion and spirituality and call out for dialog.

The following case examines the role of spirituality in a couple's attempt to deal with a devastating diagnosis. How the case evolves highlights the importance of teamwork described in Chapter 9.

Case example

Brett and Sandra had been married for four years when Brett was diagnosed with colon cancer. For Brett, aged 59, and Sandra, aged 52, the diagnosis was devastating. This was Sandra's first marriage and her commitment to Brett had been life-changing. For Brett, embarking on his second marriage meant taking a risk to care and commit deeply again. Their four years together, in conjunction with their two-year courtship, had been filled with travel, shared interests in their church, and a growing devotion to one another.

Consequently, Sandra was not prepared for Brett's response to his diagnosis of cancer. Faced with the reality of living with cancer Brett withdrew. It was a dark and safe place he entered, much like the 'emotional cave' he had sought out as a refuge after the failure of his first marriage. Indeed it had been a 'cave', a small apartment set into a mountain with windows only facing north. In his mind it was to this place, this strange respite, that he retreated when he was diagnosed.

But, for Sandra, who had unequivocally made the decision to devote herself to Brett, his withdrawal was experienced as abandonment and rejection. While distraught by Brett's diagnosis, Sandra could not quiet her anger – not at the diagnosis but at Brett. They had been so close, so connected – such kindred spirits. How could he withdraw from her at this moment?! She was disappointed that he had also turned his back on God. Their religion had been so important to both of them and now, when they most needed it, he would not discuss his feelings about his situation. When, together, they met with the surgeon to discuss Brett's treatment options they were sad, angry, confused and in conflict. The doctor was overwhelmed by their powerful display of emotions. In previous contacts with this couple he had observed their very measured and clear decision-making. Yet now they were in serious distress. Not comfortable addressing their needs the doctor referred them to the nurse clinician affiliated with the clinic. After a brief assessment she also recognized her limitations in helping this couple and contacted the team's social worker for assistance in helping Brett and Sandra.

Several sessions with the social worker, and then with a pastoral counselor, were needed to help Brett and Sandra overcome the conflict-laden behaviors they were expressing. Conversations about their shared joy of travel brought them back into conflict and disappointment because such opportunities seemed impossible now. However, exploration of other shared interests led them to express their common belief in the healing power of their spiritual world. Their sense of connectedness increased as together they regained their shared sense of faith. Recognizing and reaffirming their shared religious commitments helped them continue forward in Brett's cancer treatments and, of equal importance, to continue to share together what gave their lives meaning even in the face of his serious illness. In May's terms, they had risen to the occasion.

The person and the family life cycle

Patients may be parents, partners, sons and daughters: they all have a past, a present and a future. We are all connected on some level to a family which in turn shapes who we are as people and as patients. Relationships and kinships bind us to one another, making us feel needed, loved and connected. Illness can enhance or sever these essential ties in human relationships leaving both the sick, and the well, feeling alone and rudderless. The journey to recovery, or at best attainment of the status quo, can be experienced as an extreme effort, and for some beyond the realm of possibility.

Similar to individual development, a vast literature on family theory exists to explain and understand the intricacies and dynamics of family systems. Again, it is not the purpose of this chapter to provide a comprehensive overview of this area but to highlight the important role of the family in understanding the whole person. The reader is directed to the following texts which provide clear and thoughtful presentations of the family life cycle and family systems (Carter and McGoldrick, 1989; Hartman and Laird, 1983) and additional works, which link family systems and primary care (Christie-Seely, 1984; Doherty and Baird, 198668; McDaniel *et al.*, 1990; Sawa, 1992).

In concurrence with other authors (Carter and McGoldrick, 1989; Hartman and Laird, 1983; McDaniel *et al.*, 1990; Medalie and Cole-Kelly, 2002), we define family as two or more people related or connected either biologically, emotionally or legally. Our conceptualization extends beyond the traditional notion of the family, encompassing unions such as gay and lesbian couples, common-law relationships, single-parent families, couples without children and households composed of friends. While the composition and roles of the family have changed and expanded, the function of the family has remained constant – to provide a nurturing and safe environment that promotes the physical, psychological and social well-being of its members (Berzoff *et al.*, 1996; Woods and Hollis, 1990). In today's society this is a daunting task. The family is being buffeted by internal and external forces. The rising divorce rate, the increase in single-parent households, changes in traditional sex-role relationships, and the re-entry of women into the work force, all challenge the function of the family. The health and well-being of families is assaulted by problems such as child and woman abuse, suicide, AIDS and substance abuse. Families must also face the enormous strain imposed by unemployment, poverty and being homeless. In examining the role and influence of the family life cycle on patients' responses to the illness experience we must take heed of Candib's caution to expand our perspective beyond gender-laden perspectives (Candib, 1995). A broad definition of family must be assumed with an acknowledgment of the broader socio-cultural and political influences that shape the clinician's knowledge, beliefs and values about the family.

The additional burden of illness, either acute or chronic, may cause severe disruption to an already over-taxed family system (Mailick, 1979; Medalie and Cole-Kelly, 2002; Rolland, 1989). Illness, either acute or chronic, is a powerful agent of change. The impact of illness on the family ranges from the devastating loss of the breadwinner role caused by a cardiovascular accident to the riveting effect on a family when a child is diagnosed with cerebral palsy. In other instances, the illness may initially appear superficial and benign as demonstrated in the following case, yet the implications of the patient's injury may have a significant impact on her sense of self and her family relationships.

Case example

George Landry was considering filing a malpractice suit against the doctors who treated his daughter. His 15-year-old daughter Amy was in hospital undergoing treatment for a severe palmar space infection of her right hand. Mr Landry was extremely upset and angry. He viewed the medical care as negligent and felt that his daughter might now face a lifelong disability, one that could have been prevented.

The original injury was a puncture wound that occurred while Amy was helping her father with yard work ten days previously. Although the injury initially appeared fairly minor he took her to see the physician on call. The doctor had examined her hand, cleansed and explored the wound and determined that Amy's immunization was up-to-date. The hand was dressed in a bulky dressing. Mr Landry was reassured that the wound was not serious but was instructed to return with his daughter to have the hand rechecked in 24–48 hours.

Twenty-four hours later Mr Landry brought his daughter to see their doctor at the clinic because he was worried about possible complications. He was also anxious about whether his daughter could perform at a piano recital in a few days. There were no objective findings and Mr Landry was reassured that his daughter's hand was fine. The doctor re-dressed her hand and instructed them to have her hand rechecked in another 24–48 hours if necessary. There was no further discussion of the imminent piano recital.

When Mr Landry once again returned to the clinic with his daughter, 72 hours later, the hand and forearm were swollen and there was obvious pus coming from the wound. She was admitted to hospital and was assessed by a surgeon who recommended an exploration of the wound under general anesthesia. Amy was admitted to hospital and placed on intravenous antibiotics. The Landrys were informed that the infection was serious and there was a possibility of permanent damage to the function of the hand.

In order to understand this family's anxiety and concern, their past history and present context need to be understood. Mr Landry, aged 40, was married to Anne, aged 36, and worked in the food services industry. Anne, a teacher by profession, was currently at home with their two children. Their eldest child Amy was an accomplished pianist and considered very gifted by her music teachers, who predicted a bright future for her. The Landrys had already started a special fund for her training. They also had a second daughter, Sara, aged ten, who had Down's Syndrome. Mrs Landry had given up teaching to care for their disabled daughter. There were no plans for more children; in fact Mrs Landry had a tubal ligation after the birth of their second child. Thus, the Landrys had put all their hopes for the future in Amy. Now she was at risk of serious debilitation from a minor mishap. Their vision of the future was seriously threatened and the Landrys individually, and collectively, had to face the meaning and significance of her injury and disability.

This story illustrates many issues about the impact of a family's experience of illness, punctuated by anger, distress, a need to find someone to blame, loss and more loss. The present crisis was underwritten by past events that brought the family sorrow and put them in a position of placing much of their energy and hopes for the future on one family member – whose well-being was in jeopardy.

This case also serves as an example of how being patient-centered involves not only the 'identified patient' but the entire family; their various needs and concerns must be taken into consideration. The treatment of Amy's puncture wound was now a family affair.

Illness in the family causes a major disruption altering how families relate and may ultimately impede their ability to overcome the ramifications of the illness experience. Illness may demand a change in the family role structure and task allocation. Changes in routine may be required, such as childcare responsibilities or visits to the hospital. Major alterations may be needed, such as substantial home renovations to accommodate a wheelchair-bound family member or a return to the work force to provide for the financial needs of the family.

The disequilibrium in the family resulting from illness can also alter the established rules and expectations of the family, transform their methods of communication and substantially alter the family structure. For example, after the diagnosis of terminal breast cancer, a mother transferred her responsibilities for the care of her five children to her eldest daughter, aged 16. The daughter, in turn, quit school, assumed the full caretaker role for her siblings and became her father's confidant as he watched his wife resign herself to her cancer. The changes imposed on families by illness are limitless and are accompanied by a host of feelings – loss, fear, anger, resignation, anxiety, sadness, resentment and dependency.

Involving the family is also important given that over one-third of patients are accompanied by one or more family members during a visit to their doctor (Brown *et al.*, 1998; Marvel *et al.*, 2000). Family members may be as concerned as the patient about the problem or potential treatments. They can also provide important information about the patient and be an invaluable resource in the patient's recovery (Watson and McDaniel, 2000). But as Lang *et al.* (2002) observed involving family members in an office visit can present specific challenges, such as maintaining confidentiality and addressing family conflict. The particular needs of the patient and knowledge of the family's dynamics will assist clinicians in deciding whom to involve within the family and when to approach them.

How families have coped previously will influence how they negotiate the impact of the illness on their family roles, rules, patterns of communication and structures. Therefore in understanding the impact of the illness on the family some key questions can guide the clinician's inquiry. At what point is the family in the family life cycle (e.g. starting a family, retirement)? Where is each member in the life cycle (e.g. adolescence, middle age)? What are the developmental tasks for each individual and for the family as a whole? How does the illness affect the achievement of these multiple tasks? What kinds of illness have the family experienced? What kinds of support have they mobilized in the past to help them cope with illness? Is there currently an established support network? How has the family dealt with illness in the past? Have they responded with functional or dysfunctional patterns of behavior? For example, has the family demonstrated potential maladaptive responses, such as rejection of the sick person, or over-protection that stifles responsibility for self-care?

These latter questions are important because they elicit how families may contribute to or perpetuate illness behavior in their members (Malterud, 1998). The family may represent a safe refuge for the ill person or conversely may aggravate the illness through maladaptive responses.

The impact of the diagnosis on the patient and family will depend on what juncture in the life cycle it occurs. For example, an adult male with a pre-existing history of diabetes mellitus may find his disease has less impact on his role (as a husband and father) than a teenager who is diagnosed at the point when the family is struggling with adolescent issues of independence and identity. Similarly, the preoccupations and struggles of families in each stage may be vastly different (e.g. how does the diagnosis of multiple sclerosis impact on the childrearing responsibilities of the family system; what meaning does the death of an adult child have on aging parents who were relying on that child for support?).

Finally, while the illness of an individual family member reverberates throughout the family system, the family also plays a powerful role in modifying the illness experience of the individual. There is now a strong body of research demonstrating how families affect illness, ranging from maternal–infant bonding (Klaus and Kennell, 1976) to the consequences of bereavement (Helsing and Szklo, 1981; Kaprio *et al.*, 1987). Both McWhinney (1997), and McDaniel *et al.* (1990) provide excellent reviews of the empirical evidence documenting the significant influence of the family on the health and disease of its members.

Conclusion

Doctors develop an evolving understanding of the social and developmental context in which their patients live their lives. Usually, this information is not gathered in a single encounter as part of a formal social history but rather is accumulated over many visits that can span many months or years. As the patient and doctor have shared life experiences this understanding becomes richer and more detailed. With certain patients this information may help the doctor understand the patient's complex dynamics and idiosyncratic responses to illness or demands for care (Jones and Morrell, 1995). Specific aspects of the patient's family dynamics or developmental difficulties may not necessarily be shared with the patient, but guide the doctor in the management and care of the patient. In other instances, facilitating the patient's awareness of the origin of their conflicts or distress may help them make sense of their struggles and pain. Finally, understanding the whole person can deepen the doctor's knowledge of the human condition especially the nature of suffering and the responses of persons to sickness (Cassell, 1991; Mayeroff, 1972).

Case example: 'I don't want him to go into a nursing home!'

Judith Belle Brown and Carol L McWilliam

Mr and Mrs Latour's life together was irrevocably altered when, at 67 years of age, Jacques Latour suffered a debilitating stroke rendering him hemiplegic. Yvette, his 63-year-old partner of 30 years became devoted to his care. As Mrs Latour explained: 'Of course our way of life has changed and his world is only what he can reach. But I'm so glad he's here.' Their sense of connectedness and history together served as a foundation for their shared experience of living with his chronic illness: 'We just sit and have a glass of wine and chat and laugh and reminisce about our wonderful times together.' But as much as they attempted to work together in confronting their present situation, both Mr and Mrs Latour also described grieving the dramatic change in their relationship. Mrs Latour reflected: 'We lived such carefree lives and were able to do things, what and when we wanted, and then to have something like this is just such a tremendous change!'

Mr Latour was cognizant of the burden he placed on his wife: 'If I wasn't here, Yvette could go on with her life. I'm pulling her down.' Yet Mrs Latour, on the other hand, framed the burden of her caregiving responsibilities positively: 'What I'm learning is that the responsibility of caring for Jacques is a privilege and now this is my chance to show my love for him.'

Nevertheless, the ongoing demands of constant caregiving also gave rise to negative reactions that were damaging to the Latours' relationship. An accumulation of feelings – vulnerability, irritability, fatigue, loss and guilt – occasionally surfaced, undermining Yvette Latour's positive perspective on caregiving. She often tried to hide her frustration and irritability but the constant demands of care would sometimes become overwhelming.

At night if he's had another bowel movement before I get back to bed I think, 'Oh, no – I can't do this again!' I don't say anything but actions speak louder than words. He knows I am upset and gets feeling guilty. It's awful because he knows that now I've got to wash him again and then he starts to cry. I'm sorry that I haven't been able to put a smile on my face but sometimes it is too much to bear.

One morning when Dr Ombreck, their family doctor, was making his monthly housecall, he observed that Mrs Latour was looking particularly exhausted. 'How have things been going?' he inquired. Yvette described how Jacques had been troubled by several bouts of diarrhea over the past few days and as a result she had experienced three nights of interrupted sleep in order to attend to his needs. Although Dr Ombreck acknowledged the Latours' commitment and determination to keep Jacques at home, he was also aware of the vulnerable position they were currently in. The doctor was also concerned about Yvette's fragile physical and emotional state. Gently, Dr Ombreck broached the possibility of admitting Jacques to a respite care bed temporarily.

This was a significant turning point for the Latours as their individual and mutual emotions pushed them to accept and ultimately act on their current situation and hence to access respite care. As Mrs Latour later reflected: 'I remember saying, "What do you mean respite care? I don't want him to go into a nursing home," and Dr Ombreck just simply said, "No, it's time for him to go in so you can rest." So we made the decision and thank goodness the doctor saw that we needed it. Because you have to get out from underneath that pressure. You have to accept help and thank goodness for respite care and a doctor who could help us accept that we needed help.'

For Mrs Latour respite care offered relief – a chance to temporarily relinquish the responsibility, so that she could once again assume the privilege of caring: 'I wasn't sleeping and I could barely cope. Respite care gave me a break so I could get rested and be able to care for Jacques again.' For Mr Latour the most important aspect of respite care was that it lifted the burden of responsibility from his wife: 'Getting away gives her a chance to be without the responsibility of caring for me all the time.'

Dr Ombreck's ongoing care of this couple enhanced his knowledge of their physical and emotional needs, as well as his appreciation of their desire for independence as a couple. In making the recommendation for respite care he had walked a tightrope between undermining their independence and warding off a crisis that would perhaps permanently destroy their independence.

A priority for the Latours was finding ways to ensure that they could stay together as long as possible. Dr Ombreck's referral to respite care was one important strategy. As Mrs Latour explained: 'I've got to get away from the daily demands every once in a while and then I am refreshed when Jacques comes back. It keeps us together and that's everything to us.'

When chronic illness strikes, each partner must accept the new role of either caregiver or care-receiver and subsequently reconcile how this role change impacts on their role as a partner in a couple relationship. This necessitates renegotiation of their own, as well as their partner's, understanding and interpretation of their respective roles within a pre-existing relationship. When the illness is chronic and deteriorating, with no hope for improvement, couples need assistance in understanding and accepting the changes brought about by the chronic illness. They need guidance and new skills to help realize and express both their individual and couple needs, wants and expectations.

Healthcare professionals, like Dr Ombreck, can help couples maintain and build on their strengths of reciprocity, mutuality and concern. Supporting couples in discussing and working through feelings of guilt, anger and frustration may alleviate negative experiences and facilitate positive, reciprocal exchanges. Specific interventions, such as providing more in-home care, increasing utilization of respite services or giving the well spouse 'permission' for time out for themselves, may assist couples in shifting from instrumental needs to relationship needs.

For all couples living with a chronic illness an intervention directed at improved communication would include dialog between the partners that is sensitive, open and always patient-centered, acknowledging that both partners in the couple dyad are patients. This will result in a more positive balance of roles and function within the couple relationship and strengthen the doctor's relationship with both members of the dyad, recognizing them as both a couple and as individuals.

5

The second component: understanding the whole person, Section 2: context

Thomas R Freeman and Judith Belle Brown

Whoever would study medicine aright must learn of the following subjects. First he must consider the effect of each of the seasons of the year and the differences between them. Secondly ... the warm and the cold winds ... the effect of water on the health must not be forgotten. Then think of the soil. Lastly consider the life of the inhabitants themselves (Hippocrates, 1986).

Introduction

Consideration of contextual factors in clinical practice is a hallmark of the patient-centered clinician (McWhinney, 1997). It is understood that, just as the meaning of a word depends on the context of the sentence in which it resides, so too, the meaning of health and illness varies with the surrounding circumstances. In the clinical world, information only becomes useful knowledge when it is placed in the context of a particular patient's world. To ignore context will lead to errors in both the interpretation and application of findings. A clinician must remember that the body is made up of a number of interlocking systems and the individual, too, exists within further systems including family, community, and ecology. Complexity theory recognizes that the internal rules of elements of units in a system change with context and this is one factor that leads to the unpredictability of complex systems (Plsek and Greenhalgh, 2001).

Taking into account contextual variables in arriving at an understanding of the patient reflects the dynamic tension between two notions of ill health that have existed since antiquity (Aronowitz, 1998; Crookshank, 1926). The ontological viewpoint is that diseases are specific entities that have an existence separate from the sufferer. The task of the clinician is to categorize the patient correctly, based on the symptoms and signs. Therapeutics will, naturally, be directed at eliminating or mitigating the disease entity. The physiological or holistic or ecological view, on the other hand, sees ill health as the outcome of an imbalance or failure to adapt to the environment. In this sense, the environment is understood to include the social, psychological and economic realm, as well as the physical environment. In this approach, diagnosis consists of arriving at an understanding of these many factors and their interplay with respect to the patient's ill health. One arrives at a diagnosis of the person rather than a disease category. Therapeutics then, in the ecological approach, is multifactorial and interdisciplinary in nature.

While there have been some changes taken by the population as a whole that are consistent with the ecological approach, such as dietary changes, alcohol consumption and exercise, it would be inaccurate to conclude that the same is true of conventional medicine (Cassell, 1991). 'Even when caused by a toxin, by a microbe, or by the dysfunction of an organ, illness is a fluid process that changes as we change, enigmatic, insubordinate, subjective. It captures bodies, minds, and emotions, remains at its deepest level inaccessible to language, and alters under the influence of non-medical events from divorce to climate change. What biomedicine finds hard to recognize or to accept is that different observers – patient, spouse, doctor, pastor, insurance provider, hospital administrator, epidemiologist, to name a few – examining the same illness from their separate perspectives will observe different aspects of its truth' (Morris, 1998: 5).

Recent understandings about the lifetime effect of the socio-environmental context at key developmental times in childhood, have served to emphasize that context at critical times in people's lives can have long-lasting effects (Blane *et al.*, 1997; Guy, 1997; Smith *et al.*, 1997).

A useful categorization of the layers of context is provided by Hinds *et al.* (1992). This consists of four nested, interactive layers distinguished by these three characteristics:

- the degree to which meaning is shared, whether individual or universal
- the dominant time focus, past, present or future
- the speed with which change can occur within the layer.

The four layers of context are then: the **immediate context** focused on the individual, in the present time, and rapid changes may happen or be effected; the **specific context** oriented to the individual including consideration of the immediate past as well as the relevant present, and again change can be rapid; the **general context** including both the personal and cultural dimensions, past as well as current variables, and change, while possible, is slower to effect; and the **metacontext** which is generally shared, though rarely articulated in a clinical encounter unless explicitly sought. It is socially constructed and predominately past oriented. Only very slow change is possible in the metacontext. The clinician's task is to help the patient arrive at a shared meaning of the events, a finding of common ground or understanding that is mutually agreed upon.

Meaning comes from a purposeful interaction with various layers of the context. Each layer can act as a source of prediction and explanation but, generally speaking, the immediate and specific layers of context tend to be more predictive, and the general and metacontext more explanatory in nature. However, either of these layers can affect a patient's health and/or perception of health. Changes in context have been found to be associated, for example, with exacerbations of previously stable chronic disease states (Cortese *et al.*, 1999). Therefore, clinicians need to take into account contextual issues in helping patients to arrive at a meaning for the symptoms.

Proximal and distal factors in context

A broader categorization defines those factors that are proximal and those that are distal to the patient. Proximal factors correspond most closely with the immediate and specific categories listed above, whereas distal contextual factors are more closely aligned with the general and metacontext categories. The boundaries between these categories must be understood to be, to a great extent, artificial.

Proximal factors in context

Proximal factors include: family; financial security; education; employment; leisure; and social support. These are examined below, supported by research evidence.

Family

People linked by blood, marriage or close emotional attachment constitute a family. The field of family systems theory sees the family as a mutually interacting system which functions as an emotional unit. The interaction of family issues and health and illness was covered in the preceding chapter. As Scarf (1995: *xxii*) so eloquently states: the family unit can be viewed as 'a great emotional foundry, the passion-filled forge in which our deepest realities – our sense of who we are as persons, and of the world around us – first begins to form and take shape. It is within the enclave of the early family that we learn those patterns of being, both of a healthy and a pathological nature, which will gradually be assimilated into, and become a fundamental part of, our own inner experience.'

Financial security

The inverse relationship between household income and all cause mortality is well established (Kaplan and Neil, 1993; Kitagawa and Hauser, 1973; Pappas *et al.*, 1993). Even after controlling for known biological risk factors, social class, which is in large part determined by income levels, has been shown to be inversely related to mortality. These observations were made even where the low income people in the study were relatively well paid compared to the general population, suggesting that there are factors other than access to health-care at work (Marmot *et al.*, 1987).

Education

There is a strong positive association between the number of years of schooling and mortality (Feinstein, 1993). While education is also positively associated with income, the effects of these two variables appear to be independent.

Employment

Taking an occupational history ensures that the clinician is aware of potential toxic or other dangerous exposures to the patient. The workplace can be the source of stress as well. It must also be kept in mind that lack of employment has been recognized as having adverse effects on health. On a deeper level, as pointed out by Cassell (1991: 164): 'To know someone's occupation is to learn something about his or her social status, education, specialized knowledge, responsibilities, hours worked, income, muscular development, skills, perspective on life, politics, housing – and much more.'

Leisure

It has been shown that even activities that do not necessarily enhance physical fitness improve all cause mortality in the elderly (Glass *et al.*, 1999). Involvement in various leisure activities improves mood and widens one's social network.

Social support

It has long been recognized that there is a positive link between the strength of social support and the health of the individual (Berkman and Syme, 1979; House *et al.*, 1988). Individuals with healthy social networks are more resistant to illness and tend to have better coping strategies. It is, however, the quality of the relationships that seems to matter the most, not just the quantity. Social contacts can be a source of stress as well as support (Corin, 1994). Aware clinicians make sure that they get frequent updates on the nature of their patients' support systems.

The following case example demonstrates how the proximal factors of a patient's life context affected her response to her diagnosis and subsequent treatment.

Case example

Ruth Walker, aged 48, was at her wits' end. The recurrence of her breast cancer was too much to bear. It was not that she feared for her life or was anxious about the imminent treatment; rather she was overwhelmed by her life circumstances. Ruth's husband, Albert, had been on disability for the past two years after severely injuring his back at the car-seat factory where he worked. Although he was able to walk short distances, Ruth had to help him out with daily activities such as dressing, bathing and preparing meals because of his limited mobility. Because of his constant care needs Ruth had given up her part-time job at a local convenience store. Ruth's job had been her one outlet; her customers and workmates had been her sole source of social support. Also, finances were now very limited as the Walkers struggled to survive on Albert's meager disability pension. Tanya, their 21-year-old daughter, had recently moved back home with her 10-month old son Kyle, after separating from her husband. While Tanya was actively seeking employment she could not afford daycare and consequently had asked her mother to look after Kyle. Ruth, bound by her strong family ties, had agreed.

Ruth was extremely angry and powerless; she felt that she did not have any control over her current situation. Everyone around her seemed to have problems and they were counting on Ruth to be the support they needed. Ruth felt like she had no life of her own since she had remained at home to care for her disabled husband, and, although she loved her grandson, now she had to take care of him too. Ruth was an only child and her parents had died when she was in her teens hence her little family was invaluable to her; but at the same time she was feeling the burden of their care. Thus it was not surprising that when the surgeon began to discuss various treatment options Ruth became openly angry. 'I can't believe that this is happening again! I have a husband and grandson to take care of – and now this. How can I possibly take care of everyone else and still get through this? I have to take the bus to get here and I can't afford that every week! What will I do?'

For this patient her life circumstances, including family problems, financial difficulties and limited social support made her own health concerns a low priority. These immediate and specific contextual issues would need to be addressed as well as her health concerns.

Distal factors in context

Distal factors as examined below include: community; culture; economics; healthcare system; socio-historical; geography; the media; and ecosystem health.

Community

The concept of community refers to a group of people recognizing some commonality whether that is based on geography, religion, ethnic background, profession or leisure interests. Taking a community approach to health and disease means identifying the conditions that cause or are associated with diseases and collective ways of coping with them. Even if economically deprived, communities that have a sense of identity and belonging are generally healthier than those that do not. The feeling of belonging to a neighborhood may be more important than interpersonal support for the mental health of the elderly (Biegel *et al.*, 1980).

Culture

The increasing cultural diversity of most populations had become a characteristic of the late twentieth century. Increasing diversity of medical practitioners requires us to remember that cross-cultural issues are bi-directional. Both these trends call for the development of a culturally flexible patient interaction style. How patients conceptualize and interpret their illness is strongly determined by the culture in which they reside. Cultural norms and values influence how patients experience illness, seek care and accept medical interventions (Kleinman *et al.*, 1978). As McWhinney (1997) notes, cultural differences are not only based on ethnicity but include subcultural groups defined by age, social class, sex, sexual preference, education, occupation and religion. One might add, as well, that some disease states or disabilities help to define subcultures with strong identities, e.g. AIDS, deafness (Sacks, 1989).

There are several features to consider for each of the four aspects (disease, illness, person and context) of the whole person in the patient-centered clinical method. Although disease is explained by the conventional medical model, it is not immune to the influence of culture (Aronowitz, 1998). The conventional medical model and the scientific method are both products of Western culture, thus our cultural 'filters' affect how we, as clinicians, understand and manage diseases (Payer, 1988).

Kleinman *et al.* (1978) describe three overlapping sectors of healthcare: the popular or lay sector; the folk sector; and the professional sector. Lay care, influenced by cultural norms and values, consists of self-treatment, family remedies, and advice from friends, neighbors and colleagues. Folk care includes non-traditional healers, shamans and spiritualists – all powerful and influential figures within their specific cultural group. Each realm of healthcare – lay, folk and professional – has its own unique explanatory model of illness offering explanations of cause, onset, duration and treatment (Kleinman *et al.*, 1978).

Other factors contributing to variation in health beliefs and practices of different cultural groups include:

1 perceptions about illness causation
2 perspectives on treatment or curing practices
3 attitudes and expectations of healthcare facilities and resources deemed most appropriate for the problem
4 specific behaviors and reactions to pain and illness sanctioned by the prevailing culture (Schlesinger, 1985).

A move from one culture to another involves major upheaval and loss that can have serious effects on self-esteem. The immigrant experience is often made complicated by significant persecution and physical trauma in the country of origin. Language barriers make it even more difficult to articulate needs and to receive support.

There are different cultural responses to transitions in the family life cycle such as pregnancy, labor, childbirth and care of the elderly and dying. Cultural differences in family roles and rules may come into conflict with the expectations of the doctor. Just as it is important to recognize the role of culture in health and illness on the one hand, it is also important to avoid stereotyping on the other hand. Culture does not explain all differences and it should not be used to explain what may be class or socio-economic differences.

Case example

Mr Ali, a 50-year-old Somali immigrant presented to his physician with vague abdominal pains. Listening to his story, the physician learned that Mr Ali had recently left Somalia to join his wife and two adolescent daughters who had preceded him to this new country by five years. Mr Ali was dismayed to find that his eldest daughter had begun to adapt to her new social environment by participating in school dances and parties with friends. This was a sharp departure from his wishes. Furthermore, he expressed anger towards his wife for not enforcing the customs of their homeland. He felt angry and ashamed and sensed he was losing control over his family.

Only after listening to this man's story did his physician begin to understand the origins of his symptoms and begin to help. Somali immigrants bring a rich oral culture which values storytelling and narrative. Their trust in physicians depends in large part on the physician's ability and willingness to listen to the patients' stories – who they are, where they came from, and the meaning of the illness.

Economics

The link between socio-economic status and health has been well recognized and explored (Feinstein, 1993). More recently, debate has focused on the observation that societies that tolerate wide differences in average income, from the lowest to the highest, have poorer overall aggregate health scores than societies that demonstrate smaller differences (Daniels *et al.*, 2000; Kawachi *et al.*, 1999a). The presence of a strong primary care sector, however, mitigates these adverse effects (Starfield, 2001). Globalization of the world economy has been identified by some as creating wider economic disparities both within and between countries, resulting in significant numbers of individuals who are marginalized. The concept of core and periphery is invoked to describe first those close to the center of economic activity, the entrepreneurs, and second those who, owing to lack of ability or opportunity are not entrepreneurs and are relegated to the periphery. In general, those at the periphery are found to engage in 'retreatist' behavior characterized by increased smoking, alcohol consumption and suicide (McMurray and Smith, 2001). This has been the fate of indigenous people on many continents.

Healthcare system

It is important that the clinician remain aware that the healthcare system as a whole, including the practitioner and his/her relationship with the patient, is an important part of the context. This is particularly true for patients with chronic illness who spend much of their time interacting with various components of the larger system. Overall healthcare organization has a profound effect on whether a patient accesses healthcare, which healthcare provider is sought and what is done about their problem. The clinical context can be a source of great frustration to the practitioner as well as the patient with various barriers to accessing appropriate care. In some situations, staffing and resource problems place pressure on clinicians to change, sometimes in ways that are detrimental to patient care. These include shortened consultation times, compromised continuity of patient care and an unfortunate focus on the disease model. Chapter 9 on 'Being realistic' discusses constructive ways to deal with these situations.

Socio-historical

To some extent our concept of diseases and the experience of ill health are born of particular social and historical circumstances (Kelly and Brown, 2002). This is true of our social construction of diseases (Aronowitz, 1998; Gilman, 1988), and it is no less relevant to the social and historical factors of the individual. For example, the experience of type 2 diabetes mellitus in a North American Aboriginal is so very different from an urban dwelling Caucasian that it is a challenge to state why we give it the same name. These differences are, in part, a reflection of the social history of these two individuals.

The impact of social, economic and health policy is reflective of a country's approach to the distribution of power (Starfield, 2001). There are numerous examples of groups of people who have been marginalized, sometimes over prolonged periods of time, resulting in chronic patterns of poverty and ill health that span generations. Being aware of the history of medical experimentation on black people helps the clinician understand the reluctance of some people of color to seek medical help (Candib, 1995). Changes at the macro-level in the history and socio-cultural environment are translated into stress on the individual which can then lead to increased susceptibility to ill health. The particular manifestation of the illness will be determined by an individual's genetic make-up and environmental pressures. Early childhood experiences, for example, have been shown to be predictive of susceptibility to some chronic diseases later in life. On the other hand, social and cultural meanings and values can modify, perhaps mitigate, an individual's response to these stressors (Corin, 1994).

Geography

The field of medical geography is defined as: 'that discipline that describes spatial patterns of health and disease and explains those spatial patterns by concentrating on the underlying processes that generate identifiable spatial forms' (Mayer, 1984: 2680). This approach has evolved from the position of environmental determinism, the consideration of the physical impact of the geography on health, to a position which views human health as being interwoven with the entire biosphere (Meade, 1986). The latter line of thinking was instrumental in the recognition of the importance of the ecosystem in health and illness. Geographic Information Systems have been developed recently, stimulated by the changes in the financing of care brought about by the managed care approach. These systems make possible the linking of health outcomes with geo-statistical data (Parchman *et al.*, 2002) and serve as a bridge to considering the wider role of environmental and ecological pressures on human health and well-being.

The media

For large parts of the world, the media, consisting of print materials, television and, increasingly, the Internet, has become a pervasive promoter of a monoculture. Some have raised the alarm about the media as a disease agent (Oxford Textbook of Medicine, 2002). By promoting a high-consumption, materialistic, violence-prone lifestyle that challenges traditional social structures and values, the content of the worldwide media may undermine those dimensions of context which serve to sustain health. On the other hand, health promotion programs are greatly facilitated by information technology. Patients now attend physicians with much greater awareness of their health and options available for disease management and this can be viewed as a positive development.

Ecosystem

Since the publication of Rachel Carson's book *Silent Spring*, and spurred on by widely reported ecological disasters such as the destruction of the nuclear power generator at Chernobyl in the Soviet Union and the tragedy in Bhopal, India, there has developed a greater awareness of the impact of environment on human health. The medical literature now devotes regular attention to environmental issues (Ablesohn *et al.*, 2002a, b; Epstein, 1995; Marshall *et al.*, 2002; Patz *et al.*, 1996; Spiedel, 2000). Clinicians must now take into account the way in which air pollution and environmental toxins affect their patients. There is much greater interest in the ways that climate changes can affect human health (National Health Assessment Group for the US Global Change Research Program, 2001).

Ecosystem health problems have gradually shifted from local issues to more global issues. As urban pollution increases and higher smoke stacks are constructed, acid rain becomes a regional and even a transnational problem. The worldwide dimensions of ecosystem health problems are truly staggering, with 3 billion people malnourished, 2 billion people living in water-stressed areas and 1.4 billion exposed to dangerous levels of outdoor air pollution.

Complex relationships exist between physical conditions, ecology and human health (Garrett, 1994). For example, the outbreak of Hanta virus in the south-western USA in 1994 can be understood as occurring in a particular environmental context, as follows. The effects of El Niño caused increased rain in the region which resulted in increased desert vegetation. Under these conditions, the population of deer mice (*Peromycus maniculatus*) multiplied, with the result that humans came into greater contact with the urine and fecal material left by the mice. This material contained a particularly virulent form of Hanta virus, later named Muerta Canyon virus, that proved to be the third most lethal virus ever found in the USA (after HIV and rabies). In this way, complex environmental changes led to a set of conditions conducive to disease in humans.

The thinking fostered by the ecosystem health approach is a reminder to focus on relationships as well as individual units and, in that respect, is consistent with the basic concepts of patient-centered medicine.

Community-oriented primary care

Community-oriented primary care (COPC) began with the work of Sidney Kark and others (Gieger, 1993; Susser, 1993) and has been recognized as a method of informing and integrating the practice of medicine with knowledge of the community. As it has evolved since the work of these pioneers, it is now considered to consist of four steps:

1   defining and characterizing the community
2   identifying and prioritizing the community's health problems
3   developing interventions to address the health problems
4   monitoring the impact of programs implemented (Nutting, 1990).

The techniques of COPC are attempts to recognize contextual factors of the community as a whole rather than the individual patient. Nevertheless, such knowledge serves to improve the clinician's understanding of the problems encountered in clinical medicine.

Conclusion

Being patient-centered involves being aware of the many layers of contextual nuance in which both patient and clinician reside. In arriving at a shared understanding or common ground, meaning can only occur within a particular set of circumstances or context.

Case example: 'I just can't stop watching ...'

Thomas R Freeman

Allison Marr approached her physician with the emergence of panic attacks at the age of 45. Her physician and she had attempted over the previous eight years to help her cope with multiple musculoskeletal complaints and intermittent bouts of depression.

With the emergence of these new symptoms, Allison's physician inquired about her own ideas of why this was happening at this particular time. She responded by relating that she had been watching the daily reports of the trial of a famous individual that was at that time dominating the media. The case involved the brutal murder of the estranged wife of the celebrity. Her physician pursued this topic by asking why this particular trial was causing her so much anxiety. This opened up a deeply buried and significant part of Allison's own story. With great difficulty, she related that, at the age of 18, she had arrived home from school to find both of her parents dead as a result of murder followed by suicide. She had spent the intervening years avoiding thinking about this episode, had married and had had her own children. Though she struggled with multiple symptoms and a chronic level of unhappiness and bouts of depression, it was not until current events caused a resurfacing of her memories that she was able to begin to face the trauma. This made it possible for her to enter into therapy at last.

For Allison changes in the wider social context conveyed by a pervasive media led to the manifestation of symptoms rooted in a deeply buried past.

6

The third component: finding common ground

Judith Belle Brown, W Wayne Weston and Moira Stewart

By using a patient-centered approach, doctors can begin to explore and understand patients' feelings, ideas, the effects of their illnesses on functioning, and expectations. By this means, the patient's perceptions of the problem are defined. At the same time, by using conventional clinical methods, including history-taking, physical examination and laboratory tests, physicians establish a medical definition of the patient's problems. Through this process an integrated understanding of the whole person, including their disease, illness, personhood and context, evolves. In this chapter we will examine the third interactive component of the patient-centered method – finding common ground. This will include: the importance of patients and doctors finding common ground; a description of finding common ground; and strategies to assist the clinician in finding common ground, such as motivational interviewing and shared decision-making.

Finding common ground is the process through which the patient and doctor reach a mutual understanding and mutual agreement in three key areas: defining the problem; establishing the goals and priorities of treatment and/or management; and identifying the roles to be assumed by both the patient and the doctor. To reach common ground often requires that two potentially divergent viewpoints be brought together in a reasonable plan. Once agreement is reached on the nature of the problems, the patient and doctor must determine the goals and priorities of treatment and/or management. What will be the patient's involvement in the treatment plan? How realistic is the plan in terms of the patient's perception of their disease and illness experience? What are the patient's wishes and their ability to cope? Finally, how do each of the parties – patient and doctor – define their roles in this interaction?

The importance of finding common ground

For over 30 years research has documented how doctors have failed to find common ground (Starfield *et al.*, 1981; Stewart and Buck, 1977). In a study of primary physicians and surgeons, Braddock *et al.* (1999) reviewed audiotapes of informed decision-making and found that discussion of alternatives occurred in 5.5% to 29.5% of interactions, of pros and cons in 2.3% to 26.3% and of uncertainties associated with the decision in 1.1% to 16.6%. Physicians rarely explored whether patients understood the decision (0.9% to 6.9%).

Studies exploring physician prescribing behaviors and patients' use of medication also report a paucity of finding common ground (Britten *et al.*, 2000; Dowell *et al.*, 1996; Dowell *et al.*, 2002; Dowell and Hudson, 1997; Stevenson *et al.*, 2000). For example, in a qualitative study, Britten *et al.* (2000) found that 14 categories of misunderstanding in relation to prescribing (e.g. conflicting information, disagreement about attribution of side effects) were inextricably connected to an absence of patients' expressions of their ideas, expectations or preferences. Patients' lack of participation in the consultation was also evident in their inability to respond to 'the doctors' decisions or actions' (2000: 484). This study revealed that an essential precursor to finding common ground was an exploration of the patient's illness experience (i.e. FIFE, described in Chapter 3). However, Dowell *et al.* (2002) found that when a consultation process included an explanation of the illness experience and finding common ground, previously non-adherent patients were assisted in following their medication regimen.

Another study highlighting the centrality of finding common ground is Stewart *et al.*'s (2000) who found that the most important association with good outcomes was the patient's perception that the physician and patient had found common ground. These outcomes included patient recovery from discomfort and concern, and better emotional health two months post-encounter. As well, there was a 50% reduction in diagnostic tests and referrals. The importance of finding common ground is also reinforced by the findings of Tudiver *et al.* (2001) who explored how family physicians made decisions about cancer screening when the guidelines were unclear or conflicting. Central to the physicians' decision-making process to screen or not screen was finding common ground with patients.

A final set of studies provide additional support to the importance of finding common ground in the clinical encounter. Three separate research teams examined women's experiences regarding: the important health issues of prenatal genetic testing, specifically maternal serum screening (Carroll *et al.*, 2000); hormone replacement therapy (Marmoreo *et al.*, 1998); and the use of complementary/alternative medicine in the treatment of breast cancer (Boon *et al.*, 1999). While the medical circumstances explored in the studies were both diverse and distinct, the participants' needs and expectations regarding the decision-making process reflected a collective voice. Faced with a serious decision regarding their health, one which could have positive or negative implications on their future health and well-being, participants expressed a consistent chorus of desiring an active role in the decision-making process and ultimately in finding common ground (Brown *et al.*, 2002f). Of importance in all three studies was the sharing of information between the patient and clinician. This finding is similarly reinforced by the work of McWilliam *et al.* (2000) with breast cancer survivors, who described the inextricable link between building a relationship with their physician(s) and having the opportunity to share information, as they strived to reach common ground regarding treatment of their breast cancer.

In summary, research indicates how physicians still fail to find common ground with patients but at the same time reveals how finding common ground is important for both patients and physicians. Finding common ground may indeed be the linchpin of the patient-centered clinical method, thus further research on this component of the patient-centered clinical method is warranted.

Defining the problem

To seek an understanding or explanation of worrisome symptoms, physical or emotional, is a fundamental human need. Most patients want a 'name' or label for their disease to help them gain some sense of control over what is happening to them (Cassell, 1991; Kleinman, 1988; McWhinney, 1989b; Wood, 1991). When patients can assign a label to their problems it helps them understand the cause, what to expect in terms of the course or timeline of the problem and what will be the outcome (Cooper, 1998). It also assists them in regaining some degree of mastery over what may have been a frightening symptom. Some patients may develop quite magical notions of what is happening to them when they become ill. It may seem better to have an irrational explanation of the problem than no explanation at all. Other patients will blame themselves for the problem rather than see the disease as something beyond their control. The initial presentation of Hanna to her doctor described at the end of Chapter 3 serves as an illustration.

Patients have usually formed a hypothesis about their problem before presenting to the doctor. Failure to elicit the patient's perspective may jeopardize agreement on the nature of the problem(s). Without some agreement about what is wrong, it is difficult for a patient and doctor to agree on a treatment protocol or plan of management that is acceptable to both. It is not essential that the physician share the same perspective of the problem as the patient, but the doctor's explanation and recommended treatment must at least be consistent with the patient's point of view and make sense in the patient's world.

Problems develop when patient and doctor have different ideas of the cause of the problems. For example:

- The patient dismisses her back pain as aging and osteoarthritis, yet the doctor is concerned that it may represent metastases from her breast cancer.
- The doctor has diagnosed hypertension, but the patient insists that his blood pressure is probably only elevated because he is working overtime on a big assignment at work and refuses to see his blood pressure as a problem.
- The parent of a six-year old child thinks there is something seriously wrong because the child has frequent colds: six a year. The doctor thinks this number is within normal limits, and that the parent is overly protective of the child.

In defining and describing the problem it is essential that doctors give the information in language patients can understand, thus complex medical terms and clinical language should be avoided. If patients are intimidated by medical jargon it may limit their ability to express their ideas and concerns or to even raise important questions. Failure to elicit these patients' expressions may result in a failure to find common ground. Patients need to be encouraged to ask questions and not fear being ridiculed or embarrassed for not knowing or not understanding technical terms and procedures. Just as active listening is key to exploring the patients' illness experiences, it is also central to finding common ground. Thus it is important to understand and acknowledge patients' perspectives of their problem.

The following case example demonstrates how differing perspectives on the nature of the patient's problem did not result in conflict. The doctor acknowledged and respected the patient's perspective, while using his own understanding of the problem to guide his management of the patient's chronic pain.

Case example

Simon, aged 45, was a socially isolated and lonely man. He had suffered from chronic pain for 20 years after falling off the roof of a building at a construction site. His recovery from his life-threatening injuries had been slow and further hampered by a narcotic addiction he had to overcome. Simon's fiancée had canceled their wedding plans and many of his family members had drifted away. He long ago accepted this situation as all he could expect. But he needed his pain to legitimize his disability pension which was his only source of income. His pain also gave him an opportunity to sit down with his doctor – someone who cared about him and his suffering. Dr Rooter, the patient's family doctor, realized that the physical pain Simon experienced was also a metaphor for his intolerable life pain. But the doctor did not relate this insight to the patient, recognizing that

Simon could not bear the burden of his emotional pain. It was sufficient that Dr Rooter's insight allowed him to care more deeply for his patient and to avoid unnecessary investigations to find a disease that was not there. The doctor responded to Simon's cues and followed his lead in discussing his personal life and his feelings. Dr Rooter helped Simon to tell his own story at his own pace and avoided the risk of pushing the patient beyond his limits of endurance.

Defining the goals

Once the patient and doctor have reached a mutual understanding and agreement about the problem the next step is to explore the goals and priorities of treatment and/or the management plan; if these are divergent it may be a challenge to find common ground. For example:

- The patient requests genetic testing to alleviate her fears of having breast cancer, while the doctor knows there are no present risk factors or family history to warrant such tests.
- A patient suffering from unremitting back pain demands an MRI, yet the doctor feels that this is likely 'mechanical back' that will resolve spontaneously.
- The doctor advises the patient to adhere to a treatment regimen to prevent the advent of osteoporosis, yet the patient declines, believing that diet and exercise will suffice.

If doctors ignore their patient's expectations and ideas about treatment and/or management, they risk not understanding their patients, who in turn will be angry or hurt by this perceived lack of interest or concern. Some patients will become more demanding in a desperate attempt to be heard; others will become withdrawn and feel abandoned. Patients may be reluctant to listen to their doctors' treatment recommendations unless they feel that their ideas and opinions have been heard and respected.

Timing is important. If the physician inquires about patients' perspectives too early in the interview, patients may think that the doctor is avoiding his or her responsibility to make a diagnosis. On the other hand, if the doctor waits until the end of the interview, time may be wasted on issues unimportant to the patient. The physician may even make suggestions which will have to be retracted. Doctors need to actively engage their patients and explicitly inquire about their expectations. For example, a physician might say, 'Can you help me to understand what we might do together to get your diabetes under control?' Often, it is helpful to pick up on patients' cues that hint at their feelings, ideas, or expectations. For example, 'I have had this back pain for three weeks now and none of the pain medication you recommended has helped. I just can't bear the pain!' The doctor should avoid becoming defensive in trying to justify previous advice. Instead, it is more helpful to address the patient's frustration and the implied message that something must be done: 'You sound fed up with the length of time this pain has dragged on. Are you wondering if it is something serious?'

Often patients find it awkward or difficult to provide suggestions about the treatment or management of their diseases. Some patients may feel that their opinion lacks validity and value, while others may defer to the authority of the 'expert' clinician in the decision-making process. Physicians need to encourage patients' participation with statements such as: 'I'm really interested in your point of view, especially since you are the one who has to live with our decision about these treatments.' It is important for doctors to explain clearly the treatment and/or management options and to engage patients in a mutual discussion of the pros and cons of different approaches. It is also important to acknowledge and address patients' questions and concerns so that patients feel heard and understood. In clarifying patients' agreement with a specific plan, questions such as the following can be very useful: 'Can you think of any difficulties in following through on this?' 'Is there anything we can do to make this treatment plan easier for you?' 'Do you need more time to think this over?' 'Is there anybody you would like to talk to about this treatment?' These questions and others help forge partnerships with patients; it is, as Tuckett *et al.* (1985) described, 'a meeting of experts'.

Establishing the goals of treatment and/or management must also take into account the expectations and feelings of physicians. Sometimes doctors are concerned that patients may ask for something they disagree with, because they are not comfortable with confrontation and saying no. As a result they may prefer to avoid the issue, but then finding common ground will not be achieved. Doctors can become frustrated and disheartened when patients do not adhere to treatment protocols and management plans. But what physicians call 'non-compliance' may be the patient's expressions of disagreement about treatment goals. As Quill and Brody (1996) observe: 'Final choices belong to patients, but these choices gain meaning, richness, and accuracy if they are the result of a process of mutual influence and understanding between physician and patient' (1996: 765). The following two examples illustrate some challenges in defining the goals for treatment and/or management.

Case example

As a single mother, Tabitha, aged 32, led an active and busy life caring for her three children, aged 7, 9 and 13, as well as working part-time as a teacher's assistant. A simple slip on a small patch of ice resulted in a broken wrist requiring extensive surgery. Her entire right arm was immobilized in a cast with 'Frankenstein-like' pins protruding from her arm. Her life was turned upside-down; unable to perform routine tasks she could not care for her children or work. The healing process was slow and painful. Her confidence and hope that she would recover was becoming severely tested. Tabitha felt that she had been reduced to a disease, stating: 'I felt I was given no part in my care except to bring my arm in for appointments.' She felt diminished and excluded in decisions about her treatment and rehabilitation. Her ability to voice her concerns and expectations became weaker, in striking parallel to her damaged limb: 'I could not express how motivated I was to be included as someone who could influence my own health and healing. Also, in my view the doctor did not seem to appreciate or understand my feelings.'

The serious misunderstandings between Tabitha and her surgeon arose because there was a failure to find common ground. As Tabitha later reflected: 'I needed the physician to have a greater understanding of what I was concerned about and the relevance of my questions . . . No one asked me anything about what I needed.'

Case example

'Mary, Mary, quite contrary' she hummed silently to herself as the doctor droned on about her future need for dialysis. Mary, aged 64, smiled pleasantly as the doctor outlined the various options for dealing with her kidney failure. But she had no intention of ever going on dialysis. The very thought of being hooked up to some machine three times a week was unbearable for Mary. Just let me die peacefully and with dignity Mary thought, as she continued to silently hum 'Mary, Mary, quite contrary'.

Mary was defending herself from the terror she experienced when realizing how serious her illness was – talking about dialysis was too frightening! The nursery rhyme represented a private confession that she had not been very faithful in taking her blood pressure medication over the years. At the same time it symbolized her fierce independence and fear of disability. Until the physician could connect with some of her mixed feelings, she would not be willing to discuss the management of her renal failure.

Realizing that Mary seem distracted, Dr O'Brien, her endocrinologist, ended his 'lecture' and commented: 'You seem to have other things on your mind. Can you tell me how you are reacting to this kidney trouble?'

Mary, caught off guard by Dr O'Brien's change in direction, paused a few moments, and replied, 'Well, I don't like it one bit! But, I've had a good life and I will muddle through as best I can. I'm not ready to end my days attached to some infernal machine.'

Dr O'Brien responded, 'So, your independence is very important to you and whatever treatment I recommend must take that into account?'

Mary nodded affirmatively, 'That's for sure, Dr O'Brien.'

Agreeing on those overall goals of management was the first step in treatment planning. Mary may or may not accept dialysis but it will need to be on her terms. If she sees it as a way to provide some increased quality of life she will accept the inconvenience and distress of long-term dialysis. In the future, when dialysis becomes necessary, the doctor and Mary will need to explore the pros and cons of independence, quality of life and length of life.

In both of these examples the physician and patient needed to work together to find a treatment plan that was acceptable to both. This required that the goals and priorities of each be re-examined. Finally, when disagreement occurs it may be necessary for the doctor to explore the deeper reasons for the patient's position, as these case examples demonstrated.

Defining the roles of patient and doctor

Inherent in articulating the roles to be assumed by the patient and doctor is a definition of mutual responsibility for the actions that will follow. These may be quite simple such as: 'I want to see you again in one month to check that this new medication is lowering your blood pressure.' Implicit in this statement is the patient's use of the medication as prescribed, and the doctor's desire for future follow-up. Certain situations, however, may be more complex and therefore require an explicit statement of the roles to be assumed by the patient and the doctor. Again, referring back to the case example of Hanna, the patient with breast cancer described in Chapter 3, finding common ground was an ongoing process with the roles of the patient and doctor constantly shifting and changing in response to the patient's needs.

Sometimes there is profound disagreement about the nature of the problem or the goals and priorities for treatment. When such an impasse occurs, it is important to look at the relationship between the patient and the doctor, and at their perception of each other's roles. (The nature and characteristics of the relationship will be dealt with in depth in Chapter 8, while here we focus on problems in role definition.) Doctors, as in the example of the cancer patient, may see themselves wanting to bring about remission, and may expect the patient to assume the role of a passive recipient of treatment. Patients, however, may be seeking a physician who expresses concern and interest in their well-being, and who is prepared to treat them in the least invasive manner, viewing them as autonomous individuals with a right to have a voice in deciding among various forms of treatment. This is not such a dilemma for doctors when the various forms of treatment are equally effective, but physicians are understandably concerned when the patient chooses a treatment that they consider either less efficacious or even harmful.

Evolution of the patient–doctor relationship over time, as described in Chapters 4 and 8, allows the doctor to see the same patient with different problems in different settings over a number of years, and also to see the patient through the eyes of other family members. The physician's commitment is to 'be present' with the patient to the end. Patients need to know that they can count on their doctors to be there when they need them. This ongoing relationship colors everything that happens between them. If there are difficulties in their relationship or differing expectations of their roles, they will have problems in working together effectively. For example:

- The patient is looking for an authority who will tell him what is wrong and what he should do; the physician, on the other hand, wants a more egalitarian relationship in which doctor and patient share decision-making.
- The patient longs for a deep and meaningful relationship with a parental figure who will make up for everything the patient's own parent never gave; the doctor wants to be a biomedical scientist who can apply the discoveries of modern medicine to patients' problems.
- The physician enjoys a holistic approach to medicine and wants to get to know patients as people; the patient seeks only technical assistance from the doctor.

Finding common ground about a patient's role in the decision-making process does not necessarily imply that the patient will assume an active role. Patients' levels of participation in decision-making may fluctuate depending on their emotional and physical capabilities. Thus doctors need to be flexible and responsive to potential changes in their patient's involvement. Some patients may be too sick or too overwhelmed by the burden of their illness to actively participate in their care. Others may find decisions about treatment options too complex and confusing; hence abdicating the decision-making to the clinician. When patients are receiving care from multiple healthcare professionals, they assume different roles and relationships with each. Roles within and across the healthcare team may also influence the patient's care as we discuss in detail in Chapter 9.

Sometimes a lack of role clarity or assumptions about the patient's and doctor's roles can result in ambiguity and uncertainty. The following case serves as an illustration.

Case example

Ralph Kruppa, a 59-year-old family doctor, had suffered a myocardial infarction. The event had seriously unsettled this man, leaving him both concerned and uncertain about his future health and well-being. At the time of discharge from hospital his cardiologist suggested that Dr Kruppa look after his own warfarin, because as a doctor he was knowledgeable about managing the medication. Dr Kruppa, the patient, feeling uncustomarily vulnerable, did not challenge the cardiologist's suggestion. He subsequently ordered more INRs on himself than he had ever done before with his patients. Four weeks after his discharge from hospital Dr Kruppa had an appointment with his family doctor, who indicated that he would monitor the patient's INR to determine if it was too high or low and correspondingly alter the dosage of warfarin. There was no need for Dr Kruppa to be involved. The family doctor's office staff would call the patient if the dosage needed to be changed.

To himself Dr Kruppa thought: 'Sure, sure the lab results will go to you – but I will also arrange that I get copies of the lab results so that *I am* informed about the results! I know the system and how information can fall through the cracks.' Out loud he quietly replied: 'Sure, whatever you think.'

Neither of Dr Kruppa's physicians had asked the patient his perspective and what role he wanted to assume in the management of his warfarin. Nor had the patient's family doctor and cardiologist consulted each other; thus each physician had very different ideas about the management of the patient's warfarin. What the patient would have preferred and needed was to have the various options laid out to him as to what role(s) the cardiologist, family doctor and the patient might assume. The next important step would have been to ask him 'What option would you prefer and what role do you want to play?'

The process of finding common ground

In the process of finding common ground it is the doctor's responsibility to define and describe the problem. This may be as clear-cut as: 'You have a strep throat' or ultimately more complex and uncertain such as: 'There are several possibilities of what your symptoms suggest and what we will need to do is ...'. Next it is important to provide the patient with an opportunity to ask questions. This is not simply an 'Okay?', but an intentional engagement of the patient: 'What do you think?' Some patients may respond with, 'I don't know? You are the doctor!' Doctors need to respond with a comment such as: 'Yes, and I will provide you with information and my opinion, but your ideas and wishes are important in making our plan together.' This is when information sharing begins.

The patient and doctor can then participate in a mutual discussion of their shared understanding of the problem and how it can best be addressed. At the conclusion of their discussion of treatment options and management goals it is

Box 6.1   Finding common ground

Issue	Patient	Doctor
Problems		
Goals		
Roles		

the clinician's responsibility explicitly to clarify the patient's understanding and agreement. It is during this summation that the doctor and patient can make specific their respective roles in achieving the mutually agreed upon treatment goals. This may be as simple as agreeing on how follow-up plans will be arranged, or as complex as a discussion of how a cancer patient in the palliative phase is needing the doctor to assume a caring role versus a curative stance.

If disagreements arise doctors must avoid getting into power struggles but rather listen to patients' concerns or opinions as opposed to dismissing the patients as non-compliant or obstinate. When conflicts do arise, the grid shown in Box 6.1 may be a useful tool. How do both the patient and the doctor view the problem(s), the goals of treatment and/or management and their respective roles? Why are these divergent and can they be resolved? This grid also helps the doctor to check if important information is missing, such as the patient's experience of illness or specific issues relevant to the patient's unique context.

The next case example illustrates the key concepts of finding common ground: defining the problems, the goals, and the roles of the patient and doctor.

Case example

Mrs Asabar, aged 45, came to the office after an urgent phone call, made that same day, demanding a repeat prescription for steroid eye drops. She had experienced a painful red eye two months earlier and had seen an ophthalmologist, by referral, who diagnosed acute iritis and prescribed steroid eye drops. When similar symptoms recurred a few days previously, she started using the drops again. By the time Mrs Asabar was seen she no longer had any symptoms and her eyes looked normal. She was out of drops and was concerned about a flare-up, as she was leaving for a vacation in Bermuda that afternoon. Dr Moore, the family medicine resident who saw her had been taught in medical school that family doctors should never prescribe steroid eye drops and insisted that she see an ophthalmologist. He was concerned that the patient's history was vague and was not convinced that she had a recurrence of her iritis.

Mrs Asabar adamantly refused to 'waste two hours' in emergency and preferred to take her chance without eye drops if he would not prescribe them. Dr Moore, believing that he was in a no-win situation, was furious. If he gave her eye drops (which he was not even sure she needed) and she had complications, he would feel badly; on the other hand, if he refused, the patient might have a flare-up that would ruin her vacation and perhaps even permanently damage her eye. Dr Moore feared that this type of 'unreasonable' patient was likely to sue him either way. The staff physician who had known the patient for several years realized that she rarely backed down. Even after explaining the doctor's concerns (the uncertain diagnosis and the potential harm of treatment or non-treatment), Mrs Asabar remained adamant in her request. Dr Moore, in consultation with his supervisor, decided that, on balance and under these restricted circumstances, the patient's interests would best be served by his being flexible and prescribing the steroid eye drops. He clearly cautioned her on what symptoms to look for before she used the drops again.

In this case there was some disagreement about the nature or severity of the problems and appropriate goals or methods of treatment. There were also difficulties in the patient–doctor relationship that could easily have reached an impasse. By being clear in his explanations, by clarifying their differences of opinion while, at the same time, showing respect for the patient's point of view, and by engaging in a mutual discussion, the physician was able to avoid a harmful power struggle and perhaps sowed the seeds for a more effective working relationship in the future.

Strategies to assist finding common ground

The recent development of specific interviewing techniques such as motivational interviewing and informed decision-making provides useful strategies to assist patients and clinicians in the process of finding common ground. Motivational interviewing is a method based on a model of stages of change and is premised on the theory that persons change their behaviors in predictable stages (Rollnick *et al.*, 1999). Patients are more likely to succeed if they are helped by clinicians who tailor their interventions to patients' particular stage of change. Motivational interviewing strategies are often recommended for addictive behaviors such as smoking. A person may desire to be a non-smoker but be unwilling or unable to tolerate the struggle to quit. The traditional intervention of a physician is to point out the dangers of smoking, make a recommendation to quit and provide pharmacological aids such as nicotine patches, sticks, or bupropion. Special interviewing techniques to change behavior might be viewed with suspicion as some form of mind control or coercion. But leaving patients to their own devices to fight off the disabling effects of addiction does not encourage their free choice of treatment. Supporting patients' choice is not simply leaving all decision making up to the patient but rather providing whatever assistance is needed to learn how to cope and to strengthen their motivation to change.

Several authors advocate the importance of shared decision-making in patient care (Elwyn *et al.*, 2000; Elwyn and Charles, 2001; Godolphin *et al.*, 2001; Towle and Godolphin, 1999). For example, the Informed Shared Decision Making Model (Towle and Godolphin, 1999) provides an approach to involving patients in their own care to the extent that they wish to be involved. Using this approach, physicians determine their patients' preferences for learning more about their condition (e.g. pamphlets, Internet, videotapes or support groups) and their preferences for their role in decision-making (e.g. talking to other family members, relying on the doctor's advice, being self-reliant, comfort with risk-taking). Discussing how patients prefer to handle decisional conflict – what they do when they are confronted with opposing ideas and uncertainty – may help them to resolve such dilemmas. It is important to understand that, in this approach, the physician is not simply a servant doing whatever the patient requests but rather a partner who brings medical expertise and evidence to the discussion about management. Towle and Godolphin (1999) argue that being explicit about these issues enhances patients' opportunities for an effective partnership with physicians as they explore choices together and come to a mutual decision that best matches the patients' preferences and is congruent with the best available evidence and clinical wisdom.

The strategies described above can be very useful in finding common ground but they must always be applied in the context of patient-centered practice. As stated previously, patients may not feel well enough or confident enough to be active participants in decisions about their care. They may choose to abdicate their responsibilities and hand them over to the clinician. This is patient-centered care, as it respects the needs and preferences of the patient in that specific circumstance. The situation may change and this would necessitate that doctors be responsive and flexible to the patients' involvement in the process of finding common ground.

Conclusion

Finding common ground requires that patients and physicians reach a mutual understanding and mutual agreement on the nature of the problems, the goals and priorities of treatment, and/or management, and their respective roles. Sometimes patients and doctors have divergent views in each of these areas. The process of finding a satisfactory resolution is not one of bargaining or negotiating but rather of moving towards a meeting of minds or finding common ground.

The process of finding common ground between the patient and doctor is an integral and interactive component of the patient-centered clinical method. This is how it differs from motivational interviewing or techniques of shared decision-making: finding common ground is embedded in the patient-centered clinical method. Finding common ground may be the linchpin or place of convergence, where all of the components of the patient-centered clinical method come together. To find common ground, the clinician must take into consideration all other aspects of the patient-centered clinical method: knowing both the patient's disease and illness experience (FIFE); appreciating the person and context; recognizing opportunities for prevention and health promotion; constantly building on the patient–doctor relationship; and acknowledging the realities of the environment in which healthcare is delivered. As McLeod (1998) cogently notes:

> When we listen to, accept, and validate the illness story, when we interpret the illness in terms of its symptomatic pathophysiology, when we explain treatment plans and prognosis, and, most importantly, when we define the patient's own role in the healing process, then trust, compassion, and a human connection between the patient and doctor becomes possible. (1998: 678)

Case example: 'If you want to know a man, ask him what he cares about'

Judith Belle Brown and W Wayne Weston

> As Dr Hurst reviewed the day's schedule of appointments he was surprised to see Chris Cairns' name on the list. He also felt mildly irritated, as the patient was booked for a blood pressure recheck. 'This will be a waste of time', Dr Hurst grumbled to himself, 'and certainly take longer than ten minutes!'

Although Mr Cairns, aged 57, had been a patient of Dr Hurst's for over 15 years, he was an infrequent attender, presenting primarily with symptoms of acute disorders such as back pain or 'flu'. Over the years, when Dr Hurst had attempted to engage Chris in prevention strategies to improve his health status, such as quitting smoking, the patient had shown little interest. Indeed, he had been rather dismissive of the doctor's suggestions replying: 'I don't think it is a big deal, Doc – got more important things to worry about, like getting a paycheck.' Dr Hurst had continued to persevere in his goal to change some of Mr Cairns' lifestyle behaviors, but he was becoming frustrated and fed-up by his patient's disinterest and 'noncompliance'.

The most recent issue had arisen when Mr Cairns had been diagnosed with hypertension, one year ago. During one of his episodic visits to the office for 'cold-like symptoms', Dr Hurst had managed to check Mr Cairns' blood pressure, which was 170/100. After a lengthy discussion of what these findings could mean, and their implications, Mr Cairns reluctantly agreed to further monitoring. His other cardiac risk factor was smoking a pack a day. Over the years he had worked as a laborer and his physical activity, in spite of his poor diet, had helped keep his weight in check. At the next three visits Mr Cairns' blood pressure had remained elevated in the same range.

Convincing Chris to control his hypertension with medication was an uphill battle for Dr Hurst. From Mr Cairns' perspective there was no problem, he felt just fine. 'Well, Doc, how about I try and cut down on my smokes a bit and maybe not have a beer until sundown? That should do the trick.' Finally, after much cajoling, verging on threats of potentially serious outcomes as a result of high blood pressure, Dr Hurst had persuaded Chris to accept a prescription. He subsequently filled the prescription, only to be shocked at the cost of the medication. Mr Cairns' response has been to ration out the pills, taking them only when he felt tired or out of sorts.

Mr Cairns had never followed through on a recheck visit for his blood pressure but rather presented four months later to Dr Hurst's office with back pain. It was at this visit that the doctor learned of Chris's 'personalized' medication regime. He felt both anger and concern. Chris was not a stupid man and he should have known better than this. Now his blood pressure was 185/100.

Dr Hurst had tried to be patient as he explained how the medication worked and what might happen if Chris did not follow the proper protocol. However, Mr Cairns had appeared more interested in his back pain and how it was tough to work with such discomfort. Getting rid of his pain was his priority! Using this leverage Dr Hurst had Chris agree to return to see him weekly until the back pain resolved. Perhaps this could serve as an opportunity to educate Mr Cairns about his hypertension and, at a minimum, permit Dr Hurst to monitor closely his patient's blood pressure. Not surprisingly, Mr Cairns' back pain rapidly resolved within a month, after which his visits to Dr Hurst dwindled. He had, however, begun taking his medication daily, for the most part, yet his smoking behavior remained unchanged. His blood pressure was now 150/90.

As Dr Hurst lifted Mr Cairns' chart out of the door pocket he paused and wondered: 'Why now, why was Chris here now . . . perhaps something had changed?' With subdued optimism he entered the examination room: 'Hi, Chris, how are you doing?' he asked. Dr Hurst was taken aback to see this usually gruff man, looking sad and forlorn.

'She's gone Doc', Chris said choking back the tears, 'gone a week ago.'

The doctor sat down and was quiet, trying to review in his mind who 'she' was in Chris's life. His patient had never talked about family, let alone a partner. Dr Hurst stumbled as he asked, 'I'm sorry, Chris – she – who do you mean?' At this moment the doctor felt both guilty for his previous angry thoughts and stupid for not knowing what his patient of over 15 years was revealing to him in this clearly painful moment.

Chris roughly wiped the tears from his face with the back of his hand and replied: 'Stella, my golden retriever. She was 17. Had her since she was a puppy. God, I miss her!' He went on to describe how she had been his faithful companion all those years, helping to heal the hurt after his wife died of leukemia 18 years ago.

Chris Cairns had revealed more about himself in the last five minutes than he ever had in all the 15 years that Dr Hurst had known him. Dr Hurst no longer viewed him as a non-compliant or recalcitrant patient but as a man who had suffered significant losses. 'Doc', Chris continued, 'if you want to really know a man – don't ask him about his aches and pains or his diet, ask him about things he cares for – like his dog.'

Not only was the information about the ill and dying pet important as one potential explanation for the hypertension but perhaps also explained Dr Hurst's inability to find common ground with Chris on many health issues. Dr Hurst did not really understand this patient's experience – he did not know him as a person. This is not to suggest the doctor's more focused attempts at risk reduction were inappropriate but they were isolated from the patient's world and, hence, ineffective. He did not have a full picture, since much of the story had been untold.

Reaching a mutual understanding of the problems and involving patients as active partners in the treatment plan extends beyond the disease to include their experiences of illness and all those factors in their lives that are relevant. In the past year Mr Cairns had watched his beloved comrade, beset with old age, slowly die of a blood disorder reminiscent of his wife's leukemia. For Chris, his high blood pressure had little importance as his losses accumulated and were intensified by past memories. Knowing this assisted Dr Hurst to understand his patient and move towards finding common ground on all the issues that were important and relevant to him.

7

The fourth component: incorporating prevention and health promotion

Carol L McWilliam and Thomas R Freeman

All health professionals are currently challenged to promote health as well as to prevent disease. The patient-centered approach allows professionals to maximize their contributions to these healthcare activities, for health, like disease and illness, requires an integrated understanding of the whole person. Furthermore, disease prevention and health promotion require a collaborative effort on the part of patient and physician, who must therefore find common ground in order for these activities to be pursued. This chapter builds on the preceding four chapters to illustrate how the patient-centered clinical method facilitates focus on health promotion and disease prevention, and, in turn, how focus on prevention and health promotion incorporates the patient-centered approach.

The foundations of health promotion and disease prevention

In 1984, the World Health Organization (WHO, 1986a) redefined health as 'a resource for everyday life, not the objective of living. This concept of health emphasizes social and personal resources as well as physical capacities.' Thus, the notion of health is moving away from its former abstract focus on complete physical, mental and social well-being toward 'an ecological understanding of the interaction between individuals and their social and physical environment' (de Leeuw, 1989; Hurowitz, 1993; Stachtchenko and Jenicek, 1990). How patients and practitioners think about and, therefore, experience health continues to evolve. Therefore, both these partners in healthcare have unique and often differing understandings of health, and in turn, different understandings of health promotion and disease prevention.

The process of care has also been altered and continues to evolve in light of new definitions. Health promotion most recently has been defined (WHO, 1986b) as 'the process of enabling people to take control over and to improve their health'. The intervention strategy for promoting health has been labeled 'health enhancement' or increasing the level of good health, vitality and resilience in all people.

Unlike health promotion, disease prevention is aimed at reducing the risk of acquiring a disease. As a process, disease prevention reduces the likelihood that a disease or disorder will affect an individual (Stachtchenko and Jenicek, 1990). Disease prevention strategies fall into four familiar categories: risk avoidance (primary prevention); risk reduction (secondary prevention); early identification; and complication reduction (tertiary prevention). Risk avoidance aims at ensuring that people at low risk for health problems remain at low risk by finding ways to avoid disease. Risk reduction addresses moderate or high-risk characteristics among individuals or segments of the population by finding ways to cure or control the prevalence of disease. Early identification aims at increasing the awareness of early signs of health problems and screening people at risk in order to detect the early onset of health problems. Complication reduction comes into play after the disease has developed with the goal being to ameliorate the effects of disease.

Whether the process of healthcare is to be health enhancement, risk avoidance, risk reduction, early identification of disease or complication reduction depends upon the relationship between the timing of the opportunity for intervention and the patient's potential for disease at that time. Most importantly, both preventive care and health promotion efforts depend upon the patient's state of health and commitment to the pursuit of health. Thus, the patient-centered approach is also essential to the process of promoting health and preventing disease. As described in the preceding chapters, effective patient care requires attending to patients' personal experience of health, illness and disease, understanding patients in the context of their lives, and finding common ground regarding preventive care and health promotion.

Health promotion and disease prevention requires patient-centered care

Health promotion and disease prevention are important pillars in the 'New Public Health Movement' as described in the Ottawa Charter (Epp, 1986). Much of the energy directed toward these thrusts has been devoted to developing public policy, screening and other methods, and to addressing related ethical issues (Doxiadis, 1987; Hoffmaster, 1992). Almost all involved have taken a population-based approach to health. With notable exceptions (Audunsson, 1986; Laitakari and Asikainen, 1998; McWilliam, 1993; Pearlman *et al.*, 1997), little attention has been paid to implementing ideas of health promotion and disease prevention at the level of the individual practitioner and patient. Yet now, as never before, primary healthcare reform calls for achieving new directions that clearly hinge on individual as well as collective efforts. Viewing one's practice as a population at risk (McWhinney, 1997) requires the practitioner to utilize a population health approach in one's own practice.

Indeed, in this era of evidence-based medicine, the original concept of health as the absence of disease still demands that physicians attend to health as a product of the physician's clinical work, rendering individualized attention to disease prevention an ongoing part of medical care. Additionally however, understanding health as a state of complete physical, mental and social well-being (WHO, 1986a) demands attention to the individual's holistic potential for health. This includes attending to WHO's most recent definition of health as a process, specifically the ability to realize aspirations, satisfy needs, and respond positively to the environment (WHO, 1986b) and hence necessitates attention to the individual's everyday effort to promote his or her own health. Thus, attention to the individual in efforts to promote health and prevent disease is an essential part of primary care reform, complementary to the population health approach. The patient-centered clinical method provides a clear framework for the practitioner to apply in health promotion and disease prevention efforts, using the patient's world as the starting point.

Understanding the patient's world

A patient-centered approach to health promotion and disease prevention begins with an understanding of the whole person, as described in Chapters 4 and 5. To achieve such an understanding, the physician must assess six aspects of the patient's world: his or her experience of the broader determinants of health over his/her life course; his/her potential for health; present and potential disease; the patient's experience of health and illness; the patient's context; and the patient–doctor relationship.

Experience of the broader determinants of health over the life course

In recent years, much attention has been directed toward the broader determinants of health, adding to the usual concern about biologic and genetic determination, consideration of healthy childhood development, gender, income, social status and education, physical and social environment, lifestyle, social support networks, employment, working conditions and healthcare (Ottawa Charter for Health Promotion, 1986). Many of the broader determinants of health, including the childhood experience of income inequality, social class, limited social cohesion and related experiences of high incidence of childhood deprivation and abuse have been linked to lifestyle patterns (Lynch *et al.*, 1997; Smith *et al.*, 1997) and psychosocial factors (Anda *et al.*, 1999; Kinra *et al.*, 2000; Walker *et al.*, 1999) that contribute to chronic disease later in life. Other research has linked income inequality (Kawachi *et al.*, 1999b), social class (Lantz *et al.*, 1998; Smith *et al.*, 1997), limited social cohesion (Seeman, 1996) and related factors including high incidence of childhood deprivation (Evans *et al.*, 2000; McEwen, 2000; Power *et al.*, 2000) directly to increased incidence of chronic disease and to chronic disease-related morbidity and mortality (Bosma *et al.*, 1999; Kawachi *et al.*, 1999b). Neuroscientists suggest that adaptation to stressful life challenges such as those that accompany these broader determinants of health activates the neural, neuroendocrine and neuroendocrine-immune mechanisms to maintain homeostasis through change, and that an 'accumulated burden of adversity' (Alonzo, 2000) ultimately overtaxes the body's adaptive capacity, predisposing one to disease processes (McEwen, 1999).

Present and potential disease

In Chapter 3, disease is defined as 'a theoretical construct, or abstraction, by which physicians attempt to explain patients' problems in terms of abnormalities of structure and/or function of body organs and systems and includes both physical and mental disorders'. Dealing with the patient as a whole person invites consideration of all aspects of primary healthcare, including health enhancement, risk avoidance, risk reduction, early identification of disease or complication reduction. However, in keeping with concern about human potential for disease, much of the literature in primary care pertaining to prevention deals with appropriate screening maneuvers (Canadian Task Force, 1994; US Preventive Services Task Force, 1989) and establishing a practice infrastructure to bring these about (Audunsson, 1986; Battista and Lawrence, 1988).

The patient's experience of health and illness

To understand the perspective of the patient, the practitioner needs to explore the patient's experiential learning about health and illness, consequential personal knowledge and beliefs in relation to health and illness, and what each means to that person (Calnan, 1988). The practitioner needs to discover the patient's worldview of health and corresponding health-related values and priorities as one of many competing values in order to assess the patient's commitment to its pursuit. Fundamental to determining common ground regarding preventive behavior is the extent to which the individual feels responsible for and in control of his/her own health. Beliefs about health risks and the degree of control one has over those risks will affect the patient's actions.

Just as understanding the illness experience requires inquiry into feelings, ideas, effect on function and expectations, so too health promotion and disease prevention strategies that are patient-centered subsume the individual's self-perceived susceptibility and seriousness of disease, and ideas about health promotion, as well as the benefits and barriers to health promotion and prevention. Researchers have found a significant positive correlation between self-reported perceived health status and a health-promoting lifestyle (Gillis, 1993). Furthermore, health-valuing attitudes may buffer socio-environmental risks (Reifman *et al.*, 2001), and the image of being health-conscious may serve as stronger motivation for health-promoting activity than an internal locus of control and sense of responsibility for one's own health (Wanek *et al.*, 1999). In addition, studies have indicated that individuals who conceive of health as the presence of wellness rather than merely the absence of disease have a significantly stronger engagement in health-promoting lifestyles (Gillis, 1993). Consistent with current notions of health as a process of mobilizing resources for everyday living, other research has identified that patients with chronic illness often experience health, and do much to create their own health (McWilliam *et al.*, 1996), with positive outcomes for themselves and the healthcare system (McWilliam *et al.*, 1999). Thus, it is important to assess both the patient's own perception of experienced health and illness, and what health really means in daily life.

An individual's perceptions of the benefits and barriers to health and health-promoting lifestyle is important in determining whether or not a health-promoting strategy is adopted. Furthermore, the greater the individual's perceptions of barriers to health, the lower that person's health status (Gillis, 1993). Most importantly, research has demonstrated that a patient-centered approach to relationship building (McWilliam *et al.*, 1997) enhances the individual's health (McWilliam *et al.*, 1999).

The more illness-oriented a patient's experience, the more the patient's world calls for the doctor to act as healer or therapeutic interventionist. If, on the other hand, the patient sees great benefits to health promotion and prevention, perceives little seriousness or susceptibility to illness or is able to focus on health despite chronic illness, the patient's world calls for the doctor to be a facilitator and educator. Likewise, the less negative the individual's experience of being a patient, and the more positive his/her experience of health, including self-confidence and self-efficacy, the more appropriate is the practitioner's role as facilitator and educator.

The patient's potential for health

The patient's potential for health is determined by his/her exposure to broader determinants of health throughout his/her life course, age, sex, genetic potential for disease, socio-economic status, and personal goals and values. Perhaps the most challenging aspect of assessing a patient's potential for health lies in identifying personal goals and values. The patient's conceptualization and valuing of health cannot be assumed. Yet, his/her view of the meaning of health and his/her valuing of health is logically fundamental to a health-promoting lifestyle, and a positive correlation between the two has been demonstrated in many studies (Gillis, 1993; Reifman *et al.*, 2001; Wanek *et al.*, 1999).

Self-efficacy – the power to produce one's own desired ends – is fundamental to the patient's potential for health. Bandura (1986) suggests that self-efficacy behavior, which includes choice, effort, and persistence in activities related to desired goals or outcomes, is a function of: (a) the individual's self-perceptions of ability to perform a behavior; and (b) the individual's beliefs that the behavior in question will lead to the specific outcomes desired. Numerous studies document the positive correlation between these two factors and actual decision-making and/or action regarding health behavior (Anderson *et al.*, 2001; Martinelli, 1999; Piazza *et al.*, 2001; Rimal, 2000; Shannon *et al.*, 1997; Sherwood and Jeffrey, 2000). While research related to the influence of locus of control is contradictory, researchers have demonstrated that self-efficacy and health status are the most powerful predictors of a health-promoting lifestyle (Gillis, 1993; Stuifbergen *et al.*, 2000). Researchers have also determined that approaches that focus on increasing self-efficacy for health behaviors would improve health-promoting effort and quality of life (Burke *et al.*, 1999).

In summary, the more favorable the patient's potential for health, particularly as it relates to self-efficacy and health status, the more appropriate is the practitioner's role as facilitator of health enhancement and educator regarding risk avoidance. The less favorable the patient's potential for health, the more appropriate is the doctor's intervention with risk reduction and early identification strategies.

The patient's context

Just as the patient's context was shown to be important to patient-centered care generally, health promotion and disease prevention strategies must attend to contextual issues. The patient's context, the physical and interpersonal environment of the person, includes family, friends, job, community and culture (Epp, 1986; Watson, 1984). Mass media can influence health attitudes and beliefs in both subtle and obvious ways, and may either enhance the patient's potential for health or detract from it (National Research Council,

1989). Similarly, the availability or absence and nature of resources such as family (De Bourdeaudhuij and Van Oost, 1998; Ford-Gilboe, 1997) and social support groups (Pavis *et al.*, 1998; Sherwood and Jeffrey, 2000), as well as health promotion programs (Burke *et al.*, 1999; Feldman *et al.*, 2000), may enhance or detract from the individual's potential for health.

The doctor's office setting is an important part of the patient's context. The 'personal' element and emphasis on continuity of care may make the physician's office setting conducive to the type of patient–doctor relationship necessary for the practice of health education (Calnan, 1988) and the continuity of relationship between the physician and patient constitutes a critical element promoting health as both human potential and the daily process of mobilizing resources for everyday living (McWilliam *et al.*, 1997). Yet doctors have found that lack of time, space and necessary staff are barriers to both health promotion and preventive activities (Becker and Janz, 1990; Bruce and Burnett, 1991; Pommerenke and Dietrich, 1992). Office hours, location and physical structure have the potential to represent real barriers from the patient's perspective. Ease of access, proximity to screening resources such as mammography sites, and the privacy and comfort of the doctor's office all constitute contextual factors which influence the patient's receptivity to using the physician as a resource for health promotion and disease prevention (Carter *et al.*, 1981; Godkin and Catlin, 1984). Furthermore, the skills, perceptions, and attitudes of office staff, particularly the office nurse, affect patients. Staff need to be supportive of the doctor's health promotion and disease prevention efforts by providing positive reinforcement to patients, especially reinforcing patient perceptions that changing health-related behavior is possible, and where interdisciplinary teams exist, all need to work together toward such aims. Evidence to date suggests that when interdisciplinary teams provide health promotion programs, positive outcomes can be achieved (Fries *et al.*, 1993; Leigh *et al.*, 1992). Chapter 9, 'Being realistic', provides more details on interdisciplinary teamwork.

In summary, the patient's context is an essential component of any effort to promote health or prevent disease. A supportive social context is particularly important for successful health enhancement. The doctor's office context can be intentionally designed to enhance all strategies to promote health and prevent disease.

The patient–doctor relationship

In the same way that the patient–doctor relationship is the foundation of patient-centered care generally, health promotion and disease prevention strategies are built on a strong patient–doctor relationship. Very much a part of the patient's context and potential for health is the nature of the patient's relationship with the doctor and personal experience of care. Built over time, the physician's approach determines how much and what kind of trust the patient places in the physician, what the patient's expectations of the roles of doctor and patient are, and what kind of power relationship exists between them (Brody, 1992). The patient's approach to assuming or relinquishing power to the physician shapes the physician's approach to patient care, and, ultimately, the patient–doctor relationship. Thus, the doctor's power to intervene both shapes and is shaped by the patient's world.

Investigation of the impact of the patient–doctor relationship on health promotion and disease prevention has been limited. Nevertheless, several authors (Pommerenke and Dietrich, 1992; Quill, 1989; Sanson-Fisher and Maguire, 1980) note that poor physician communication skills may be one of the most important and overlooked barriers to preventive care, and building a trusting relationship has been found in other research to be an essential component of promoting health as a resource for everyday living (McWilliam et al., 1997). A regular source of primary care has been associated with greater likelihood of provision of preventive medicine services (Forrest and Starfield, 1998; Sox et al., 1998;).

In summary, health promotion and disease prevention require a patient-centered approach. Knowledge of the patient's present and potential disease, the patient's experience of health, as well as of illness, and the patient's experience of the context of health and healthcare, facilitates the choice, implementation and success of health promotion and disease prevention strategies. The physician's patient-centeredness ensures greater success in promoting health and preventing disease.

Applying a patient-centered approach to health promotion and disease prevention

Applying the patient-centered approach allows the practitioner to find the methods of health promotion and preventive care which most appropriately match the patient's world. The patient's world may be viewed as an integrated system, and the components of this system together create a whole which is different from the sum of the parts. The practitioner's knowledge of this world helps in making a judgment about which health promotion or disease prevention strategy provides the most appropriate fit.

The doctor and patient together find common ground arriving at decisions about the goals and priorities of care, and their respective roles in it. If the most recent definitions of healthcare are to be enacted, strategy selection in health promotion and disease prevention calls for special attention to appropriately sharing power. Being alert to the sense of powerlessness which patients often experience, supporting and encouraging the patient's own exercise of power 'so long as it is consistent with a good therapeutic outcome and with the patient's long-term goals and interests' (Brody, 1992: 65), and using 'the physician–patient relationship as a primary therapeutic tool' (Brody, 1992: 65) are all a part of the process of finding common ground. Through this process, the physician and patient together decide the health promotion and/or prevention strategies to be pursued.

Strategy selection within the patient-centered clinical method also requires the doctor to adopt more current thinking about adult learning, and to approach health promotion with adult patients accordingly. The patient-centered educational approach in health promotion is a learner-centered social process (*see* Chapter 11). The doctor precipitates the patient-learner's critical reflection about health through dialog which makes the patient aware of his/her own potential for health and health promotion and the potential threats to health inherent in the individual's current life. The physician guides the patient through exploration of the personal meaning of current practices, and the personal values, needs, motives, expectations and understanding which underlie these life elements. Over time, the process of guiding the patient-learner also includes exploring alternative ways of looking at current practices, and finding and trying new ways of fulfilling personal values, needs, motives and expectations. A supportive role is also part of this process: listening, empathizing, validating changed perspectives through rational discourse, and working out new relationships with the patient-learner, consistent with changes in perspective.

The learning is self-discovered, and cannot be directly communicated (Rogers, 1961) by the physician. Rather, the physician is guided by the conditions of learning (Rogers, 1961). The commonly known strategies of health education, most of which emphasize information giving and behavior modification, comprise only a small part of the process of health promotion. In order for true personal growth and change to transpire, the patient-centered approach is critical.

The patient's world is understood as a dynamic situation that varies with each patient at different points in time and with each healthcare issue. The doctor's aim is to find the best fit with the patient's world. Sometimes, for some issues, the patient requires a health enhancement strategy. At other times, for other reasons, the patient requires prevention strategies. Evidence to date suggests that individuals move dynamically across five potential stages of change (Prochaska *et al.*, 1992). The following case examples illustrate how the doctor uses the patient-centered approach in choosing and implementing a strategy for health promotion and/or disease prevention.

Case example

George Applebee was a 35-year-old insurance adjuster who had been found to have blood pressures ranging between 130–135/90–95 over three successive visits. He had smoked a pack of cigarettes a day for the past 15 years and had consumed 8–10 bottles of beer a week, usually on weekends. He had also led a sedentary lifestyle. Recently, George's father underwent coronary bypass surgery at the age of 64, having had symptoms of angina for about five years. George had never taken much interest in his health until his recent marriage. Generally, he had viewed physicians with some suspicion but his current family physician, Dr Modell, had earned his respect when she attended him following an appendectomy five years ago.

When George presented at the office, the doctor used a preventive medicine model, screening him for other risk factors of heart disease and end-organ damage. Being patient-centered, she recognized that the new marriage could play a significant role in motivating George to a healthier lifestyle, and that George's new wife could also be included in health teaching regarding diet and exercise. Capitalizing on George's receptivity to health teaching and newly acquired social support, Dr Modell therefore also addressed the need to quit smoking, exercise more regularly and optimize weight.

Case example

Shauna Bright was 16 years old and, while in the doctor's office for her monthly allergy shot, noticed a waiting room poster designed to draw attention to the disadvantages of unplanned pregnancy. She had been dating another student in her high school and was aware that their relationship may involve sexual intercourse soon. Shauna had been in good health all her life and because of her interest in sports and physical fitness, took the maintenance of her health very seriously. She was aware of the importance of a balanced diet and regular exercise. She had been going to her current family doctor since her childhood and was on generally good terms with him. However, approaching him regarding the birth control pill raised fears that her parents may eventually find out, since they also attended the same doctor. Shauna therefore decided to make an appointment for knee pains which had been bothering her in any case. If it seemed safe enough, she intended to bring up the issue of birth control on the same visit.

When Shauna presented in the office, the patient–doctor relationship was tested in the crucible of adolescence. Using a patient-centered approach, the physician maintained a non-judgmental attitude and openness to discussing Shauna's concerns, and thereby facilitated Shauna's verbalization of her wishes. Acting as health educator, the physician provided information about birth control as well as prevention of sexually transmitted disease.

Using health enhancement strategies, he also explored with Shauna the psychosocial aspects of sexual behavior. Subsequent visits emphasized the need for regular screening procedures such as Pap smears, once she became sexually active. The encounter served to empower this young woman with respect to her health and gave her a sense of self-worth and heightened self-esteem.

Case example

Mrs Bell: Doctor, my husband and I thought about having Jason vaccinated, but after reading some books, we're not so sure that it is the right thing to do.
Doctor: Tell me about your concerns.

The Bells, responsible and conscientious parents of 6-month-old Jason, were new to their family doctor's practice. The doctor was surprised to find that the child had received no vaccinations.

A bright and well-educated couple, Mr and Mrs Bell had taken time to inform themselves on infant and baby care. The Bells had invested in a good quality baby car seat and were very interested in planning for the baby's future, yet they were reluctant to have Jason immunized. They had been aware of sensational media reports of presumed vaccine adverse effects resulting in permanent neurological damage. This had left them doubtful about the benefits and risks of vaccination for their son. In contrast, their family physician saw vaccination as a basic investment in Jason's future health.

It may be difficult for a physician to understand a patient's opposing viewpoint given the clear benefits that have been made possible by vaccination programs. There are many reasons why the lay public may evaluate medical risks differently from the 'experts'. Research in the field of decision-making has found that people's perceptions of risk are not determined by rational processes but that greater weight is given to risks if the issue is perceived to be involuntary, dreaded, immediate, appears to be uncontrollable, puts children at risk or is unfamiliar (Whyte and Burton, 1982).

Media attention has played a significant role in shaping the public's perception of vaccinations and in some countries has been instrumental in the decline in vaccination rates and has resulted in the resurgence of previously controlled infectious diseases (Cherry, 1984). Perceived risk has been found to be one variable in a person's decision about whether or not to participate in a program of disease prevention (Adjaye, 1981; Carter and Jones, 1985; Morgan *et al.*, 1987).

The Bell family had serious reservations about allowing vaccination of their child. Their family physician listened carefully to their concerns and answered them respectfully. She was able to put the small risks of vaccine side effects into perspective by comparing the published risks of adverse vaccine reactions with the risks of everyday events. After careful consideration of these points, the Bells eventually decided to have Jason immunized, which proceeded without any side effects.

In this case the family physician was able to find common ground with the parents and come to a mutually satisfactory agreement by recognizing that it is possible to have legitimate opinions that differ from those of the 'experts', and then listening carefully to the concerns raised by those opinions and addressing those concerns in a forthright manner.

The strategies that physicians employ will vary from patient to patient and from time to time with the same patient, depending on the circumstances, the life stage of the patient and the presence or absence of health risk behavior. Deciding on an appropriate strategy ultimately means finding common ground. Of course, no strategy is pursued without the patient's informed consent (Lee, 1993).

Achieving informed consent presents a particular challenge in the areas of health promotion and disease prevention. Since the benefits or risks of a preventive procedure are generally determined on a societal rather than an individual level, it is not possible to predict the consequences for any one person (Hanckel, 1984). The tendency has been to weigh the benefits and potential harm of a preventive procedure (e.g. immunization) on a societal rather than an individual level (Rose, 1981). However, the physician has a moral and ethical responsibility to present the risks and psychological costs of proposed prevention programs to the patient (Marteau, 1990). Additionally it must be made clear that the problems are difficult to predict in advance and that little is known about the prognosticators of health (Schoenbach et al., 1983). Even when problems and prognosticators are correctly predicted, known treatments only work for a portion of patients, and that portion cannot be identified. Thus, physicians cannot tell patients how certain they might be that the preventive treatment will produce the desired effect (Hanckel, 1984).

Clearly, health promotion and disease prevention necessitate increased physician effort to address the ethical issues of care (Strasser et al., 1987). Ultimately, patients have the right to choose, and, in so choosing, share the responsibility for outcomes. This, too, is an important parameter of health, health promotion, and disease prevention.

Conclusion

There is compelling evidence that health promotion and prevention efforts can be effectively applied by physicians. Yet both physician education and attitudes

(McPhee *et al.*, 1986; McPhee and Schroeder, 1987), and patient education, expectations, motivations, and attitudes (McGinnis and Hamburg, 1988) can undermine such interventions. Overcoming such barriers to achieve success in health promotion and disease prevention efforts can be achieved through using a patient-centered approach.

Case example: 'I should write a letter to the editor!'

Carol L McWilliam

Mrs Samm was an 80-year-old widow with chronic obstructive pulmonary disease and hypertension. Both the physiological incapacitation and the accompanying need for oxygen by nasal cannula severely limited her mobility, leaving her largely confined to her eleventh floor apartment, where she lived alone. Mrs Samm managed from day to day with the assistance of her only 60-year-old daughter, Gloria, who lived on a farm 40 minutes outside of town, but dutifully visited every Wednesday afternoon to clean her mother's apartment, to grocery shop, to assist with managing the household finances and to organize meals, which she froze as individual meals for easy preparation by microwave. Additionally, Gloria visited every Sunday afternoon along with her farmer husband. Both reluctantly pursued this family routine, despite the 24 hours a day, 7 days a week demands that the farm placed on them as an aging, childless, self-sustaining couple. Every week they listened to Mrs Samm's incessant complaining about everything from the weather to her lot in life.

Dr Aronson, Mrs Samm's aging family physician, had cared for her for many years, supporting her through a life-threatening diagnosis of meningitis that Gloria had contracted as a teenager, through her husband's two-year bout with terminal lung cancer, and through her own struggle to quit smoking at the age of 75 years, as her own COPD worsened. Now, he made a house visit to her once a month to monitor her condition and treatment.

In the past, Mrs Samm had managed to amuse herself by watching television, reading, and talking on the telephone. However, Mrs Samm's condition had begun to deteriorate in recent months. Increased difficulty in breathing, loss of appetite and anxiety related to a fear of developing lung cancer had begun to take its toll. Mrs Samm had become preoccupied with the fear of having to go to a nursing home, or, worse, the possibility of death. As her preoccupation intensified, Mrs Samm had begun to make regular visits to the hospital emergency room, seeking urgent medical attention for chronic symptoms that were clearly being adequately mana- ged at home under her family physician's care. In response, Emergency Department physicians were urging Dr Aronson to consider admitting Mrs Samm to a nursing home.

Familiar with Mrs Samm's larger life context and her personal goal of avoiding admission to a nursing home, Dr Aronson decided to explore the broader notions of health with her. He knew from his routinely provided care that her condition had not really deteriorated. Dr Aronson needed to know more about how Mrs Samm viewed health, and what personal resources she might have to optimize her health, despite her chronic ill- ness. Also he needed to learn what her commitment to the pursuit of opti- mizing her health, despite the chronic illness, might be. He recognized that there might be broader determinants of health entering into Mrs Samm's current inability to maintain the level of wellness and quality of life that she had managed to have for the past several years. He decided to see if he might promote health by engaging her as a partner in its enhancement.

Accordingly, during his next visit, the following conversation transpired:

Dr Aronson: While I see no change in your physical condition over the past year, you seem to be experiencing more illness in recent months. Can you tell me about your experience of health right now?
Mrs Samm: I've lost my confidence. I'm afraid I will end up in a nursing home. Now, every time I feel a little down, I think I've just got to get help! I go to the hospital's Emergency Department and they check me out and just send me home. That makes me angry and upset, and I begin to worry even more and get very frightened that I will end up in a nursing home. It's a vicious circle, and I don't know what to do, don't know what will happen, don't know where I'll end up.
Dr Aronson: You are afraid because you don't know what to do, don't know what will happen, and don't know where you'll end up.
Mrs Samm: Yes, that's it.
Dr Aronson: So it's fear of the unknown, isn't it.
Mrs Samm: Yes, that's it. And it's affecting my health.
Dr Aronson: So is there anything that can be done about this fear of the unknown in order to help your health?
Mrs Samm: I don't know, I just want to be able to do the things I want to do.
Dr Aronson: Yes. And what might some of those things be?
Mrs Samm: I don't know. I guess I'll have to think about it.

Following this lead, Dr Aronson agreed and suggested he would come again to monitor her condition next week. At the next visit, following his routine examination, Dr Aronson resumed his effort to engage Mrs Samm in health enhancement.

Dr Aronson: So have you come up with a list of things you'd like to do yet?
Mrs Samm: Well, for one thing, I'd like to able to be more actively involved in the community like I used to be, but that's out with this bad breathing problem!
Dr Aronson: Maybe, maybe not. I wonder if there is anything in particular you think you might like to do?
Mrs Samm: Well, I'd sure like to do something about the mess City Hall have made of our water bills! The latest billings are outrageous, and it's all because they've increased the rates to offset the cost of new housing developments!
Dr Aronson: I wonder what you might be able to do about it from here?
Mrs Samm: Well, I should write a letter to the editor. Someone should tell them what this means to people like me on a fixed income!
Dr Aronson: Yes, that's a great idea. I think you should do that.

Dr Aronson made a commitment to check up on Mrs Samm in two weeks, and followed up accordingly.

Dr Aronson: How is your health today, Mrs Samm?
Mrs Samm: Well, I'll tell you, my blood pressure must be back to normal because I did write that letter to the editor, and I've since had telephone calls from many seniors who happen to agree with me, and from my city council member, who has agreed to address it at the next council meeting. I'm glad you helped me to get onto this. When the councilor called, I also told him what I thought he should do about the problem of vandalism in our parks, and I've written a letter to the editor about that too!
Dr Aronson: Sounds like you've found a new niche in the world.
Mrs Samm: (*Chuckling*) Well, perhaps I have. I certainly am going to keep on to these problems. Somebody has to!

Dr Aronson agreed, and proceeded to check Mrs Samm's vital signs, review her medication adherence, and make his usual assessment. Dr Aronson observed that Mrs Samm had not been making her usual trips to the Emergency Department and he and Mrs Samm agreed that she was well enough for him to go back to the routine of visiting once a month.

This case illustrates how patient-centered practice can facilitate the promotion of health as a resource for everyday living. Dr Aronson sought a broader understanding of Mrs Samm, and her experience of health, illness and disease. He determined that health to her meant being able to do the things she wanted to do. He helped her explore her commitment to and options for achieving her notion of health. He also facilitated her determination of what and how much she might do to experience health more positively, despite her debilitating chronic medical problems, and within the broader parameters of her larger life context. He used a patient-centered approach and built on the continuity of his relationship with her to enable her to use her full resources for everyday living, thereby optimizing her ability to realize her aspirations, giving her a renewed a sense of purpose in life, to satisfy her needs for social cohesion within her community, and to respond positively to the environment, despite her chronic medical problems.

The fifth component: enhancing the patient–doctor relationship

Moira Stewart and Judith Belle Brown

The relationship is the bedrock or the basis for all interchanges between two people and could be described as a primal exchange between the two individuals. Relationships, in general, involve caring, feeling, trust, power and a sense of purpose. In a patient–doctor relationship the purpose is to help the patient, i.e. to be a therapeutic relationship and frequently to foster healing.

We begin with a quote from Sir William Osler: 'I would urge upon you ... to care more for the individual patient than for the special features of the disease. ... Dealing as we do with poor suffering humanity, we see the man unmasked, exposed to all the frailties and weaknesses, and you have to keep your heart soft and tender lest you have too great a contempt for your fellow creatures. The best way is to keep a looking-glass in your own heart, and the more carefully you scan your own frailties, the more tender you are for those of your fellow creatures' (Cushing, 1925). How do doctors put into practice the concepts described by Osler? In this chapter we discuss compassion, power, constancy, healing, self-awareness, transference and counter-transference.

Compassion, empathy and caring

Brian McDonald, a young man in his early twenties, had already had two visits to the family doctor and had been diagnosed with mononucleosis. After three weeks he became too weak to get out of bed and the doctor made a housecall to the patient's home where he lived with his parents. Even before examining Brian, the doctor stated: 'If I had a room like this I'd want to stay here all the time too!'

Anne Montgomery, a young pregnant woman, was in her eighth month when she developed signs of toxemia of pregnancy. When entering her bedroom at her home, the doctor remarked, 'So you've taken to your bed already, have you?'

The lack of respect, compassion, empathy or support reflected in these two cases may have negative consequences for patients' self-respect and inner resources just when patients need them most. Our self-absorption as professionals, whether it is recognized or not, can interfere with care in so many ways. Further, arrogance among physicians is unfortunately common, possibly because of the unconscious collusion between the vulnerability of the patient needing an all-powerful caregiver and the invisible hubris of the doctor. Current emphasis on technology and efficiency in medical practice provides fertile ground for this problem to grow: 'This distancing of the doctor from the patient breeds a kind of "system arrogance", in which the patient is no longer seen as a human being but simply as a job to be done cost-effectively' (Berger, 2002: 146). Doctors are mistaken if they think that compassionate care is more difficult and more taxing. On the contrary, sometimes our difficulty is that we fail to understand that what the patient wants is something very simple: a *recognition* of his or her suffering or perhaps only our *presence* at a time of need.

Turning now to the positive side, caring has been defined in a series of qualitative studies as a process encompassing eight concepts. These can be found to reverberate throughout the chapters of this book; they are: time; being there; talking; sensitivity; acting in the best interest of the other; feeling; doing; and reciprocity (Tarlow, 1996). Caring implies that the doctor is fully present and engaged with the patient. The notion of the detached clinician who keeps a safe emotional distance is replaced by the notion that doctor and patient are interconnected in such a deep way that the doctor can fully immerse him or herself in the concerns of the patient (Montgomery, 1993). Intense caring moments in relationships involve mutual recognition on the part of patient and practitioner and a reciprocal learning of both individuals (Frank, 1991; Suchman and Matthews, 1988; Watson, 1985). Boundaries may be much more blurred than in the traditional, distanced, one-way relationship. However, the closeness restores the patients' sense of connectedness to the human race, a connectedness which may have been broken by their physical or emotional suffering (Belenky *et al.*, 1986; Candib, 1988; Cassell, 1991).

For generations, medical students have been taught: 'don't get involved'. In the conventional clinical method, the doctor is assumed to be a detached observer and prescriber of treatment. Remaining uninvolved may protect doctors from some very disturbing things, especially as they encounter the depth of a patient's suffering. But it also has a personal price. To remain uninvolved, physicians have to build up protective shells to suppress their feelings. This lack of openness creates difficulties in relationships, not only with patients, but also with colleagues. To suggest that one can remain uninvolved is also a fallacy. One cannot help being affected in some way by the encounter with suffering, even if the result is avoidance and denial.

Candib (1987) has spoken about not only the inherent intimacy of patient–doctor relationships but also their reciprocity. She noted that doctors' sharing their own story with a patient can go awry but it also can be healing for the doctor as well as patient. The question then becomes one of what it means to be involved. Perhaps what the conventional teaching intended to say was: 'Don't get involved at the level of your egoistic emotions.'

Enid Balint and colleagues (1993) point out that for doctors it is important to move back and forth from objective observation to empathetic identification in the same sort of 'biphasic structure' that we recommended in Chapter 3 and replicate here in Figure 8.1 (Virshup *et al.*, 1999). In a similar vein, we are reminded by Rudebeck (2002) that, while empathy today implies an emotional connection, earlier definitions included 'the whole inner world of the speaking voice' in which 'perception, emotion and cognition are integrated dimensions of any experience' (2000: 452).

The following story, recounted by McWhinney illustrates this multifaceted connection.

> I have never forgotten a brief experience I had as a medical student. When at home (during school holidays) I used to do rounds with the surgeon at the local hospital. After the round (one day), he was asked to see an old vagrant who was complaining of abdominal pain. The experience made a deep and lasting impression on me. The patient was exactly as one would have expected; his face red and blotchy; several days' growth of beard on his chin.

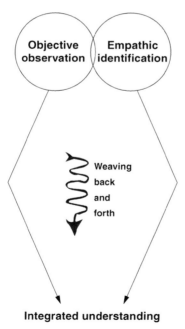

Figure 8.1 Connecting with patients.

For those few minutes, this old vagrant seemed to be the most important person in the world for the doctor. All his attention was focused on the old man, whom he treated with the utmost respect – a respect that showed in the way he talked and listened and the way he examined him. The word that perhaps describes it best is presence; for those few minutes the doctor was a real presence in the patient's life. (McWhinney 1997: 6)

Redelmeier *et al.* (1995) conducted the only randomized trial, to our knowledge, of compassionate care for the homeless. This care was provided by well-trained volunteers who listened attentively, and spent time and shared common experiences with the patients who visited emergency departments. The study found that the homeless patients who were randomly assigned to receive compassionate care were significantly more satisfied and took significantly longer to return for another visit than patients receiving usual care.

Perhaps the kernel of the caring relationship from the patient's point of view is trust. Breast cancer patients have difficulty understanding the vast amounts of information they need to assimilate before treatment decisions can be made, especially in their understandable state of anxiety and fear. Women with breast cancer say that they cannot make sense of all the facts and figures regarding options, unless they work with a trusted physician (McWilliam *et al.*, 1997). The sources of trust in medical practice include: a just society; moral integrity; continuity of care; sharing power; compassion; authenticity and competence (Fugelli, 2001). 'Trust is an individual's belief that the sincerity, benevolence, and truthfulness of others can be relied on. Trust often implies a transference of power, to a person or to a system, to act on one's behalf, in one's best interest' (2001: 575).

Power in the patient–doctor relationship

Case example

Janet Sutherland, a healthcare worker in her late thirties, recently broke her arm in a car accident. Her world was shattered as were the bones in her arm. For ten weeks she was unable to care for her two preschool children, or drive the car, or work. By this time, her confidence in herself was deteriorating because she felt responsible, not only for the accident, but also for the fact that her bones were not healing as quickly as expected. Moreover, her confidence and trust in her family doctor were also waning because the decisions they made together (regarding the type of surgeon she would be referred to, the type of anesthetic she would receive, and the type of follow-up care) were never realized. The information about the surgery too was conflicting. Janet expressed these fears, 'Why is nothing as it should be? Why am I not recovering? Is something being hidden? Why can't I get better – I need to get better!'

The central issues of lack of control over the recovery and over the healthcare created a sense of powerlessness. As angry as Janet became at herself, she was doubly angry at the doctors, including the family doctor. The ebbing trust and the increasing powerlessness united in a crisis of care. It took weeks of work on the part of this patient to gain insight into her own issues. It took a new willingness on the part of all the physicians to listen and to solve problems mutually with the patient, before both the healing of the person and the healing of the bones became evident.

Much has been made of power and control in the patient–doctor relationship in the literature in the past 20 years. There is no doubt that the relationship which is the foundation for patient-centered care, compared to the traditional relationship, demands a sharing of power and control between the doctor and the patient (Brody, 1992). Other authors who have proposed models of patient–doctor relationships have variously described the state of high patient control of decision-making as: mutuality (Szasz and Hollender, 1956); the contractual relationship (Veatch, 1972); the consumerist approach (Haug and Lavin, 1983; Roter and Hall, 1992; Stewart and Roter, 1989). These approaches are similar but not identical to component 3, 'Finding common ground', described in Chapter 6. The quality of a relationship within which finding common ground is possible includes a readiness of doctor and patient to become partners in care. Their encounters are truly meetings between experts (Tuckett *et al.*, 1985). Each partnership is unique and may include permutations and combinations employing varying degrees of control along many dimensions and changing over time. One example would be the adolescent, who needs information (from the expert doctor) but who also maintains control of management (envisioning herself as expert on her life) because she yearns to be treated as an adult, but at the same time needs guidance. An ability on the part of the doctor to remain open and alert to these shifting needs for control is an essential aspect of a partnership.

The resulting therapeutic alliance is related in complex ways to enhancing patients' sense of self-efficacy, i.e. sense of control over themselves and their world or, to put it another way, a sense of omnipotence. We will see later in this chapter that these desired outcomes are considered key dimensions of health and wholeness (Cassell, 1991). The connection between the dimension of trust in the therapeutic alliance and the taking and giving of control is best illustrated in the following qualitative longitudinal study. Bartz characterized the evolution of relationships of nine Native diabetic patients with one physician over time, in terms such as disease-focus, misunderstandings, mistrust, detachment and hopelessness (Bartz, 1999). 'To control the environment, the doctor adopted various strategies that constrained the interactions, including use of a diabetic protocol form and a medicalized way of knowing patients. Paradoxically, these strategies produced varying degrees of mistrust, clinical nihilism, interpersonal distance, and loss of control in relationships with these patients' (Bartz, 1993). One sees the negative implications of continued attempts to exert medical control.

Another alternative in situations of misunderstanding and mistrust may be consciously to share power, to move away from medical conversation and to be curious about patients' lives and beliefs (Brody, 1999; Suchman, 1998). 'By facilitating the telling of their life-stories over time, doctors share with their patients the process whereby they reconstruct themselves through the experience of their suffering. In sharing this, doctors are also open to change, experiencing their own vulnerability and powerlessness ... [an acknowledgment of which] may be one of the most powerful things doctors do to facilitate healing in patients ... the strength borne from the awareness of shared weakness' (Goodyear-Smith and Buetow, 2001: 457). The conscious choice of such an approach is considered 'new to medicine ... the doctor must initiate this transformation in the unequal relationship' (Candib, 1995: 252).

Case example

> Mrs Patrick was an elderly woman who had arthritis, irritable bowel syndrome and had had a cancer of the breast six years ago. Her doctor, in his late thirties, had been Mrs Patrick's family physician for the past year. This insightful patient and doctor found a way to accommodate her seemingly contradictory needs. On the one hand, her advanced age and physical problems left her insecure enough to require explicit reassurance. The doctor provided the reassurance after appropriate questioning and physical examination and by exploring the nature of her symptoms. On the other hand, she needed to maintain control over some aspects of her life and health; this manifested itself in her controlling the choice and the order of topics during the encounter with her family doctor. She was one of those patients who brought in a written list of her complaints. Although this family physician thoughtfully interpreted her behavior, other doctors might have been offended by her somewhat bossy manner and might have failed to see it as an important coping mechanism.

Continuity and constancy

Continuity of care is longitudinal care delivered over time within the context of a long-term relationship between patient and physician: 'the words themselves emphasize the importance of a connected unbroken course, of inherent qualities that continue without essential change' (Loxterkamp, 1991: 354). He described the power of continuing relationships in this way: 'Doctors who remain deeply connected to their patients will know the privilege, as will those who retain the capacity to listen, touch, tether ourselves to the wounds of others. In modest ways, we accomplish the utterly profound long before the prescription is filled or the blood test is taken. We profit by the patients' periodic return and by the mutual exchange of friendship, intimacy and trust' (Loxterkamp, 2001: 247). Continuity of relationships have been shown to accrue many benefits (Ettner, 1999; Hjortdahl and Borchgrevink, 1991). Nonetheless, in all medical disciplines and in most Western countries, policy decisions have resulted in marked disruptions in continuity of care.

Not only does the system put barriers in the way of continuity of care, but also physicians themselves consciously or unconsciously close doors or at worst abandon patients. Nonetheless, it remains the doctor's responsibility to be constant in his or her commitment to the well-being of the patient. As Stephens (1982) explains 'physicians do not have the luxury of limiting their involvement to those patients who can make and keep promises' (1982: 164). The required commitment is not easily achieved because the doctor may experience feelings of failure and have to encounter a patient's anger or other expressions of mistrust. Cassell (1991) describes constancy in the following way:

> Constancy to the patient is necessary. Constant attention and maintained presence are not difficult when things are going well. It requires self-discipline to maintain constancy when the case is going sour, when errors or failures have occurred, when the wrong diagnosis has been made, when the patient's personality or behaviour is difficult or even repulsive, when impending death brings the danger of sorrow and loss because emotional closeness has been established. When constancy is absent or falters, too frequently, patients lose that newfound part of themselves – the doctor – that promised stability in the uncertain world of sickness arising from their relationship. (1991: 78)

Healing

The attributes of the doctor and the characteristics of the relationship are what make the patient–doctor relationship therapeutic. Like many other helping professionals, doctors are experienced as instruments (agents) of healing. This image of the doctor is contained in numerous stories of patients (Stephens, 1993). In particular, Arthur Frank wrote in his book, *At the Will of the Body: reflections in illness* (1991), about his own experience as a patient:

> Medicine has done well with my body and I am grateful. But doing *with* the body is only part of what needs to be done *for* the person. What happens when

my body breaks down happens not just to that body but also to my life, which is lived in that body. When the body breaks down, so does the life. Even when medicine can fix the body, that doesn't always put the life back together again. (1991: 8) (emphasis in original)

Healing the body and healing the person are not identical and do not even necessarily go hand in hand. The healing of a patient involves a process of restoring the patient's lost sense of connectedness, indestructibility and control. The healing process is 'no more than allowing, causing or bringing to bear those things or forces for getting better that already exist in the patient' (Cassell, 1991: 234).

Physicians for the most part see themselves as curers of patients' physical ills. They are less conscious of the need to restore patients to wellness by embracing the mandate to care and to heal. The words heal, health and whole all come from the same linguistic root in Old English. To heal is to restore a sense of coherence and wholeness after the disruption in a person's life that is caused by a serious illness. After a heart attack at the age of 39 and cancer at 40, Arthur Frank wrote about his experience in a healthcare system which was technically proficient but essentially uncaring. It was a system that seemed to have lost the capacity to heal the patient as well as treat his body.

In an ongoing patient–clinician relationship the process of healing has been described as following certain paths. For a group of patients who suffered alcoholism and/or suicide attempts but survived, the steps in their healing relationships were: listening, trust, willingness to change, acquisition of life skills and control (Seifert, 1992). For a group of chronically ill older persons, the process included: trust, connecting, caring, mutual knowledge and mutual caring (McWilliam et al., 1997). One sees a synergistic benefit to both patient and clinician in these accounts of healing.

Examples of the work of a doctor who recognized his healing role are contained in Berger and Mohr's (1967) story of a country doctor, *A Fortunate Man*. Because illnesses and crises separate people from the ordinariness of the rest of humanity, one requirement of the doctor is to recognize accurately the pain of the patient in order to help restore the patient's lost sense of connectedness and therefore promote healing (Stephens, 1982). This is not only difficult to do, but it also takes courage, a fact that often goes unacknowledged.

[The country doctor] is acknowledged as a good doctor because he meets the deep but unformulated expectation of the sick for a sense of fraternity. He recognizes them. Sometimes he fails – often because he has missed a critical opportunity and the patient's suppressed resentment becomes too hard to break through – but there is about him the constant will of man trying to recognize. 'The door opens,' he says, 'and sometimes I feel I'm in the valley of death. It's all right when once I'm working. I try to overcome this shyness because for the patient the first contact is extremely important. If he's put off and doesn't feel welcome, it may take a long time to win his confidence back and perhaps never. I try to give him a fully open greeting. All diffidence in my position is a fault. A form of negligence'. (Berger and Mohr, 1967: 76–7)

Self-awareness

Whatever use doctors make of themselves, and the relationship, in caring for patients, it affects them as well as their patients. The use of self, and attending to the impact on self, both require a well-depth of self-knowledge. To truly be a healer the physician must always strive for self-awareness and self-knowledge.

Over the past decade experts on the patient–doctor relationship have published articles elucidating the importance of self-awareness in medical education and practice (Kern *et al.*, 2001; Novack *et al.*, 1997; Novack *et al.*, 1999). Their writings emphasize how personal insight is integral to the clinician's use of self in the patient–doctor relationship. Novack *et al.* (1997: 502) state: 'Because physicians use themselves as instruments of diagnosis and therapy, personal awareness can help them to "calibrate their instruments", using themselves more effectively in these capacities.'

Self-awareness can be a natural outgrowth of reflection on experience and sharing these reflections with colleagues, friends, and family. It can be further enhanced by supervision or consultation, professional and personal development. Medical education must provide a safe and nurturing environment that fosters students' self-awareness, personal growth and well-being (Novack *et al.*, 1999). This topic is addressed in more depth in Chapter 12.

Epstein *et al.* (1993) propose three possible venues for developing self-awareness: Balint groups which were conceived by Michael and Enid Balint (Balint, 1957); family of origin groups, stemming from the work of Murray Bowen (1976, 1978) which examine how individuals' families of origin influence their relationships with patients; and personal awareness groups which have evolved from the contributions of Carl Rogers (1961). Other authors endorse the important knowledge and understanding imparted in the classical literature or the insights offered by narratives of illness (Borkan *et al.*, 1999; Brody, 1992; Brown *et al.*, 2002d; Greenhalgh and Hurwitz, 1998; Kleinman, 1988; McWhinney, 1989).

Kern *et al.* (2001), in their qualitative study of how personal growth and self-awareness is experienced by medical faculty, identified the following process. Personal growth or self-awareness was often prompted by a powerful experience, either personal or professional, that evoked strong feelings and altered the physician's sense of self. Helping relationships, either one-on-one or in a group setting, were another venue for personal growth. Both led to the physician being introspective and hence more self-aware.

Stephenson's (2002) rather poignant encounter with a patient, served as an opportunity for self-awareness. In brief, Stephenson arrived to see his last patient in the surgical admissions clinic. He was tired and running late; it had been a busy day with many difficult patients. This particular patient was an elderly gentleman who was reading a large leather-bound book. The doctor assumed it was the Bible and feared he would be the recipient of a sermon. In fact, the book was the complete works of Shakespeare which led the patient and doctor into an animated discussion of the Bard. But their lively exchange came to an end as they explored the patient's symptoms and their sinister implications. At that moment of uncertainty regarding the diagnosis, the patient's anxiety and fear were palpable but he quoted: 'Thy best of rest is sleep; And that thou oft provok'st, yet grossly fear'st, Thy death, which is no more.' In the end the patient's symptoms were found to be benign but this encounter had an indelible influence on Stephenson who concluded:

> On quiet nights now you can find me hidden away in the duty room, reading the complete works, still trying to fathom the lessons of that episode. Something about not judging a book by its cover, perhaps, but I believe there may have been another lesson, a lesson about stories – how one shared story could brighten up my entire week, how a well thumbed book could provide my patient with enough armour that he could look serious illness in the eye and not so much as blink. (Stephenson, 2002: 713)

Whatever the source, self-awareness and self-knowledge are imperative. As Howard Stein (1985a) observed, 'one can truly recognize a patient only if one is willing to recognize oneself in the patient'. McWhinney (1989: 82) had a similar message: 'We cannot begin to know others until we know ourselves. We cannot grow and change as physicians until we have removed our defences and faced up to our shortcomings.'

The development of self-awareness requires clinicians to know their strengths and weaknesses. What are potential blindspots or emotional triggers that elicit a negative response to certain patients? As Longhurst (1989) noted, self-awareness means confronting the emotional baggage emanating from our families of origin and conflicts in current relationships. Self-awareness and self-knowledge also have a positive value in that they promote and nurture the qualities of empathy, sensitivity, honesty, compassion and caring in the physician. Because acquiring self-knowledge is often a painful process, this form of knowledge is the most difficult of all to acquire. It is perhaps best seen as a lifelong journey, a process which is never complete. Epstein's (1999) conceptualization of 'mindful practice' raises the concept of physician self-awareness to a new level that is more complex and multifaceted. He states: 'This process of critical self-reflection depends on the presence of mindfulness. A mindful practitioner attends, in a nonjudgmental way, to his or her own physical and mental processes during ordinary everyday tasks to act with clarity and insight' (1999: 833).

Transference and counter-transference

All human relationships, and in particular therapeutic relationships, are influenced by the phenomena of transference and counter-transference. Thus any discussion of the patient–doctor relationship that excluded these important psychological processes would be remiss. We do not intend to provide the reader with a detailed examination of transference and counter-transference, but rather with a brief description. We feel that this is essential in order to define the parameters in which many of the dimensions (i.e. compassion, power, constancy, healing and self-awareness) of the patient–doctor relationship frequently occur.

Transference is a process whereby the patient unconsciously projects, onto individuals in his or her current life, thoughts, behaviors and emotional reactions that originate with other significant relationships from childhood onwards (Dubovsky, 1981; Goldberg, 2000; Woods and Hollis, 1990). This can include feelings of love, hate, ambivalence and dependency. The greater the current attachment, such as a significant patient–doctor relationship, the more likely that transference will occur. Transference, while often perceived as a negative phenomenon, actually helps build the connection between patient and doctor. Frequently, doctors are intimidated by the concept of transference, which has its roots in psychoanalytic theory, viewing it as something mysterious and to be avoided. As Goldberg (2000: 1165) notes: 'Many physicians intuitively and successfully use positive transference manifestations without necessarily being aware of them, negative, hostile transference manifestations in the patient may be more problematic.' However, knowledge of the patient's transference reaction, either positive or negative, assists the doctor in understanding how the patient experiences his or her world and how past relationships influence current behavior.

Transference can occur during any stage of the patient–doctor relationship and be activated by any number of events. For example, when the capabilities of seriously ill patients are impaired or when patients are overwhelmed by the ramifications implied by a specific diagnosis, they may respond to their doctor in an uncharacteristic manner. They may return to a position of dependency and neediness which is more a reflection of unresolved past relationships than of their current relationship with the physician. Patients may seek the care and comfort which was absent in the past, during this time of crisis. Conversely, they may respond by becoming distant and aloof indicating the return to a stoical stance adopted in their early years when they were forced to assume a position of pseudo-independence and self-sufficiency. A doctor's inadvertent failure to respond to a patient's need or request may evoke unwarranted anger or hostility. Again it is imperative to understand the genesis of the patients' response which may originate from years of feeling misunderstood and uncared for.

Understanding the patient's transference reactions enhances the doctor's capacity for caring and can provide an emotionally corrective experience.

Stein (1985b) has noted 'how rarely the issue of physician countertransference was addressed in medical school, residency training, or continuing education'. He believes that 'most of the problems in clinician–patient relationships did not have to do with technical or procedural issues in patient management but with those unconscious agendas which physicians and patients brought to the encounter' (1985b: xii). Like transference, counter-transference is an unconscious process which occurs when the doctor responds to patients in a manner similar to significant past relationships (Dubovsky, 1981; Goldberg, 2000; Woods and Hollis, 1990). Doctors need to be alert to what triggers certain reactions, i.e. unresolved personal issues, stress or value conflicts. It is here that self-awareness, coupled with the ability for self-observation during the consultation, is paramount.

Some of the commonly agreed-upon signs of counter-transference are touched on in our description of the first three components of patient-centered practice, e.g., not listening attentively, interpreting too soon, misjudging the patient's level of feeling, becoming too active in giving advice, becoming overly identified with the patient's problem, gaining vicarious pleasure in the patient's story, engaging in power struggles with the patient, running late, running overtime or covering the same material with the patient over and over (Dubovsky, 1981; Hepworth and Larsen, 1990).

The origins and significance of doctors' counter-transference are as varied and complex as their patients. As noted earlier in this chapter we all struggle with unresolved issues from our past. For example, the doctor who finds himself repeatedly giving advice to depressed female patients may be attempting to rescue the patient from her sorrow in a way similar to how he responded to his own mother's chronic angst. The constant inability to listen to a patient's painful story of failed relationships may relate to parallel experiences in the doctor's own life. The demanding and obstinate behaviors of a patient may in turn activate behaviors on the part of the physician such as running late, avoidance or engaging in power struggles, all responses that may have been characteristic of the doctor's relationship with her domineering father.

Stein (1985b) observes that the most common subjects of medical counter-transference are: 'intensely personal ones that correspond to the culturally most vexatious emotional issues as well: aggression, death, loss, grief, separation, sexuality, intimacy, control, autonomy, dependency, self-reliance, time, and integrity of the self (for example, self/other boundaries)' (1985b: 28).

The primary tool for effectively using transference and counter-transference to aid and deepen the patient–physician relationship is physician self-awareness. Such self-knowledge is a requirement for the doctor's accurate recognition of both transference and counter-transference. Self-evaluation and working with others may help doctors gain valuable insights which will ultimately strengthen relationships with patients and also increase their own comfort and satisfaction with the practice of medicine (Goldberg, 2000).

Conclusion

The interactive components of the patient-centered clinical method occur within the ongoing relationship. The relationship serves the integrating function and is accomplished through a sustained partnership with a patient which includes compassion, sharing power, constancy and healing.

Case example: 'Can I trust you?'

Judith Belle Brown and Moira Stewart

For several months Renee had been experiencing fatigue and trouble swallowing. She had dismissed these symptoms, attributing her fatigue to the accelerating demands at work and her swallowing difficulties to persistent allergies. As a junior lawyer at a large and prestigious law firm, Renee could not afford time off from her grueling schedule to seek medical advice. She ploughed through each day, fighting her overwhelming fatigue. Her inability to swallow impeded her ability to eat, and consequently her weight rapidly declined to just over 100 pounds. Eventually her co-workers began to notice her state of exhaustion and significant weight loss. Concerned, they urged her to seek help. Renee was reluctant, but ultimately decided to take the time to see a doctor about her symptoms.

Renee was a new patient for Dr Dupont. This 26-year-old woman presented herself as confident and self-assured. She was an attractive young lawyer who had been the gold medallist in her class. Renee explained to the doctor that she thought her symptoms were just the result of overwork. All of her classmates and current colleagues were exhausted. Why should she be any different?

After exploring the history of her problem, Dr Dupont could not find an immediate explanation for Renee's symptoms. Subsequently, he ordered relevant blood work and asked her to return for a complete physical exam. She appeared to agree and although she did go to the convenient laboratory in the doctor's office building, she did not book the appointment for the physical exam. Instead, she telephoned on two occasions anxiously requesting same-day appointments to discuss her difficulty swallowing. Dr Dupont, consciously suppressing his impatience at her anxious but controlling behavior, offered a calm and supportive demeanor, accepting her symptoms as important and repeating twice the need for a complete physical exam. Repeated cues of her anxiety about such an exam registered with Dr Dupont and he made a mental note not to request the physical exam on a next visit. However, relaxing into Dr Dupont's calm support, Renee finally found her resistance to the physical exam diminish and she made the appointment.

At the subsequent consultation, Dr Dupont inquired how things were going. Renee replied, 'Much the same.' During the physical exam, Dr Dupont stood behind her to examine her thyroid. Renee suddenly began to shake uncontrollably and tears welled out of her eyes. The doctor, surprised by her response, stood back and said, 'Renee – what is happening – why are you upset?' The patient continued to cry but as her tears subsided, she began to reveal a painful family secret.

What allowed Renee to reveal and ultimately disclose the well-kept secret was the doctor's sensitivity and empathy. Although they had not known each other for long, Dr Dupont had openly expressed his concern and respect for Renee. As her story unfolded, he came to understand a history of abuse that had existed in her early adolescence when her 18-year-old stepbrother had repeatedly attacked her from behind, fingers around her neck, threatening to strangle her and then fondling her as she tried to catch her breath. Because her mother did not act on her disclosure, the attacks only ceased when her stepbrother left home at the age of 20. Each stage of her life had been haunted by her past. Her current symptoms were compromising her life, yet she felt terrified to face their origin.

It took many visits with Dr Dupont for Renee to explore her past experiences. It was difficult for her to trust that he would not, like others in her past, betray her confidences or minimize the reality of her experience. Each recollection of the abuse she had suffered, and the lack of support she had received at the time, was excruciatingly painful for Renee. At times, she felt she could not continue this painful journey. Yet, her growing therapeutic relationship with Dr Dupont gave her strength and hope. He validated her experiences and helped her make sense of her symptoms. He was compassionate, caring and, most important, he believed her. While at times Dr Dupont was overwhelmed by the intensity of Renee's pain, he remained committed to helping his patient heal the wounds of the past.

9

The sixth component: being realistic

*Judith Belle Brown, W Wayne Weston
and Carol L McWilliam*

Patient problems are increasingly complex and multi-faceted. The public expectations of care are influenced by the rapid advances in medical research juxtaposed against fractioned delivery systems. Time is scarce, resources are at a premium, doctors' physical and emotional energies are constantly taxed and the increasing demands of bureaucracy are often overwhelming. Back in the late eighties and early nineties, when we first conceived the sixth and final component of the patient-centered clinical method, 'Being realistic', we had no sense of how managed care organizations would proliferate and dominate medical care in the USA. A decade ago few could have predicted how technological advances, such as the Internet, would rapidly change the nature of medical practice. Nor did we foresee the radical reforms in the delivery of primary care, many of which are still in the early implementation phase, including the implementation of interdisciplinary teams. Thus our understanding and appreciation of this specific component of the patient-centered clinical method, being realistic, has taken on new meaning and been enhanced by this accumulated knowledge. This has led us to view this component of the method as one that will always be fluid and responsive to the multiple changes and advances in medical practice and society at large.

On a global level the provision of healthcare is in flux. Nations side by side, such as Canada and the USA, are struggling to find the 'right answer' to the difficult and complex problem of equitable healthcare for all. While we will not endeavor, in this chapter, to enter into that discourse, we do acknowledge the healthcare delivery challenges that we are facing around the world. In this chapter, we will address the following issues: time and timing; teamwork and teambuilding; and the importance of wise stewardship in accessing resources.

Time and timing

Time

Do patient-centered consultations take more time? First let us establish what is the length of an average visit, for example in primary care. The length of consultations in primary care varies around the world, being as brief as 5 minutes or less in the United Kingdom (Howie *et al.*, 1991), as long as 21 minutes in Sweden (Andersson *et al.*, 1993), 12 minutes long in Australia (Wiggers and Sanson-Fisher, 1997), 11 minutes in South Africa (Henbest and Fehrsen, 1992), and 9.4 minutes in Canada was a sufficient time frame to achieve a patient-centered consultation (Stewart *et al.*, 1989). Concern has been voiced that managed care, a reality in the USA healthcare system, has resulted in primary care physicians spending less time with patients (Gordon *et al.*, 1995). However, recent studies demonstrate that the length of time family physicians are spending with patients has increased by at least two minutes, between 1989 and 1998, placing their consultation length at approximately 17 minutes (Blumenthal *et al.*, 1999; Mechanic *et al.*, 2001; Stafford *et al.*, 1999).

The following studies provide evidence supporting the belief that patient-centered consultations do not result in longer office visits. For more information on the studies of time, refer to Chapter 17. Marvel *et al.* (1998), comparing the interviews of exemplary family physicians (physicians who had received postgraduate training in family therapy) versus community family physicians (physicians who had no additional training), found there was no difference in the length of the office visits between the two physician groups. Of note, however, was that in the same length of time, the exemplary physicians engaged the patients in more patient-centered activities, including exploration of patients' personal and social issues (i.e. understanding the whole person) and patient collaboration (i.e. finding common ground).

Consultations described by both physicians and patients as being positive were reported as taking less time, while also exploring patients' ideas and concerns more than negative consultations (Arborelius and Bremberg, 1992). Greenfield *et al.* (1988) observed that while the total volume of conversation between experimental group patients (who were educated to improve their information-seeking skills) and their physicians was greater than control group patients, there was no corresponding change in the length of the visit. Henbest and Fehrsen (1992: 316) found that the 'frequent assumption that it takes longer to conduct a patient-centered consultation was not supported. Lack of time cannot be legitimately offered as an excuse for not conducting patient-centered consultations.' Finally, Williams and Neal (1998) found that when booking appointments were extended from five to ten minutes patients reported more satisfaction with the consultation, a better understanding of their illness and improved coping strategies.

These studies document evidence supporting the viewpoint that patient-centered visits are not longer and do improve patient care. In addition, there are the real experiences of patients and physicians as described in their narrative accounts. In the past several decades there has been a resurgence in the medical literature of a historical form of storytelling, the narrative, which provides a different and richer perspective of both patients' and physicians' experiences of time (Borkan *et al.*, 1999; Greenhalgh and Hurwitz, 1998). As Heath notes, in Greenhalgh and Hurwitz's (1998) compilation of narratives:

> Stories can only be told when people have time to talk and time to listen and to hear . . . The magnificent advantage of general practice as a mode of clinical care is its longitudinal dimension and the opportunities this gives both doctor and patients to develop and respond to complex narratives in relatively short instalments but over a sustained period of time. (1998: 90)

Timing

One of the strong points of primary medical care is the possibility of using several visits, over time, to explore complex or deeply personal issues (Stewart, 1995). Often, after a close and trusting relationship has developed, doctor and patient can get to the heart of a matter very quickly. Thus, time and timing are two key interrelated factors.

While it is not realistic to deal with all the problems of every patient in each visit, doctors must be able to recognize when a patient requires more time, even if it means disrupting their schedules. When a patient presents with multiple symptoms and concerns, the physician must learn how to establish which are the most pressing issues at that time and to pave the way for the patient to explore the remaining concerns in the near future. This requires that the doctor learn how to prioritize the patient's problems, guided by the patient's expressed concerns and the potential seriousness of the problems. When the patient's or another's safety may be at risk, the clinician may need to take a more assertive role in this process, e.g. child abuse, suicidal ideation, woman abuse, or a life-threatening medical situation, such as ketoacidosis or asthma.

In adopting this prioritizing approach, clinicians must learn how to create quickly an atmosphere in which patients feel heard and understood and feel that their problems are important and worthy of further exploration. If patients leave the visit feeling frustrated, they may not pursue their remaining concerns during subsequent encounters. Alternatively, a patient's symptoms may intensify and be presented through multiple visits in an attempt to cue the doctor about unresolved concerns. In either scenario the interactions that transpire will be unsatisfactory and unfulfilling for both patient and doctor.

Essential skills needed by clinicians are flexibility and a readiness to respond in a manner that expresses both concern and a willingness to work with the patient in the future. They need to work with patients to establish mutual agreement as described in Chapter 6. This applies to both defining the problem and deciding on the most realistic treatment or management plan that avoids misuse of resources. The following case illustrates some of these key points.

Case example

Mr Palumbo was a 75-year-old man admitted to hospital with pneumonia, a complication of long-standing chronic obstructive pulmonary disease. His physical symptoms had necessitated nebulized ventolin therapy by mask. Just prior to discharge from hospital, the specialist and his team had decided to switch Mr Palumbo's treatment to a self-administered inhaler which was more practical for use at home. Mr Palumbo, distressed by this new treatment approach, tried unsuccessfully to make his physicians understand his concerns. 'I just can't get this stuff in ... I can't inhale!' he exclaimed. Even after the use of a spacer was carefully explained he still felt overwhelmed. As the time to return home approached, he became increasingly anxious, expressing fear that he would not be able to breathe well enough to resume the daily chores he undertook as part of caring for his frail wife.

At home, Mr Palumbo continued to suffer from his respiratory symptoms. Ever conscious of his family responsibilities, Mr Palumbo struggled unsuccessfully to follow medical instructions to regain weight. Eating had become a 'tremendous chore', because of his respiratory problems. Unable to resume his customary homemaking duties, Mr Palumbo became progressively demoralized. He felt totally misunderstood by his physician who explained: 'The puffers haven't been shown to be any less effective ... the only difference is psychological!' Mr Palumbo disagreed, saying, 'I know you can't tell the doctors how to treat you, but ... I don't think it is psychological. The problems I have with trying to clear phlegm from my throat before I can eat my meal is certainly not psychological! ... I will tell you one thing for sure. It rules out all of the relatively simple things that you used to be able to do.' Mr Palumbo's lack of confidence in his ability to use the hand-held nebulizer was aggravated by his feeling that the doctor did not understand his problem. He became more anxious and his general condition deteriorated.

As a consequence of the doctor's failure to grasp the implications of his prescribed treatment plan precious time and resources were consumed. Additional professional home care services were required, and Mr Palumbo eventually had to be rehospitalized. Following guidelines without addressing the individual patient's unique concerns does not translate into effective patient-centered care.

Timing also speaks to the issue of the patient's readiness to share certain concerns or experiences with the doctor. Reluctance to present concerns may arise for any one of a variety of reasons. Here the clinician's knowledge of the whole person can be of vital importance in understanding patients. For example, patients may be reluctant to disclose family problems because disclosure runs counter to family norms and values. Some patients may feel an intense loyalty to family members and, as a result, feel that seeking help is an act of betrayal that could lead to rejection or isolation from the family. But keeping the family secrets denies them what they need most – help and understanding.

Patients are often reticent to share their concerns or problems for fear of reprisal or abandonment by their doctor. They may experience their inability to independently resolve their problems as a failure or a loss of face. As a result, patients often feel shame, embarrassment or anxiety when seeking help. Especially in the primary care setting it may take them several visits with the doctor, frequently marked by undifferentiated physical complaints, before they can reveal the actual source of their concern. When they finally do share their understanding of the problem with their doctor, it may be on an occasion when the doctor is pressed for time or emotionally worn by the demands of the practice. Again, it is important for the doctor to acknowledge the patient's concerns, and to provide an environment which lends itself to further exploration of the problem. It may not be realistic, or even wise, to delve extensively into the problem at this time. But it is essential that patients feel understood and know the doctor is prepared to work with them on their problem during future visits. This will be supported and enhanced by the strength of the patient–doctor relationship.

Teamwork and teambuilding

At the outset of this book we stated that while many of the concepts of the patient-centered clinical method originated from work in family practice, the method has broad applicability and transferability to multiple healthcare professions at the primary, secondary, tertiary and quaternary levels. It is a model of practice – a mindset and methodology of placing the patient at the center of care. This is important, indeed essential, when we consider using interdisciplinary teams to provide patient care.

Before we embark on a brief synopsis of teamwork and teambuilding it is important to anchor the place of patient-centered practice in this discussion. The patient-centered model and clinical method provides the team with a theoretical framework for practice and a common language for communicating. The team's ability to communicate is a basic and fundamental function, without which the team is doomed to failure. Payne (2000) notes that each discipline has a unique language with specific linguistic traditions (i.e. medicine, psychology, nursing, social work, etc.) and although some language is similar (i.e. medicine and nursing) interpretations may differ. This is where the language of the patient-centered clinical method may offer all professions a common medium of communication that enhances the team's interaction and subsequently patient outcomes. The fundamental principles of patient-centered care, we have found over the years, are core concepts within all healthcare disciplines. Hence from our perspective patient-centered practice can serve as a unifying and binding framework for interdisciplinary healthcare teams.

In the past several years there has been a proliferation of publications in the UK, USA and New Zealand on teamwork and teambuilding, particularly in the primary care setting (Drinka and Clark, 2000; Elwyn and Smail, 1999; Havelock and Schofield, 1999; Lilley *et al.*, 1999; Opie, 2000; Payne, 2000; Suchman *et al.*, 1998). The number of refereed articles and commentaries on this topic since 1995 is too many to cite. Clearly a team approach to healthcare delivery is becoming the expected standard of care.

The tradition of multidisciplinary teams dates back almost a century. Cabot, a physician working at the Massachusetts General Hospital in the early 1900s, advocated that patient care should be provided by teams of doctors, social workers and educators (Schlesinger, 1985). But interest and commitment to teamwork has waxed and waned over the past 100 years. Teamwork in hospital and community settings has expanded and contracted in response to the economic dictates of a particular time and place. In the seventies the community health center movement strongly endorsed teamwork, and in the eighties there was strong ideological and conceptual support for teamwork, particularly in primary care. But economic barriers meant that teams were not sustainable.

However, with the social, economic and political changes that have occurred in the past decade and resultant health services reform and restructuring, teamwork in primary care has become an essential component of integrated healthcare delivery. For example, dramatic changes in the National Health Service (NHS) in the United Kingdom introduced the concept of Primary Care Groups and Trusts to serve as the vehicles for delivery of health and social care (HSC, 1998). In addition, the Royal College of General Practitioners in 2001 created a document operationalizing the standards and criteria for quality team development in the UK (Royal College of General Practitioners, 2001). In New Zealand, governmental and policy reform gave priority to patients' involvement in decision-making within the context of the team (Opie, 2000). In describing the resurgence of interdisciplinary healthcare teams in the USA, Drinka and Clark (2000) observed how support for collaborative teamwork is being articulated by national organizations and government commissions.

Definitions of teams

Most authors, when writing about teams, struggle with how best to define them; are they multidisciplinary, interdisciplinary or transdisciplinary? Multidisciplinary teams are as Opie (2000: 39) notes 'characterized by parallel work' and in many instances maintain a hierarchical structure with one discipline (i.e. doctor, case manager) delegating tasks and responsibilities appropriate to each discipline. Multidisciplinary teams serve to coordinate care among independent, autonomous practitioners and promote the achievement of multiple tasks and goals. But each discipline's tasks remain separate and distinct from the others. This approach serves as a useful strategy when healthcare professionals seek to avoid unnecessary competition or duplication in their care of patients. However, the coordination approach of multidisciplinary teams has several disadvantages. This manner of care compartmentalizes healthcare delivery, assigning each group specific tasks or responsibilities. The drawback for the busy practitioner may be the demands of coordinating such an effort. In the absence of full knowledge of the involvement of other health and social service professionals, duplication of services or gaps in service may result. From the patient's perspective, the consequences may be fragmented care and confusion about accessing and using the appropriate resources.

Numerous authors have described interdisciplinary teams (Anderson and West, 1998; Campbell *et al.*, 1998; Drinka and Clark, 2000; Lockhart-Wood, 2000; Opie, 2000; Payne, 2000; Poulton and West, 1999; Stapleton, 1998; Stichler, 1995; Suchman *et al.*, 1998; Yaffe *et al.*, 2001). Collaborative interdisciplinary practice is a negotiated process among equals, characterized by mutuality, respect and trust that enables appropriate self-disclosure without discomfort. Thus interdisciplinary teams are composed of two or more disciplines which, actively and continuously, participate in a process of communicating, planning and acting together toward mutually shared goals. They have shared values, goals and visions enhanced by an understanding and valuing of each team member's perspective and scope of practice.

Team members need to expect and accept differences and have a willingness to acknowledge and discuss diversity. They must confront conflict and seek an equitable and fair resolution. Fostering resolution of differences is assisted by open and frank communication including information-sharing, evaluation and constructive feedback. With open discussion and ongoing dialog, the interdisciplinary team is comfortable with permeable boundaries. Listening and learning are key.

Because the collaborative interdisciplinary approach tends to be more flexible and crosses disciplinary boundaries, it capitalizes on the talents and expertise of all professionals involved thus providing opportunities for creativity and innovation. Consequently this approach requires a more equitable distribution of responsibility, accountability and power. Professional activities will cross traditional roles and functions and ultimately lead to increased comprehensiveness of patient care. Critical to the collaborative interdisciplinary approach is the active involvement of patients in all phases of planning and implementing their care – they are viewed as an equal participant on the healthcare team.

Transdisciplinary teams reflect the highest level of integration and complexity. They are characterized by a common and shared knowledge base and a language unique to the team. Equality is a cornerstone and role overlap is both anticipated and expected. In many regards the concept of transdisciplinary teams remains at the theoretical and conceptual level. The development and implementation of interdisciplinary teams for providing patient-centered care is both realistic and advantageous, perhaps even essential.

Team composition

McWhinney (1989: 343) notes: 'No one profession can meet all of patients' needs, hence the need to work together in teams. There are strengths, but also pitfalls, in teamwork. There are also misconceptions about what teamwork is.' He also suggests that there should be a distinction between the core team and the extended team. Today the role of nursing as an integral part of the care team is now well documented and seen by many as essential. Nurse–physician teams are viewed as the core team (Elwyn and Smail, 1999; Kernick and Scott, 2002; Way *et al.*, 2001; Zwarenstein and Bryant, 2001). The extended team reflects a wide range of professionals who can respond to individual patients' needs (i.e. social workers, physiotherapists, psychologists, occupational therapists, nutritionists, speech pathologists and pharmacists). Patients and their families are also important members of the team and need to be embraced as partners in care when they are willing and able to do so (Campbell *et al.*, 1998; Opie, 2000; Saltz and Schaefer, 1996; Suchman *et al.*, 1998).

Team composition will also depend on the setting, the patient population and the key disciplines. Thus, the issue is not one of knowing the specific resources, but of knowing the key personnel who can locate, motivate and promote change. For example, who can advocate for the patient about housing; who can recommend an appropriate support group; who can facilitate a referral to a local rehabilitation program; who can mediate between the bureaucracy of the welfare system and their patient; who can provide patient education about lifestyle changes. Few, if any, individuals would have all the skills needed to respond effectively to all these needs; teamwork is essential. Thus collaborative interdisciplinary teams are in prime position to best serve the needs of patients and offer patient-centered care.

Challenges for interdisciplinary teamwork

In the previous chapter, on enhancing the patient–doctor relationship, we highlighted the importance of practitioners developing self-awareness. Being aware of one's own strengths and weaknesses guides the clinician in seeking help and support with problems that are baffling or difficult. Requesting assistance or consultation with other team members should not be viewed as a deficit in knowledge or ability, but as an opportunity for further learning and growth. This approach can also provide the practitioner with new information and offer a different perspective on the problem. While a collaborative interdisciplinary team approach may initially seem time-consuming, and not particularly cost-effective, seeking guidance can reduce the clinician's frustration, confusion and emotional depletion. Ultimately, both practitioner renewal and improved patient care often result.

For example, working in collaborative interdisciplinary teams may be the most effective means of caring for patients with chronic disease. Such an approach can improve the transfer of information among healthcare professionals and therefore enhance communication between patients and their caregivers. Teamwork may also offer support and relief from the emotionally draining nature of the work which is inherent in caring for patients with chronic illness. Only by preserving emotional well-being can clinicians sustain the capacity to be truly patient-centered in the care of patients with certain chronic illnesses such as cancer.

The success of collaborative interdisciplinary teams is challenged by numerous factors. There are bureaucratic, logistical and fiscal problems that must be overcome. Additional problems are exemplified by turf issues, role blurring, boundary confusion, ambiguity of function and task, and lack of a common framework. However the era of niche-seeking and turf protection by healthcare professionals should be a thing of the past. Collaborative interdisciplinary practice may be a *sine qua non* of effective care.

To promote and support interdisciplinary practice, educational programs need to be developed to provide an opportunity for various disciplines to work together as team members (Boaden and Leaviss, 2000). Participation in common seminars or lectures, shared cases, and joint supervision can create an environment that fosters collaboration. Under the guidance of their teachers, students can have an opportunity to learn how to appropriately and effectively deal with the conflicts and struggles that are inherent in the collaborative process. Through frequent interaction and discussion of ideas and philosophies, students can become more familiar with their colleagues' skills and competencies. They will be exposed to the ideas of other disciplines and come to appreciate and accept differences. Armed with this knowledge, the groundwork will be established for the development of trust, respect and mutuality, which are the cornerstones of successful collaborative interdisciplinary teams.

There are challenges for teachers promoting collaborative interdisciplinary practice. It takes time and commitment to develop a common and complementary curriculum. Developing a common language to use in team teaching and supervision will be a key to success. Finally, teachers must role model collaborative practice for their students, particularly the qualities of humility and grace. In summary, education and exposure will facilitate collaborative interdisciplinary practice.

The following case serves as an illustration of the challenges in attaining collaborative interdisciplinary practice and providing patient-centered care.

Case example

Forty-two-year-old Martina Morgan had denied the symptoms she had been experiencing over the past several months, including weight loss, frequent urination and occasional blurred vision. When she finally went to the doctor she declared, 'I have diabetes.' Mrs Morgan was in fact very familiar with diabetes as her mother had been diagnosed with diabetes over 30 years previously and had suffered from numerous related complications.

However, Mrs Morgan refused to accept the doctor's recommendation that she begin insulin injections to control her very high blood sugars. Furthermore, Mrs Morgan adamantly declined a referral to an endocrinologist because, from her perspective, interventions from such specialists had hastened her mother's deterioration. In response, the doctor, serving in the role of coordinator, notified several other healthcare professionals including a dietician, a visiting nurse, and a social worker to assist in addressing Mrs Morgan's serious health problems. Because the team's focus was primarily on getting Mrs Morgan's diabetes under control, efforts to coordinate care leaned towards the medical model, such as modifying her lifestyle by attending to tight diet control, providing education about proper footcare and exploring options for financial aid. In spite of each individual team member's best intentions, Mrs Morgan remained reluctant to follow their recommendations and attempts at coordinating services faltered.

The more she didn't 'comply', the more the healthcare team intensified their efforts to 'educate' her. Also each team member was focused solely on achieving their own professional goals, specific to their discipline. While they were not engaging in 'turf wars' there was a lack of shared language and indeed a shared vision for Mrs Morgan's overall care plan. What the team, collectively, had failed to ascertain was Mrs Morgan's experience of illness.

Mrs Morgan had been raised in a very dysfunctional family. Her father had often been out of work and he would frequently 'disappear for months' leaving the family destitute. When Mrs Morgan was 16-years-old her mother had a below-knee amputation due to complications of diabetes. Her progressively deteriorating eyesight meant she could no longer administer her insulin injections and this responsibility fell on Mrs Morgan. While administering the injections into her mother's stumped limb repulsed her, Mrs Morgan dutifully assumed this task. The entire experience had been very difficult for her.

Thus the diagnosis of diabetes was overwhelming for Mrs Morgan. She was afraid and uncertain about her future. She had witnessed the effects of diabetes on her mother and was convinced that she would suffer the same long-term consequences of the disease. For Mrs Morgan, this was the 'final blow' from her family of origin.

It was only when some members of the team began to question and then listen to Mrs Morgan's other issues, as well her medical problems, that change began to occur. In visiting with the patient's husband, the social worker learned that although Mr Morgan was supportive and understanding, he was struggling to cope. Further exploration by the social worker revealed that Mr Morgan was worried that his wife was going to have a hypoglycemic reaction in her sleep and die in bed next to him. Consequently he was awake most of the night. He found it difficult to talk to his wife about his fears and was reluctant to reveal his terror that she might die.

In her work with Mrs Morgan on diabetic self-care issues, the visiting nurse learned that Mrs Morgan desperately needed to regain some control over her life. The nurse began to appreciate the strong link between Mrs Morgan's struggles with her own diabetes and her past family relationships. She was not unwilling to assume responsibility for self-care of her diabetes, rather she was immobilized by what she perceived the future would bring. Her past experiences had propelled her to future possibilities and her ability to exercise current options was frozen. The nurse's task, along with other members of the team, was to help weave the past, present and future together into an acceptable and achievable care plan for Mrs Morgan.

Eventually, the social worker and visiting nurse began to move towards a more collaborative and interdisciplinary team approach regarding Mrs Morgan's care. They now understood the multiple reasons for her non-adherence but it was still a hard sell to the rest of the team. Until each clinician could relinquish their entrenched position in their discipline silo, practicing collaborative care would be difficult to achieve.

This case example illustrates some of the challenges in team functioning when each discipline becomes entrenched in their own care plan and belief model. The fear of role blurring, rigid adherence to their own disciplinary goals and boundary issues, stifled the communication among the team members and the potential for team synergy and creativity. Once they recognized their need for a collaborative approach to patient care they were able to assist each other as a team in caring for Mrs Morgan and her family.

The use of wise stewardship in accessing resources

The topics covered in this section include managed care, information technology and clinical practice guidelines. How do healthcare professionals effectively and efficiently access necessary resources and simultaneously practice wise stewardship in the provision of patient-centered care? Contrary to some misconceptions, patient-centered care is related to efficiencies in care, i.e. fewer subsequent visits, few diagnostic tests and fewer referrals (Stewart *et al.*, 2000). It can therefore be argued that being patient-centered is an avenue to wise stewardship.

The rapid penetration of managed care organizations into the USA healthcare system serves as one example of both patients and healthcare providers fearing the deleterious effects of the corporatization of medical care (Dudley and Luft, 2001; Emanuel and Dubler, 1995; Goold and Lipkin, 1999). In 1999 Simon *et al.* (1999b) reported their findings of a nationwide survey on views of managed care. Collectively, the sample of medical students, residents, faculty members, program directors, chairs and deans from USA medical schools expressed negative views about managed care. Noteworthy were their views about the detrimental impact of managed care on the patient–doctor relationship. Of equal interest was the flurry of letters to the editor published in the *New England Journal of Medicine* in response to this study, demonstrating the controversy and conflict about the role of managed care in the USA healthcare system (Brett, 1999; David, 1999; Michels, 1999; Norman and Scherger, 1999; Wald and Brody, 1999; Simon *et al.*, 1999a).

But all systems of remuneration (salary, capitation, incentive plans, fee-for-service) can be viewed as suspect, leaving patients uncertain of their physicians' motivations in providing, or not providing, care (Dudley and Luft, 2001). As Goold and Lipkin (1999) observed: 'Managed care organizations thus have conflicting roles and conflicting accountability. . . . This ambiguity erodes trust, promotes adversarial relationships, and inhibits patient-centered care' (1999: S27). Yet patient-centered care and managed care are not necessarily in conflict if the following principles of practice are ensured and hence promote patient-centered practice. These include: attending to patients' preferences and particulars in the application of evidence-based medicine; exemplary communication; promoting continuity of care via integrated systems and teamwork; preserving the patient–doctor relationship; and addressing both prevention and health promotion (Goold and Lipkin, 1999). To achieve these goals and find balance between patient-centered care and managed care may require more time than some managed care organizations support; however as Goold and Lipkin (1999) note: 'A penny of good communication time may avert a pound of unnecessary or even harmful spending used to reassure an anxious patient or substitute for a sketchy history' (1999: S29).

Yet as healthcare delivery systems become corporatized, physicians will be called upon to be both advocates and wise stewards of patient-centered care. A lack of attention to how medical care is provided, and how contractual obligations can erode the patient–doctor relationship, may result in scenarios like the following described by Scherger (1996):

> Just as the frog about to be boiled does not jump out of the water if the heat is turned up slowly, so might the family physicians in a large medical group or delivery system experience erosion of the personal physician role without realizing the loss until it is gone. (1996: 67)

Patients also expect and trust that their physicians will be more than gatekeepers of the healthcare system; they will be advocates and work in the best interest of their patients (Grumbach et al., 1999; Mechanic and Meyer, 2000).

The provision of healthcare is also being shaped by other powerful changes in society. There is growing interest in the use of information technology (IT) as an important resource for enhancing patient–doctor communication. For example in New Zealand, a country known to be an early adopter of new technology, Internet use by physicians and patients is widespread (Eberhart-Phillips et al., 2000). Patients frequently arrive at their doctor's appointments armed with information from the Internet. Physicians are now developing practice-related websites for patient education (Friedewald, 2000). Rapid changes and innovations in information technology such as videoconferencing, are also providing new ways for patients and clinicians to interact, particularly in remote or underserviced areas (Jadad, 1999).

But with the advent of IT use in medical practice comes debate. For example, some authors strongly encourage the use of e-mail (Mechanic, 2001) while others caution that it may further erode the patient–doctor relationship (Baur, 2000; Eberhart-Phillips et al., 2000). Mechanic (2001) contends that e-mail communication can 'facilitate information flow, allow better scheduling of appointments to prevent discontinuity, and avoid gaps in communication. It may also reduce unnecessary appointments, save the patient and doctor time and inconvenience, and contribute to health education and patient responsibility' (2001: 268). Baur (2000), however, argues that use of e-mail may further the deterioration of the patient–physician relationship if the focus shifts to technically-oriented interactions with patients. In addition, she highlights current flaws in e-mail technology such as violation of confidentiality due to potential third-party access, lack of informed consent by patients about how e-mail information will be used and the impact of delayed responses to messages on timely diagnosis and treatment.

Regardless of that debate, there is no question that the Internet is transforming healthcare. As Jadad (1999) states, 'It is creating a new conduit not only for communication but also the access, sharing, and exchange of information among people and machines' (1999: 761). Do the rapid advances in information technology threaten patient-centered care? Maybe, if IT becomes the center of care and not the patient. However, in providing patient-centered care clinicians may find the use of e-mail and other IT services useful adjuncts to practice that enhance continuity and reduce fragmentation of care (Glick and Moore, 2001). But IT will not replace the face-to-face encounter where the patient-centered clinical method is enacted and learned.

Clinical practice guidelines (CPGs) and evidence-based medicine are major themes in medicine today. Do they pre-empt patient-centered care? Are evidence-based medicine and patient-centered medicine polar opposites? We think not. In Chapter 1 we describe the confluence between evidence-based medicine and patient-centered medicine, pointing out that proponents of evidence-based medicine recognize the importance of patients' preferences and characteristics in using practice guidelines (Haynes *et al.*, 2002; Sackett *et al.*, 2000), thus acknowledging the illness experience as important in treating the disease. Recent research supports this perspective, extending it further to include the role of the patient–doctor relationship and finding common ground in the process of CPG applications (Tudiver *et al.*, 2001). Another component of the patient-centered clinical method, understanding the whole person, is supported by Sobel's (2000) contention that: 'Mind/body medicine is not something separate or peripheral to the main tasks of medical care but should be an integral part of evidence-based, cost-effective, quality health care' (2000: 1705).

There are limitations to the fiduciary role assigned to physicians, yet they need to practice wise stewardship of the limited community resources. Meeting the needs of all constituencies demands creating a balance between the needs of the individual patient and the needs of the community. Doctors cannot avoid the conflict of interest inherent in resource management. Therefore, part of being realistic is constantly making a conscious choice in exercising professional judgment in making value trade-offs between patient's needs and wants and the resources available. It is a taxing part of professional judgment but should not occur by default.

Case example

> It had been a busy morning for Dr Hawquin in the Saturday morning on-call clinic. She had seen 20 booked patients, as well as ten walk-ins. Now she has received a phone call from the orthopedic resident in emergency

about her 82-year-old patient, Mrs Braun, who had a suspected fracture of the sacrum. In discussing the next steps in Mrs Braun's management the orthopedic resident stated: 'Admission to an ortho bed is out of the question. A CAT scan will be booked for next week and the patient will then be seen in the ortho clinic.' Dr Hawquin responded by suggesting that she would try to locate a bed in the family medicine ward and for the next hour set about that task. But she was thwarted at every turn. There were no beds available.

Yet she still had Mrs Braun, an elderly woman, in severe pain, with a suspected fracture. This patient could not sit or stand and her pain was unremitting. Dr Hawquin knew that Mrs Braun lived with her 85-year-old husband who would do his best to care for his wife, but now, after a week constantly attending to her needs, his health was being compromised.

Even more determined, Dr Hawquin called the ER doctor to request assistance in locating a bed. After briefly outlining the situation, the ER physician interrupted Dr Hawquin stating: 'It's not my problem and I don't care.'

'Pardon me?' said Dr Hawquin.

'I've had a busy morning and this is not my problem,' replied the ER physician.

Dr Hawquin responded: 'Well look – let's not get confrontational – let's try and solve the problem.'

'It's not my problem – it's *yours*,' retorted the ER physician and slammed down the phone.

Dr Hawquin was flabbergasted. Never in all her professional years had she experienced such an uncaring response by a physician. Nor had she ever been treated with such disrespect by a colleague.

Many important points are raised by this story that are relevant to the final component of the patient-centered clinical method – being realistic. First, it demonstrated the family doctor's commitment to provide the best available care for her patient. Second, it illustrated how the system can undermine such goals. Thirdly, it presented a sad commentary on how many health professionals perceive the healthcare needs and well-being of the frail elderly as being easily dismissed. Finally, it showed how an overburdened healthcare system fails to meet the needs of both patients and healthcare professionals resulting in patients receiving sub-optimal care and placing professionals in combative positions.

Conclusion

Being realistic about patient-centered care necessitates mastery of several elements of the art of medical practice. Learning the best timing and time allotment for problems is essential. Teamwork and effective teambuilding also contribute to practicing realistically. Awareness of one's own abilities and priorities both as a practitioner and as a person is critical in participating in interdisciplinary teams. Currently, issues of cost-containment and increasing demands of bureaucracy create the need for wise stewardship of the healthcare system's resources. Ongoing advances in the area of information technology and evidence-based medicine will continue to influence the practice of patient-centered care.

We do not pretend to have all the answers. This would be impossible given the rapid and radical changes continuously occurring in the healthcare system. Flexibility and a willingness to explore the most appropriate options available for practice are a neverending necessity. The ideas we present are relevant to today, but will need to adapt to the changing environment, and all of the societal, economic, cultural and health issues that confront us in the future.

Case example: 'How soon will I be in a wheelchair?'

Judith Belle Brown and Carol L McWilliam

'What is happening to me?' Gadish Omar, aged 38, felt panic as he thought back on the events of the past six months. It had all started one morning after a celebratory evening when his amateur baseball team had their first victory of the season. His legs had felt stiff and numb – which he attributed to being out of shape. More disturbing was that when he and his wife Ima, aged 36, had tried to have sex he could not have an erection. Gadish's leg symptoms resolved but he remained impotent – which he attributed to fatigue and stress at work. Although concerned, he feigned disinterest in sexual relations with Ima, causing some strain in their marriage. But their busy schedules distracted them, including daily demands and responsibilities which included their two active sons, 10-year-old Jidah and 8-year-old Said, and Ima's elderly parents.

Almost six months to the date of Gadish's initial episode he once again experienced leg weakness, stiffness and numbness. His impotence had persisted over the past six months. Upon contacting his family doctor he was referred to a neurologist in the urgent care clinic to be assessed for query of a herniated disk.

As Gadish proceeded through the history, physical examination and MRI he focused on the possibility of a surgical intervention to relieve his problem.

Yet in the back of his mind he was nagged by the memory of an uncle who had multiple sclerosis (MS) and had been wheelchair-bound for most of his life. This memory was intolerable for Gadish and he actively tried to squelch it until the neurologist inquired about his past medical history.

As Gadish and Ima waited for the results of the MRI his fear and panic grew. Perhaps, yes perhaps, he had MS. How could this be happening to him? Gadish had come to see Dr Ing, the neurologist, to be assessed for an operable condition and now within a brief five-hour period he would learn he had MS – a progressive chronic disease.

While Dr Ing attempted to break the bad news to Gadish and Ima in a caring and compassionate manner, she was not prepared for the outpouring of grief and sadness. 'How soon will I be in a wheelchair?' asked Gadish. For Ima, a nurse who worked at a chronic care facility caring for advanced MS patients, her husband's future looked dismal and without hope. Devastated by the diagnosis of this unpredictable and often unrelenting chronic disease Gadish and Ima were overwhelmed. Their personal and professional experiences foreshadowed only the worst case scenario.

Dr Ing acknowledged the couple's response to the devastating news of the diagnosis and spent a considerable amount of time with them laying out +the facts and future for Gadish as best she could. The doctor had spent half an hour with the Omars and in that time realized that they needed emotional support to adjust to living with a chronic illness, detailed recommendations regarding physical functioning and employment, and ongoing support as a family. Dr Ing also knew that the depth of the couple's emotional response, given their personal and professional histories, was beyond her skills and expertise. A team approach would be essential in this case including the family doctor, a social worker, a physiotherapist and an occupational therapist. These professionals would be pivotal in helping Gadish cope with his diagnosis and aid Ima in caring for her husband.

Each professional would bring their unique expertise and set of skills to assist Gadish and Ima. The neurologist would monitor Gadish's MS and provide treatment when appropriate; the family doctor would be critical in offering continuity and ongoing care for all the concerns relevant to Gadish and his family; the social worker would attend to the instrumental and emotional needs of Gadish, his wife and his children; the physiotherapist would help the patient retain his mobility and independence, and the occupational therapist would assist the Omar family in accommodating their environment to accommodate Gadish's current and future needs.

Central to the enterprise of caring for Gadish and his family would be teamwork. At times, the various team members' roles might overlap, hence communication between and amongst team members would be essential. Clear and consistent communication would be the basis of all interchanges between the healthcare team and the patient and his family.

Flexibility and collaboration would be core team skills, as the professionals responded to the changing needs and concerns of the Omar family.

As the day came to an end, Dr Ing reflected to her resident: 'I spent more time than usual today with Mr and Mrs Omar. But their situation was so tragic and they needed that time. Hopefully the team we have here at the clinic will be able to give them all the time they need to help them in the future.'

Time, being present to our patients' needs and concerns – that is what patient-centered care is.

PART THREE

Learning and teaching the patient-centered clinical method

Introduction

Judith Belle Brown and W Wayne Weston

In this section of the book, we examine how to learn about and teach the patient-centered clinical method. The first chapter explores the theoretical concepts that underlie the human dimensions of learning, with a specific view to the patient-centered clinical method. The second chapter explores the parallel process between being patient-centered and learner-centered, with a matching of each of the six components. In the third chapter of this section, some of the challenges confronted by both learners and teachers are addressed. This leads to two chapters describing some basic and essential elements required to teach the patient-centered clinical method such as the patient-centered case report. The concluding chapter of this section examines the development of a patient-centered curriculum and offers the experience at The University of Western Ontario as a case example.

10

Teaching the patient-centered clinical method: the human dimensions of medical education

W Wayne Weston and Judith Belle Brown

Luke Fildes[1] famous painting, 'The Doctor', shows a physician at the bedside of a seriously ill child with her distraught parents worrying in the dark shadows in the background. It depicts a mythological image of the country doctor waging war against disease single-handed, with no tools but what can be carried in the doctor's bag. It is a popular image of caring and compassion which appeals to our longing for an all-powerful healer.

But there is another way to see this picture – through the eyes of a young physician. What does he or she see? A doctor, without a laboratory or CT scan to confirm the diagnosis; no drugs to cure the problem; impotent to alter the natural course of the disease and no one to refer the patient to. It is a terrifying prospect for many graduates who carefully avoid moving to small communities where they fear they might face situations like this.

This is ironic because, even in large medical centers, physicians frequently confront the limits of medical science. Ingelfinger (1980) stated that 90% of the time, when a patient consults a doctor, the patient's condition is either self-limited or there is no treatment which will alter the natural history of the disease. Much of the time, the most important thing that doctors have to offer to their patients is themselves – their time, their caring and their understanding.

In a study of 272 patients presenting to their family doctors with headaches in London, Canada, The Headache Study Group (1986) looked for what would

---

[1] The painting by Luke Fildes, 'The Doctor' can be seen on the Internet at http://www.victorianartinbritain.co.uk/fildes_doctor.htm

predict a favorable outcome one year later. The best predictor of a good outcome was when patients felt they had been given sufficient opportunity to tell the doctor all they wanted to say about their headaches on the initial visit. Another predictor of good outcome was the doctor's statement that he or she liked the patient.

Glasser and Pelto (1980) present the dilemma for medical educators who recognize that physician effectiveness often relates to their personal qualities:

> It is rather tragic: modern physicians are a type of shaman without the proper upbringing. It is rather like being Jewish as a third generation American and not knowing how to read or sing Hebrew. It is as though we physicians do not know the prayers and chants. (1980: 24)

How can physicians learn these 'prayers and chants'? What does educational theory offer to guide educators who are responsible for the development of the modern 'shamans'? The patient-centered clinical method describes a different way of doctoring; consequently, education about the method requires a different way of teaching. In this chapter, we describe a framework which addresses this challenge – a framework which builds on the distinction between traditional conceptions of teaching and several ways of understanding the human experience of learning a profession.

Two metaphors used in teaching

Teaching is too complex to be embraced by a single model. Medical education, like medicine itself, embraces opposing theories. Tiberius (1986) outlines two common metaphors used to describe teaching.

- The **transmission metaphor** dominates all levels of education. In this metaphor, teaching is telling, and learning is listening. The emphasis is on the efficient flow of information down the pipeline to the students. Examples of this metaphor in common speech are:
  - It is hard to get that idea across to him.
  - Your reasons come through to us.
  - Delivery of material.
- The metaphor of **dialog or conversation** has roots in the Socratic method and the humanist tradition. In this metaphor, students and teachers are 'inquirers, helping one another in the shared pursuit of truth ... they are engaged in a common enterprise in which the responsibility for acquiring knowledge is a joint one' (Hendley, 1978: 144). 'Education ... is not a bunch of tricks or even a bundle of knowledge. Education is something we neither

"give" nor "do" to our students. Rather, *it is a way we stand in relation to them'* (emphasis in the original; Daloz, 1999: *xvii*).

The dialog metaphor recognizes that becoming a physician is more than simply learning a set of knowledge, skills and attitudes; medical training not only teaches a body of knowledge but changes the person. In this sense, medical education is as much about the acquisition of values and character development as it is about learning a discipline. Unfortunately, although these issues have been acknowledged for generations, medical education is often inimical to healthy personal development.

The following example illustrates the challenges inherent in the application of the dialog metaphor. One of us (WW), many years ago, learned the hard way about the importance of personal factors in teaching and learning:

> One of my postgraduate students had a very different idea of what he wanted to learn to what I wanted to teach. He worried about being able to deal effectively with emergencies but I wanted him to learn more about interviewing and the patient–doctor relationship. We often debated the proper role of family doctors and each of us stubbornly clung to our own point of view. While he was away doing hospital rotations, he sent me a book to read, a book which he told me had meant a great deal to him in his adolescence. He thought it might help me to understand him better. I started to read it but found it so at variance with my own worldview that I could not finish it. Later, he urged me to see the movie *Chariots of Fire*. He explained that he strongly identified with the main character in the film at the point when the Prince of Wales was called in to persuade him to 'bend' his strong Christian principles by running a race on Sunday. I felt he must be exaggerating and had trouble equating his struggles with the moral issues in the film. He then shared with me how he grappled to assert his identity in his conflict with his authoritarian father. Despite our attempts to understand each other, we continued to disagree about what he should learn. He eventually graduated and set up a successful rural practice. A few years later I met him at a dinner party where we immediately struck up a conversation, talking for over an hour about his experiences since graduation. He told me that I had been right – he handled emergencies without trouble but still experienced difficulty helping patients with emotional problems. On his own, he was gradually learning how to help them. It was an emotional and very special meeting for both of us. We learned a lot from each other about our stubbornness and need to be in charge. Through our struggles with each other, we were challenged to re-examine the roles of the physician and the goals of postgraduate education. But, more importantly, our encounters showed us a different way for teacher and learner to relate to one another – we had to

move beyond an authoritarian model which provoked resistance to a model of dialog which respected the contributions of each person.

This change, this different way of relating, illustrates a learner-centered approach which is a conceptual parallel with the patient-centered method. Both approaches seek a partnership between the protagonists – patient and doctor or student and teacher – characterized by mutual respect which leads to finding common ground.

Understanding the human dimensions of learning

In becoming physicians, students pass through three phases: gaining technical competence in dealing with disease; developing a professional identity; and learning to heal.

Gaining technical competence in dealing with disease

This is the principal preoccupation of the four years of medical school. Students are immersed in the biological sciences and quickly learn the value system of the medical establishment – the primary task of medicine is the recognition and treatment of disease. Everything else – communication, psychological, social and environmental factors – becomes peripheral. One result of this is the deterioration of students' ability to communicate effectively with patients as they progress through medical school (Barbee and Feldman, 1970; Cohen, 1985; Helfer, 1970; Preven *et al.*, 1986).

Developing a professional identity

This is usually begun during the clinical clerkship and completed during residency training. It is only when students work as part of the clinical team and have responsibility for patient care that they begin to feel like doctors. The metamorphosis is dramatic – students usually become comfortable with their strengths and limitations, develop a clearer sense of their professional roles and refine their ability to critically appraise their own performance (Brent, 1981).

Learning to heal

During this phase physicians learn to be instruments of healing – accepting with humility and wisdom the power to heal bestowed on them by their patients. This phase takes at least five to ten years and is not accomplished by all physicians. Cassell (1991) challenges us to address the responsibility of medicine to heal:

> It has been one of the most basic errors of the modern era in medicine to believe that patients cured of their diseases – cancer removed, coronary arteries opened, infection resolved, walking again, talking again, or back home again – are also healed; are whole again. Through the relationship it is possible, given the awareness of the necessity, the acceptance of the moral responsibility, the understanding of the problem and mastery of the skills, to heal the sick; to make whole the cured, to bring the chronically ill back within the fold, to relieve suffering, and to lift the burdens of illness. (1991: 69)

It is important to note that learning to be a healer continues after formal education is completed. The seeds are planted during the training period but only grow and develop as physicians experience the power of the healing relationship in practice. When teachers introduce the concept of healing they need to be cautious about the expectations they place on their students. These young physicians often find the tasks of diagnosing and treating the biological dimensions of their patients' problems challenging enough; pushing them to become therapeutic instruments of healing may leave them overwhelmed. They need frequent encouragement, support, effective role-modeling, and opportunities to discuss their feelings and internal struggles to adopt the healer's mantle. Ways *et al.* describe the personal challenges posed by the clinical years of medical school:

> Many clerkship experiences can be repugnant, sad, or painful. They can stimulate difficult memories and feelings, resurface unresolved personal issues, remind you of a loved one now dead, or all of the above. These impacts may be conscious or unconscious. *Of all aspects of clerkship education, students least expect the magnitude of its psychological and spiritual impact.* We see students initially open and outgoing toward their patients become self-absorbed, isolated, or depressed during a difficult clerkship. In contrast, on the rare clerkship where they receive appropriate support and attention, students can become more self-assured and open. (Ways *et al.*, 2000: 13–14, original emphasis)

To help their students negotiate these three phases of development, teachers need a conceptual framework that will guide their understanding of the human dimensions of medical education. A confluence of writings from several directions provides us with valuable insights:

- Personal descriptions of the **journey through medical school**: a remarkable number of students have described their personal experiences and struggles in medical school, including a former professor of medicine (Eichna, 1980), an educational psychologist (Eisner, 1985), an anthropologist (Konner, 1987) and others (LeBaron, 1981; Klass, 1987, 1992; Klitzman, 1989; Little and Midtling, 1989; Reilly, 1987). A number of self-help books provide useful insights into the struggles of student doctors (Coombs, 1998; Kelman and Straker, 2000; Myers, 2000; Sotile and Sotile, 2002; Ways *et al.*, 2000).
- **Developmental theory**: the recent works of psychologists in adult development (Brookfield, 1986; Chickering, 1981; Knowles, 1984, 1986, 1989; Merriam and Caffarella, 1999) provide valuable frameworks for understanding the professional development of physicians.
- **Mentoring**: Levinson (1978), Daloz (1999) and others (Baskett and Marsick, 1992; Freeman, 1998; Murray, 2001) describe the teacher–learner relationship as a mentoring relationship. This concept leads to a number of practical suggestions for improving one-to-one teaching.
- **The nature of the professional task**: Schön (1983, 1987) introduces a new educational paradigm rooted in a practical analysis of the professional's role. He argues that learning to think like a professional requires a new approach to teaching and curriculum design that addresses the 'messiness' of daily practice in the real world.

The remainder of the chapter will elaborate on each of these four areas.

Learning as a transformational journey

One of the central tasks in our development is to find the meaning of our lives. One way to do this is by telling stories. 'Within the narrative structure lies one of the most basic ways through which we make sense of our experience' (Daloz, 1999: 23). Common to hundreds of myths and legends across numerous cultures and times is the tale of the heroic quest:

> The hero ventures forth from the world of common day into a region of supernatural wonder; fabulous forces are there encountered and a decisive victory is won; the hero comes back from this mysterious adventure with the power to bestow boons on his fellowman. (Campbell in Daloz, 1999: 26)

Through the 'heroic quest' of medical school, the student conquers many 'fabulous forces' and becomes a physician; he or she is transformed. Perri Klass (1987) describes her experience at Harvard Medical School in these terms:

The general pressure of medical school is to push yourself ahead into professionalism, to start feeling at home in the hospital, in the operating room, to make medical jargon your native tongue; it's all part of becoming efficient, knowledgeable, competent. You want to leave behind that green, terrified medical student who stood awkwardly on the edge of the action, terrified of revealing limitless ignorance, terrified of killing a patient. You want to identify with the people ahead of you, the ones who know what they are doing . . . One of the sad effects of my clinical training was that I think I generally became a more impatient, unpleasant person. Time was precious, sleep was often insufficient, and in the interest of my evaluations, I had to treat all kinds of turkeys with profound respect. (1987: 18)

Another medical student, Melvin Konner, had been a professor of anthropology prior to medical school. He describes his experiences as follows (Konner, 1987):

And of course, last but hardly least, I now tend to see people as patients. I noticed this especially with women. It is often asked whether male medical students become desexualized by all those women disrobing, all those breast examinations, all those manual invasions of the most intimate cavities. I found that to be a rather trivial effect. What I found more impressive was the general tendency to see women as patients. This clinical detachment comes not from gynaecology but from all the experiences of medicine. During my medicine rotation, on a bus, I noticed the veins on a woman's hand – how easily they could be punctured for the insertion of a line – before noticing that she happened to be beautiful. (1987: 366)

Both examples illustrate how the journey through medical school may desensitize students to human suffering – they become more impatient and detached. The experience of postgraduate training may be even more brutalising, leaving young physicians feeling abused. There is evidence that students who feel abused by their teachers are more likely to abuse their patients (Baldwin *et al.*, 1991; Silver and Glicken, 1990). Such an environment is inimical to learning to be patient-centered.

Developmental theory

Developmental theory provides a way of understanding learning, not simply as the accumulation of knowledge but as a transformational experience. Klass (1987) and Konner (1987) describe their own experiences of being changed, of no longer being able to see the world 'through preclinical eyes'.

Perry (1970) provides a theory of intellectual and ethical development in adult students which is helpful to make sense of these changes in thinking and perceiving. According to Perry, students progress from thinking that is simplistic and 'black and white' to where they recognize and can accept different points of view. In the first stage, students view knowledge as dualistic – there is one right answer, determined by the authorities. Next, students recognize different perspectives to issues, but are unable to evaluate them; then students develop an ability to critically compare different viewpoints and make their own judgments. Finally, a stage of commitment is attained in which the learners are willing to act according to their values and beliefs, even when plausible alternatives are recognized. Students recognize that they must take the risk of making their own choices.

In Perry's approach, learning requires the student to make sense of his or her own experience. As students grow and develop, they discover new and complex ways of thinking and seeing. He argues that this often demands a 'loss of innocence' which may be painful and difficult.

> It may be a great joy to discover a new and complex way of thinking and seeing; but yesterday one thought in simple ways, and hope and aspiration were embedded in those ways. Now that those ways are left behind, must hope be abandoned too. (Perry, 1970: 108)

He cautions us that it takes time for students to come to terms with their new insights – 'for the guts to catch up with such leaps of the mind' (Perry, 1970: 108). Time is needed to mourn the loss of simpler ways of thought. This may explain why development is stepwise rather than steady.

Mentoring

Mentors lead students along the journey of their lives. They are trusted because they have been there before. According to Levinson (1978), mentors are especially important at the beginning of people's careers or at crucial turning points in their professional lives. Mentors are people who have already accomplished the goals sought by the students. A mentor is typically an older, more experienced member of the profession who takes the student 'under his or her wing'. The role of the university, as a parent-substitute is reflected in our reference to the university as our 'alma mater' and in the term 'in loco parentis' – in the place of the parent. In the beginning, the student often experiences the mentor as a powerful authority – a parental figure with almost magical skill.

This is also a common source of trouble in the relationship especially with students who have a long history of problems with authority figures. It is in

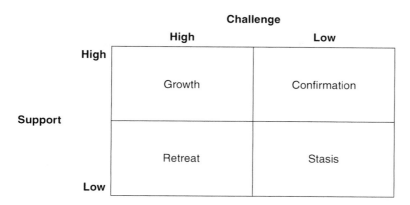

Figure 10.1   Framework of the tasks of mentors. From: Daloz (1999).

the context of this relationship that students grow into their professional identity. In the early stages of their intellectual and personal development, students look to the mentor as all-knowing and expect to be given the right answers to questions. They are not ready to see the mentor's clay feet. As the students learn and develop, they recognize that authorities are not always right and that even their mentor is human. Eventually, with a growing sense of their own professional identity, students recognize mentors as colleagues.

Daloz (1999) provides a valuable framework for understanding the tasks of mentors. Effective mentors provide a balance of support and challenge and, at the same time, provide vision (*see* Figure 10.1).

Support

Mentors should 'be with' the students. Let them know that they are understood and cared for. Such support promotes the basic trust needed to summon the courage to move ahead. The mentor is tangible proof that the journey can be made. Listen empathically – what is it like in the students' world; what gives it meaning; how do they view themselves; how do they decide among conflicting ideas; what do they expect from their teachers? Note the similarities between these learner-centered questions and those we suggest that doctors ask of their patients to explore the illness experience (*see* Chapter 3).

Setting aside time indicates that students' ideas matter and that they are important as people. Preparatory empathy is helpful. Before the student arrives, remind yourself what it was like to be a student starting a new rotation. Prepare yourself to respond to indirect cues. Students are generally wary at first and will rarely be direct with authority figures. Express positive expectations. Whenever possible, build self-esteem and confidence.

Challenge

'Mentors toss little bits of disturbing information in their students' paths, little facts and observations, insights and perceptions, theories and interpretations – cow plops on the road to truth – that raise questions about their students' current worldviews and invite them to entertain alternatives to close the dissonance, accommodate their structures, *think* afresh' (Daloz, 1999: 217, original emphasis). Daloz justifies this approach by reference to the work of Festinger (1957) on cognitive dissonance – a gap between one's perceptions and expectations – which creates an inner need to harmonize the apparent conflict and thus motivates new learning.

In setting tasks, the mentor brings learners to see a world they might not otherwise have observed. Examples of tasks are projects or reading assignments. The purpose may be clear or unclear. Asking pointed questions, pointing out contradictions or offering alternative points of view may help push students past the stage of dualism; encouraging them to take a stand on a difficult issue or to criticize an expert may help them to develop a commitment. Engage in discussion. College learning involves the construction of new frames of meaning, therefore students need the opportunity to try out their understandings and clarify contradictions. Hearing the views of their peers is often helpful.

Heat up dichotomies. Pushing different points of view and challenging students to comprehend not only the differences but to deeply appreciate contrasting points of view stimulates personal development.

Vision

Inspire learners to see new meaning in their work and to keep struggling despite confusion and discouragement. Vision sustains learners in their attempts to apprehend a fuller, more comprehensive image of the world.

One way of providing vision is through being a role model for the student. Parker Palmer presents a view of the importance of inner strength and courage in teaching:

> Teaching, like any truly human activity, emerges from one's inwardness, for better or worse. As I teach, I project the condition of my soul onto my students, my subject, and our way of being together. The entanglements I experience in the classroom are often no more or less than the convolutions of my inner life. Viewed from this angle, teaching holds a mirror to the soul. If I am willing to look in that mirror and not run from what I see, I have a chance to gain self-knowledge – and knowing myself is as crucial to good teaching as knowing my students and my subject. (Palmer, 1998: 2)

Provide a framework for understanding the developmental tasks facing the individual student. Offer a vision of the role of the physician which goes beyond the enumeration of skills to be learned and which acknowledges the personal and spiritual qualities inherent in becoming a healer.

Suggest a new language. According to Fowler (1981), a mentor's primary function is to 'nurturize into new metaphors'. They give us new ways to think about the world. The good teacher helps students not so much to solve problems as to see them anew. To think in new ways requires us to learn a new vocabulary and especially to develop new metaphors. Physicians may be constrained by the dominant military metaphor in medicine that implies we are always 'doing battle' with disease and must adopt an aggressive, interventionist approach. To see physicians as 'witnesses' to their patients' illnesses, who help give that suffering some meaning, frees physicians to be more imaginative in their approaches to healing. Some of these approaches are described in Chapter 8, 'Enhancing the relationship'. For example, in *A Fortunate Man*, Berger (Berger and Mohr, 1967) describes John Sassall, a country doctor working in a remote and impoverished English rural community:

> He does more than treat them when they are ill; he is the objective witness of their lives . . . He keeps the records so that, from time to time, they can consult them themselves. The most frequent opening to a conversation with him, if it is not a professional conversation, are the words 'do you remember when . . . ?' He represents them, becomes their objective (as opposed to subjective) memory, because he represents their lost possibility of understanding and relating to the outside world, and because he also represents some of what they know but cannot think. (1967: 109)

> . . . it is the doctor's acceptance of what the patient tells him and the accuracy of his appreciation as he suggests how different parts of his life may fit together, it is this which then persuades the patient that he and the doctor and other men are comparable because whatever he says of himself or his fears or his fantasies seem to be at least as familiar to the doctor as to him. He is no longer an exception. He can be recognized. (1967: 76)

The nature of the professional task

Donald Schön (1983, 1987) provides valuable insights into the nature of clinical problem-solving. Learning to be a physician is learning to recognize, analyze and manage clinical problems. Common sense implies that the nature of these problems should influence the nature of medical education. Schön (1987) makes a distinction between 'the high ground' and 'the swamp'. In the high ground, patients present with problems at least partially defined. The clinician's task is to rule in or rule out a few clearly defined disease entities. If disease is identified, the standard therapy is prescribed; if no disease is found, the patient is reassured with the expectation that he will be satisfied and not bother the physician again. In the swamp, where most clinicians work, the job is not so clear-cut. Much of the time no disease can be identified to explain the patient's suffering; even when disease is found, there is often no effective treatment. Frequently, it is more helpful to explore what the patient is worried about and to provide understanding and support, even when diagnosis is possible.

How can we teach this? To deal with problems on the high ground, students are taught about basic science and how to apply basic science knowledge to defined clinical problems. But for the messy situations which clinicians manage, this approach often is unhelpful. To learn how to handle these situations, students must 'jump in' and try their best with the support and guidance of a skilled practitioner. Schön points out that professional training often involves an inherent paradox – students can only learn to be professionals by doing; but they do not yet know how to do it and the task is too complex to fully describe in words. Consequently, the teacher cannot tell them exactly what it is they must do; they function more as coaches, helping them along each step of the way, guiding their students' eyes, hands, heads and hearts in doing. They will challenge their students with questions like: What will you do now? Why? How? Did you notice that . . . ? What happened when you . . . ? For example, in teaching interviewing skills, the teacher can give rules of thumb regarding question style but needs to get the learner doing things and observing what happens and making sense of it. Sometimes it is helpful for students to observe teachers thinking out loud as they try to make sense of a problem.

Meno describes this paradox of learning in the dialog of Plato named after him (Hamilton and Cairns, 1961):

> But how will you look for something when you don't in the least know what it is? How on earth are you going to set up something you don't know as the object of your search? To put it another way, even if you come right up against it, how will you know that what you have found is the thing you didn't know? (1961: 363)

Inherent in this paradox of learning is the learner's dependence on the teacher. For example, in order to learn the patient-centered approach, students must give up their old ways of doing things and perhaps even their old ways of seeing things. The conventional clinical method, which gave them a sense of competence, autonomy and security will no longer suffice. In learning this approach, they must be willing to suspend their disbelief in the teacher's point of view. This can make students too vulnerable and the cost of dependency may be too high. Schön (1987) notes:

> As he willingly suspends disbelief, he also suspends autonomy as though he were becoming a child again. In such a predicament, he is more or less

vulnerable to anxiety . . . If he is easily threatened by the temporary surrender of his sense of competence, then the risk of loss will seem difficult or even impossible. (1987: 95)

Students cannot be *taught* what they need to know, but they can be *coached* (Schön, 1987):

He has to *see* on his own behalf and in his own way the relations between means and methods employed and results achieved. Nobody else can see for him, and he can't see just by being 'told', although the right kind of telling may guide his seeing and thus help him see what he needs to see (Dewey in Schön, 1987: 17; emphasis in original).

Guidelines for teachers

- Help learners develop sufficient skill and comfort with the conventional clinical method to be ready to move ahead to the next phase of learning.
- Show examples during training. Even if they are unable to transcend the conventional medical model, the idea that there is more to medicine than diagnosis and treatment may become apparent and serve as a model for future learning. It is important for teachers to share their struggles and challenges, modeling the ability to learn from their experience.
- Help them learn how to attend to what the patient wants to talk about and to realize that listening may be more therapeutic than any biomedical intervention.
- Help them develop survival strategies to avoid becoming overwhelmed. For example, physicians need colleagues with whom they can discuss difficult or emotionally draining encounters with patients.
- Help students to reflect on their experiences and to discover how to learn from them. This provides the tools for a lifetime of learning.
- Use the relationship between teacher and learner to demonstrate aspects of the patient–doctor relationship. There should be the same caring and attention to the humanity of the learner that we expect the learner to demonstrate with patients.
- Remember how stressful medical education can be and attend to the personal struggles of students as well as to their learning needs. Watch for signs of unhealthy coping strategies, or frank mental illness, and be prepared to intervene. Faculty, like students, have a tendency to deny the seriousness of these problems and may assume the student is 'just having a bad day'. Don't procrastinate; explore the problem promptly and sensitively and be prepared to provide modified work responsibilities or sick leave and the appropriate professional help.

Conclusion

Learning to be a patient-centered doctor challenges young physicians to develop their skills and, more importantly, themselves. The task can feel overwhelming at times and may awaken feelings of vulnerability and terror as students grapple at the growing edges of their abilities. Their teachers must be responsive to their struggles and address the learners' needs and concerns. Teachers must model, in their behavior with students, the quality of interaction they expect students to demonstrate with patients.

We have woven several strands of educational thought which provide the fabric of the dialog metaphor of education. Medical education is a 'journey through a swamp' guided by a wise mentor who is sensitive to the issues involved in human development. At the same time, teachers must be skilled in the use of a variety of teaching strategies illustrated by the transmission metaphor, e.g. able to teach specific interviewing and history-taking skills. Combining this repertoire of teaching methods into a seamless whole will provide the learning environment needed to foster the human dimensions of medical education. It is only in such a setting that the patient-centered clinical method can be mastered.

11

The learner-centered method of medical education

W Wayne Weston and Judith Belle Brown

The setting for learning in a medical school is molded by many things, but the major artisan is the teacher whose work penetrates to unnumbered patients who profit or suffer from encounters with his students. This responsibility is too heavy for tradition, inertia, or ennui to be allowed to dictate his actions – as a scientist he can do no less than prepare himself for this responsibility as carefully as he prepares to be a physician or investigator. The means are at hand. All he need do is use them. (Miller *et al.*, 1961: 296)

In this chapter we describe the learner-centered method of education, a conceptual framework for teaching, which parallels the patient-centered clinical method. In the same way that patient–doctor relationships have changed, so have the relationships between learners and teachers. These parallels provide a framework to understand the changing roles of teachers and learners in medical education. This framework also serves as a tool; learners' experiences of their relationships with their teachers help them understand their relationships with patients. For example, when teachers interact with learners as autonomous adults responsible for their own learning, they illustrate the kind of relationship teachers expect learners to develop with patients. Analogous to the patient-centered clinical method, the learner-centered method consists of six interactive components (*see* Box 11.1 and Figure 11.1):

1 exploring both learning needs and aspirations
2 understanding the learner as a whole person
3 finding common ground
4 building on previous learning
5 enhancing the learner–teacher relationship
6 being realistic.

Box 11.1 The learner-centered method of education: the six interactive components of the learning/teaching process

1 Exploring both learning needs and aspirations
   - Prescribed needs (the 'official curriculum', requirements for competency)
   - Aspirations – felt needs (self-assessment, expectations, feelings, level of performance)

2 Understanding the whole person
   - The 'person' (life history, and personal and cognitive development)
   - The context (opportunities and constraints of the learning environment)

3 Finding common ground
   - Priorities
   - Teaching/learning methods
   - Roles for teacher and learner

4 Building on previous learning
   - Pre-existing learning needs
   - Strengths

5 Enhancing the learner–teacher relationship
   - Empathy, respect, congruence
   - Sharing power
   - Self-awareness
   - Transference and counter-transference

6 Being realistic
   - Time
   - Resources
   - Teambuilding

Exploring both learning needs and aspirations

In the learner-centered approach, teachers and learners collaborate in defining the objectives for learning. These are based on an assessment of two potentially divergent sets of learning objectives. On the one hand, there are the prescribed needs – the 'official curriculum' or the core requirements for competence – and on the other hand, the learner's aspirations or felt needs – their special interests, perceived weaknesses and concept of their future practice needs. Effective

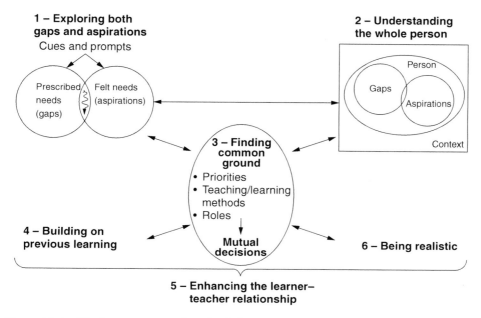

Figure 11.1 The learner-centered method of education: six interactive components.

education requires learners and teachers to find common ground regarding both sets of objectives.

Weimer (2002) describes a valuable approach to learner-centered teaching in which she outlines its challenges and values, common reasons for resistance by students and faculty alike and practical strategies for implementation. The learner-centered approach shares many features with self-directed learning (Brookfield, 1985, 1986; Candy, 1991; Cheren, 1983; Chovanec, 1998; Grow, 1991; Hammond and Collins, 1991; Knowles *et al.*, 1998; Merriam, 1993; Mezirow *et al.*, 2000; Tough, 1979) but also requires an active role on the part of the teacher. Cheren points out that self-direction in learning is not an all-or-none phenomenon but rather a continuum with self-directed at one end and teacher-directed at the other. He points out seven major aspects to a learning experience that can be expressed as a series of questions:

1 What is to be learned (both in general terms and specifically)?
2 How is the learning to be used?
3 How is the learning to be accomplished?
4 How is the learning to be consolidated, demonstrated or shared?
5 How and by whom is the learning to be assessed? (And what criteria are to be used to determine that a satisfactory, or better, level of learning has been achieved?)

6 How, if at all, is the learning to be documented?

7 What is the time limit, or schedule, for the effort? (Cheren, 1983: 26)

Learners who are completely self-directed will answer all of these questions on their own. But often this task is too daunting, especially for students who are unfamiliar with the content to be learned. '[S]o much work is required to exercise complete control over every aspect of a learning project that it is not practical or worth the effort to try to exercise all that control all the time' (Cheren, 1983: 27). For these learners, the questions will need to be answered by the students in consultation with their teachers. There are many reasons to begin by determining students' deepest-felt concerns about what matters most in their education. This enhances motivation (Lucas, 1990; Forsyth and McMillan, 1991; Spiegel, 1981) and personal responsibility for learning. Furthermore, it gives them practice in self-assessment – a critical skill for lifelong learning. But students may not be aware of all the requirements for competent practice and may have blind spots regarding their own abilities. Addressing these issues is a paramount responsibility of their teachers who must have a clear conception of the requirements for practice and the skill to assess students on each of these. In addition, teachers must be able to articulate these learning needs in a manner which is constructive and practical. Teachers will help students understand what is important for practice, not by threatening them with difficult exams, but by providing opportunities to experience the need to know. Such motivating experiences can take many forms: stories of teachers' own struggles to learn; role-play with simulated patients; seminars with previous students who discuss the evolution of their own understanding of their discipline; discussion with patients about qualities they most admire in physicians.

Case example

Joshua Stewart, a first year family practice resident, after seeing his patient recovering in hospital from a myocardial infarct, wanted to focus his learning on the pharmacological management of cardiac risk factors. The resident had seen this patient in the office about a week before the infarct and wondered if he had missed some subtle warning signs. Joshua was determined to provide optimal care of his patient's cardiac problem and failed to recognize the major adjustment the patient was now experiencing. The initial reaction of his supervisor, Dr Green, was to address the importance of understanding the patient's illness experience and the value of good communication in improving adherence and recovery. But, knowing that this might not match the resident's learning needs, Dr Green decided to explore the resident's experience with this patient. He discovered that Joshua felt somewhat guilty that he had not addressed all of his patient's risk factors before the infarct and was determined to make up for it now. Dr Green asked Joshua to tell him more about the office visit – in hindsight, had he in fact missed anything important? Together, they reviewed the chart. The resident had checked the patient's blood pressure and ordered a serum cholesterol and asked about diet, exercise and smoking. The patient had mentioned being more tired than usual but had no chest pain or shortness of breath. He was working longer hours than usual but was planning to take a vacation in the near future. The resident agreed that a vacation would be a good idea and asked the patient to return in three months to see how he was doing. Dr Green stated that he agreed with his assessment and plan and complemented him on his thorough review.

Dr Green commented: 'Even when we have done everything right, we can feel upset when things turn out badly for our patients. Our feelings may lead us to overreact by ordering too many tests or by not tending to the patient's other needs. You are feeling badly for your patient's predicament. How do you think he feels?' By supporting Joshua, Dr Green modeled the kind of concern he hoped the resident would demonstrate with his patient. This encouraged Joshua to recognize that his preoccupation with the biomedical issues was related to vague feelings of guilt and to realize that the patient would benefit from a discussion of his personal reaction to his serious illness.

In a survey of third year medical students, Hajek and colleagues assessed their common concerns about communicating with patients and derived a list of 16 issues ranked in order of importance from the students' perspective:

- the patient starting to cry or becoming angry with me
- the patient being in pain or emotional distress
- not understanding the patient
- the patient telling me something important but wanting to keep it confidential
- not knowing the answer to a patient's questions
- appearing nervous or incompetent
- drying up, not knowing what to ask next
- being so concerned about what to ask next that I don't take in what the patient is saying
- making a fool of myself or being humiliated when presenting a patient
- the patient not wanting to talk to or be examined by a student
- being embarrassed about asking certain questions or by the patient's response
- the patient rambling on and not being able to interrupt them
- being unsure about shaking the patient's hand. When is it all right to touch the patient?

- the patient asking me personal questions
- being unsure how to introduce myself
- being unsure how to dress, e.g. should I wear a white coat? (from Hajek *et al.*, 2000: 657)

It is ironic that student manuals often offer advice about dress, an issue at the bottom of the students' list of concerns, but often do not address more important issues such as 'drying up' and not knowing what to ask next. The list above may assist teachers to be more attentive to students' learning needs.

Understanding the whole person

Akin to the two important dimensions of understanding the patient as a whole person (the patients' stage in their life cycle and their context), there are two dimensions to understanding the student as a whole person: the student's life history, and personal and cognitive development; and the learning environment.

In the same way that physicians oversimplify their patients' complex problems by focusing on the pathophysiology of disease, so, too, do teachers oversimplify their students' educational needs by concentrating on their major learning deficiencies. Teachers may speak of making a 'learning diagnosis' in terms of the gaps in students' knowledge, skills and attitudes compared with the objectives of the program. This may be very helpful, as far as it goes, but it may fail to convey an accurate understanding of what the learner, as a person, really needs. Students are different in so many important ways: in previous life experience, courses taken, preferred learning styles, willingness to take risks, self-confidence and resistance to change (Curry, 2002).

Case example

Ted, a first year resident in internal medicine, was a former soccer star. A catastrophic injury had ended his career and his prior interest in science led him into medicine. When he discovered he had a latex allergy he was forced to abandon his first choice of a career in surgery and ended up in internal medicine. Ted was big, bombastic and loved being right. For his 5'2" female supervisor he was a daunting presence. Early in Ted's life, he had learned to mask his self-doubt with an artificial aura of confidence. When his supervisor would question his choice of management, he would often respond in a combative manner, defending his diagnosis and treatment decision.

Dr White, his supervisor, recognized that his aggressive manner was a defense against his deeper feelings of fear of failure. Questioning Ted on his decisions threatened him and increased his defensiveness. Dr White needed another approach, one that would help Ted begin to reflect critically on his behavior. She discussed the value of 'reflection on action' (Schön, 1984, 1990) – thinking about our prior actions and discovering the reasons for our decisions – and suggested a strategy for working together to enhance his clinical reasoning. Instead of the usual quizzing, which often feels like a test of competence, Dr White suggested that she probe Ted's thinking to help him understand how he made clinical decisions. In the process, Ted would recognize his strengths and weaknesses as well as the unconscious factors that might influence his thinking. Ted found the idea intriguing and appreciated being treated as an adult learner and colleague.

Even students from the same school and the same class have vastly different abilities and learning needs. It is crucial to identify these so that the students are not put into situations where they are out of their depth. It is also essential to identify strengths so that valuable time is not wasted practicing skills already mastered while ignoring areas of deficiency. Students differ in their stages of personal, cognitive and professional development as described in Chapter 10, 'The human dimensions of medical education'.

Case example

Dr Kumar was concerned – this was the third complaint from patients about her new resident, Andrew Garcia. The complaints all had a common theme – he was aloof and did not seem to care. Dr Kumar was surprised because he had been near the top of his class and, in case discussions, was always up-to-date on the latest evidence-based recommendations for treatment. In addition, he always seemed genuinely concerned about his patients. Upon reflection, Dr Kumar wondered if Andrew's quiet and reserved manner was being misinterpreted. Some students are fascinated by people and seem to be able to interact comfortably with anyone; others are more at ease in the world of ideas and things. Perhaps this explained Andrew's difficulty relating to patients. Dr Kumar pondered how she would address such a personal issue with her resident. She was tempted just to wait and see if more experience would increase Andrew's comfort with patients but she realized that this would be avoiding the issue and deprive Andrew of an important opportunity for self-awareness. And it would be unfair to his patients.

Dr Kumar approached Andrew privately, when they both had time for discussion. She explained to him that there had been some concerns expressed by patients about his 'bedside manner'. Andrew expressed surprise – he enjoyed family medicine and several patients had expressed their appreciation for his interest and time. Dr Kumar complimented him on his ability to connect with these patients and asked him if he had any thoughts about what would explain why some patients were so happy with his care and others were complaining. He was confused about this and commented: 'I guess you can't satisfy everyone!' Dr Kumar agreed but suggested that this was an opportunity to learn more about his interactions with patients and discover the behaviors that made the difference. She offered to sit in on some of his interviews to observe his interviewing techniques and provide him with feedback.

The student population has changed dramatically in many medical schools with the entrance of more women and greater ethnic diversity. These changes have the potential to alter the focus and priorities of the curriculum. Some authors have commented on the impact of the 'feminization' of medicine. For example, Gilligan and Pollack comment on the impact of increasing numbers of women entering medicine:

> [W]omen medical students in their heightened sensitivity to detachment and isolation often reveal the places in medical training and practice where human connection has become dangerously thin . . . women physicians may help to heal the breach in medicine between patient care and scientific success. For this reason the encouragement of women's voices and the validation of women's perceptions may contribute to the improvement of medical education. Since humanism in medicine depends on joining the heroism of cure with the vulnerability of care, reshaping the image of the physician to include women constitutes a powerful force for change. (Gilligan and Pollack, 1988: 262)

Another important issue is the effect of stress, substance abuse and mental illness on the performance of medical students. In a study of burnout in residents in internal medicine programs, Shanafelt and colleagues (2002) found 76% of respondents met the criteria for burnout using the self-administered Maslach Burnout Inventory. Burned-out residents were more likely to self-report providing at minimum one type of suboptimal patient care at least monthly. For example, 40% of burned-out residents, compared with less than 5% of non-burned-out residents, reported that they had 'paid little attention to the social or personal impact of an illness on a patient' weekly or monthly (Shanafelt et al., 2002: 363). Several studies of substance use among medical students report worrisome levels of abuse. In a survey of seven medical schools in Great Britain, Webb and colleagues reported that, of those who drank (85% of the students), 48% of men and 38% of women exceeded sensible weekly limits of alcohol consumption, and high-risk levels of consumption were reported by 12% of men and 7% of women (Webb et al., 1998). In a survey at nine USA medical schools, Roberts and colleagues (2001) found one quarter of students suffered from symptoms of mental illness, including 7–18% with substance abuse disorders, and 90% reported needing care for various health concerns, including 47% having at least one mental health or substance-related health issue. In a study of family practice residents, Hawk and Scott (1986: 82) reported that trying to balance both a professional life and personal life is the 'most outstanding stress of all'.

Kumar and Basu (2000) present a useful taxonomy of predisposing factors for resident and physician substance abuse:

1 Stress:
   a situational stress – sleep deprivation, fatigue, inflexible time, excessive workload, burdensome clerical and administrative responsibilities
   b personal stresses – stress of family, lack of social relationships and leisure time, marital difficulties
   c professional stresses – workload, difficult patients, career planning, dissatisfaction with specialty, fear of professional incompetence.

2 Medical student abuse – 72% of students reported at least one abusive experience, the most common was being yelled at by faculty, residents and other staff (reported by 54% of students) (from Kumar and Basu, 2000: 448).

Although teachers should generally not take on the role of therapist with their students, they need to know when their students are struggling with personal issues which might be interfering with their learning, help them to recognize the problem and direct them to appropriate professional care.

In addition to understanding the cognitive, developmental and personal struggles of students, a whole-person approach requires the teacher to comprehend the student's learning context. The environment of medical education strongly influences what can or will be learned. In the first two years of medical school, the course structure, content and evaluation will steer students' learning. In clinical teaching, case mix, quality of teaching and practice setting – inpatient, outpatient, primary, tertiary – will be the principal influences. Medical education is not just about learning a set of knowledge, skills and attitudes; it is also about changing lay persons into physicians – a profound and awesome transformation, as we described in Chapter 10. The syllabus defines the course of study that students must digest, but does not describe the intimate personal interactions that bring about this important change. To understand how this occurs we need to examine medical school as a cultural institution. Roff and McAleer (2001: 333) comment:

> In addition to the documented curriculum, students and teachers both become aware of the 'educational environment' or 'climate' of the institution. Is the teaching and learning environment very competitive? Is it authoritarian? Is

the atmosphere in classes and field placements relaxed or is it in various ways stressful, perhaps even intimidating? These are all key questions in determining the nature of learning experience.

For example, many medical schools have developed courses on communication in the preclinical years and espouse the importance of the patient's role in decision making. However, students often report that their role models – residents and faculty – do not exhibit these skills. In fact, the culture of many clinical settings is inimical to the values of patient-centeredness. For more discussion of the context of learning, *see* Chapter 15, 'Developing a patient-centered curriculum'.

Finding common ground

There are three key elements in finding common ground in the learner-centered approach: establishing priorities; choosing appropriate teaching/learning methods; and determining the roles of both learner and teacher.

Establishing priorities

Difficulties arise when there is a conflict between what a student wants to learn and what a teacher wants to teach. Also, students may become frustrated when there are so many required objectives that there is no time left to address topics of particular interest. When the official curriculum reflects the realities of practice, rather than being a difficult hurdle for students to jump in order to 'prove themselves', such conflict is less likely. A learner-centered approach does not hand over the curriculum to the students but it does respect their intelligence, common sense and good intentions by involving them in decisions about what to learn, when to learn it, how deeply to focus and how to evaluate their learning. For example, the value of understanding the family situation of patients may only become relevant to students when they are faced with patients whose family dynamics are central to management.

Case example

Roger Fenway, a first year resident in family medicine, had been an infrequent attender at behavioral science seminars. He argued that 'most of this stuff is common sense and I need more time learning about heart failure and COPD'. But then he met Pat! Pat was a 75-year-old crusty woman with metastatic lung cancer who challenged all of her healthcare providers. She seemed to anticipate rejection and was determined to reject them before they rejected her. Roger could not understand why she insisted on being so difficult. Despite her rough edges, he liked her hard-nosed determination and stoicism. When he was discussing discharge plans with her, he learned that her family had sold all of her belongings and canceled the lease on her apartment. They had even sold off her clothes and jewellery. Roger was furious at Pat's family and wondered how they could behave in such a cruel manner. He explored the family dynamics further and discovered that this was not the first time they had acted this way. He started to understand why Pat kept people at a distance – it would be too dangerous to risk trusting anyone based on a lifetime of betrayal. The seminars on family dynamics started to have more interest for Roger as he realized how a better understanding of family functioning could help him to provide better care to his patients.

Teaching and learning methods

There are several studies defining the characteristics of excellent clinical teaching that support the use of a learner-centered approach (Beaudoin *et al.*, 1998; Irby, 1978; Schwenk and Whitman, 1987; Wright *et al.*, 1998). Whether done from the point of view of learners, teachers, or both, these studies agree that clinical teachers should demonstrate:

- *Clinical competence* including demonstrating good skills, procedures and patient-care abilities: They have a humanistic orientation, stressing the social and psychological aspects of patient care. They possess an excellent fund of knowledge and are able to present information in a clear and well-organized fashion. They are prepared to share with students their struggles and success with patients as a model of continuing learning.
- *Enthusiasm for teaching*: They obviously enjoy associating with students and make themselves accessible to them.
- *Supervisory skills*: They are sensitive to patient and student needs simultaneously and involve students actively in patient care and in their own learning. They provide clear and appropriate direction and give frequent constructive feedback. Helpful feedback is the teacher's description of students' effective and ineffective behaviors that shows them how to improve their ineffective behaviors. (*See* the outline of constructive feedback in Chapter 13, 'Teaching the patient-centered clinical method: practical tips'). They emphasize problem-solving by challenging students to discuss their thinking processes and give students an opportunity to practice skills and procedures. They are open to criticism from students, using it to enhance mutual learning.

- *Effective interpersonal skills*: They are sensitive to student concerns, such as feelings of inadequacy, and demonstrate a genuine interest in students through a friendly manner. Whenever possible, they build the self-esteem of students. Schwenk and Whitman (1987) argue that the most important thing an effective teacher does is to form a good relationship with each student and to give of themselves.

Roles of teacher and learner

McKeachie's outline of teachers' roles helps us understand the many and varied responsibilities of teachers (McKeachie, 1978: 68–82). On the one hand, teachers function as facilitator, ego ideal and person; they support and encourage students by the force of their own personality. Students incorporate aspects of their teachers into their own developing professional identity and often form close personal relationships with them. On the other hand, teachers are experts, formal authorities and socializing agents; they are guardians of the traditions of the profession and stand as trustees who decide whether or not each student measures up for admission into the ranks. In this sense, no matter what else they represent in the minds of their students, they are powerful and sometimes intimidating authority figures. Thus, teachers wear many hats and have complex multidimensional relationships with their students.

Building on previous learning

In the patient-centered clinical method, it is important for the physician to acknowledge patient's pre-existing problems so that current issues will be managed in the context of all of the patient's problems. In the same way, teachers need to be cognizant of their students' prior learning experiences. Students are not blank slates. Previous knowledge of learners' strengths, weaknesses and special interests accelerates the learning process and increases the potential intensity and complexity of the knowledge, skills and attitudes that can be mastered. The curriculum can be viewed as a spiral; the same content may be encountered on several occasions but each time it is assimilated in greater depth. Sometimes such repetition is misunderstood and students complain about unnecessary repetition. They need to understand the purpose of revisiting some topics and may need to be challenged by their teachers to dig deeper.

Pacing is also important. When students become overwhelmed by the emotional intensity of a learning experience, they may need a break. Then, restored, they return to the learning environment ready to proceed with the next learning task. For example, helping dying patients come to terms with their mortality is often psychologically draining and students may need an emotional respite. This may only happen with the support and permission of their teachers. Finally, continuity allows the whole process to be more efficient and effective. The important personal and contextual issues, so critical in determining what will be learned, cannot be easily communicated from one teacher to another.

Case example

Nelson Martin, a second year resident in family medicine, came to his supervisor with questions about his patient, a 27-year-old attractive woman with vague symptoms. After asking a few questions, the supervisor quickly realized that Nelson had not explored possible psychological sources of her problem. This was not surprising to the supervisor who had previously recognized and discussed with Nelson his discomfort with relationships, especially with young attractive women. He asked Nelson if he had any theories about why he had not inquired about this patient's personal life. Nelson was able to immediately recall their previous discussion of this issue. Together they explored how he could approach this particular patient and also decided to set aside some time to examine further this perplexing issue for Nelson.

Enhancing the learner–teacher relationship

Above all else, the relationship between teachers and learners is the single most important variable affecting the outcomes of learning (Tiberius *et al.*, 2002). Good teachers have a desire to help others learn which transcends the problems that teaching creates. Teaching interferes with physicians' intimate one-to-one relationships with their patients. It slows them down. It exposes their weaknesses and areas of ignorance. It demands a positive regard for the learners even when their behavior may frustrate or upset the teacher. It is essential that there be congruence between the patient-centered clinical method and the process of teaching it. For example, just as our commitment as doctors is to the person and not the disease, so, too, our commitment as teachers is to the learner and not to the subject matter. This commitment transcends individual learning problems or specific skills to be learned. It extends into the very being of the learners and challenges them to stretch themselves to their limits. Such learning may require students to experience painful self-discovery or to make difficult personal changes.

Case example

Fionella MacLean had wanted to be a child psychiatrist since her youth. She had loved caring for young children and had served as an aide at a children's psychiatric facility during her teens. Fionella had also battled with bulimia throughout her late teens and early twenties; hence she was very familiar with the process of psychotherapy. Upon completion of her Bachelor of Education, aged 22, Fionella decided to apply to medical school. It had been an uphill battle conquering the basic sciences she lacked in her undergraduate education and keeping her bulimia at bay. But she had succeeded and now was embarking on her child psychiatry residency. Fionella was both excited and anxious. She was eager to work with the younger children but doubted how she might relate to the adolescents, particularly the females who had an eating disorder like hers. Yet as time went by Fionella became both skilled and assured in her work with adolescents. It was not until her rotation on the inpatient adolescent unit when she was assigned two seriously ill patients with anorexia nervosa that she began to question her ability to work with this patient population. Their issues were too close to her own and she struggled to keep clear what were their issues and what were her own demons.

Dr Tillman had been her supervisor and mentor since Fionella had joined the residency program. While she had not disclosed her bulimia to him, she realized that it was time to share this information. Her own personal problems were beginning to impact on her ability to care for her patients.

What allowed Fionella to expose her feelings about this situation was the trust and respect she experienced in the learner–teacher relationship with Dr Tillman. She knew from her past experiences with him that he would not judge her past behavior or question her current situation. He would listen and be there for her. Dr Tillman would invite her 'to wonder' what might be causing her present difficulty and how she would overcome this problem. He would not cross the bridge and become her therapist but remain her teacher, all the while knowing when referral for further professional counseling would be important for Fionella both personally and professionally.

Students will often defend against such self-awareness and may find themselves in conflict with their teachers over the need for change. At this stage in the development of their professional identity they often experience ambivalent feelings about their teachers: on the one hand they wish for a dependent relationship where their obligations are spelled out and clearly limited; on the other hand they resent the imposition of control and long for independent responsibility. Their feelings may vacillate from one extreme to another depending on the complexity and volume of patient care, fatigue and feelings of self-efficacy.

It is not surprising that intense emotions may develop in the student–teacher relationship, replicating similar feelings with other powerful authority figures from the student's past. Working through this transference may enhance the student's self-understanding and prevent similar reactions from occurring in the future. It requires the development of an intimate and trust-based relationship before such intensely personal learning and growth can occur. Supervision of psychotherapists shares many similarities with clinical teaching, especially regarding the importance of the relationship between teacher and learner. Alonso (1985) summarizes this aspect as follows:

> ... the development of a clinician from novice to expert is primarily an emotional, maturational process, much like the development of a child from infancy to adulthood ... It is assumed that a transference relationship will develop between therapist and supervisor and that this transferential field will become a primary vehicle for influencing the student's clinical growth ... there is a concerted effort to shore up and strengthen the supervisee's healthiest defences, either by reducing the ambiguity or by helping the trainee to tolerate the inevitable confusion of clinical work ... When difficulty occurs ... this regression is seen as a healthy and expectable rite of passage ... In fact, the clinician who never regresses in the course of training is probably avoiding the more difficult levels of learning that occur in the unconscious merger of patient/therapist and may be keeping too great a distance between self and patient. (1985: 47–8)

There are a number of teacher behaviors that contribute to the creation of an impasse with their learners: the need to be admired; the need to rescue; the need to be in control; the need for competition; the need to be loved; the need to work through unresolved prior conflict in the supervisor's own training experience; spillover from stress in the personal or professional life of the supervisor; tension between supervisor and the administration of the institution (Alonso, 1985: 83–104). This highlights the importance of a healthy and open relationship between teachers and learners characterized by empathy, genuineness and positive regard (Rogers, 1951). It is one of the special privileges of teaching to share in the struggles of students for growth and self-actualization.

Being realistic

Teachers must recognize that they cannot be all things to all people. The destructive myth of faculty members as 'triple threats' (Mundy, 1991), expected to be exemplary clinicians, outstanding researchers and superb teachers, casts faculty into impossible situations of role overload. Not only is this behavior self-destructive but also it demonstrates poor role-modeling for students. As a consequence, students may set unachievable objectives for themselves. Conversely, to avoid replicating their teachers' lifestyle and to prevent role strain, students may impose inappropriate limitations on the responsibilities they will assume. One outcome of the establishment of rigid boundaries between their personal and professional lives is lost opportunities for learning and growth. Examples of such behavior in primary care include: working in settings where the hours of work are limited, interactions are superficial and all complex problems are referred (e.g. walk-in clinics); and limiting hours of practice or range of services provided (e.g. refusal to provide home visits, hospital visits, intrapartum care or palliative care). In specialist care, physicians may reduce their office hours or limit their scope of practice.

The patient-centered clinical method requires doctors to become involved in the full range of problems which their patients present but acknowledges the importance of setting reasonable limits on how much time and energy will be expended. While more effective time-management will ease some of the problems, the answer is not that simple. Each doctor must discover how to juggle competing demands while maintaining openness to both patients' needs and personal and family needs. Thus it is important for teachers to strike a balance for themselves and to create a learning environment where students can discover how to be realistic.

An important feature of modern medical practice is teamwork, as discussed in Chapter 9. Students need opportunities to work in effective interdisciplinary teams and to collaborate with other healthcare professionals. They need to learn how to be effective team members and team leaders. Doctors have traditionally seen themselves as team leaders and have been reluctant to learn from other healthcare professionals. This 'medical chauvinism' is anachronistic and counterproductive. Young doctors in training have an opportunity to complement their traditional medical education by learning from teachers in other health disciplines. Team teaching is a powerful method for faculty members to model collaborative teaching and learning. Another valuable way in which medical students learn about the roles and functions of other professionals is by sharing learning experiences with students from other healthcare disciplines.

Case example

Allison Tsui, a first year resident in internal medicine, was consistently an hour late at the end of her outpatient clinics. Patients and staff were complaining and the Chief Resident, Russ Johar, arranged to meet with her to discuss these mounting concerns. Dr Tsui attributed the problem to overbooking. She felt that she was expected to see too many patients in the time allotted – they all had many complex medical problems and many of them also had personal problems that were very time-consuming. She felt overwhelmed. Dr Johar wondered how he would address his junior colleague's difficulty. He decided to approach Dr Tsui as an adult learner and asked what she thought they could do together to address these issues. He offered to meet with her in one of the clinics to review the bookings and to observe her with a few patients. He discovered that she was doing complete assessments on many of the patients and that she was spending a lot of time in patient education and counseling rather than referring patients to the nurse educator, social worker or other appropriate staff. Her prior experience had not prepared her to work collaboratively with other team members and as a junior she did not feel she could ask other team members, who all seemed so busy, to assist with her patients. Dr Johar realized that he had failed to provide Dr Tsui with an adequate orientation to the role and function of the interdisciplinary team in the outpatient clinic. He apologized to Dr Tsui for this oversight and, in doing so, role-modeled open and direct communication as an important aspect of good teamwork.

Conclusion

In this chapter we have described the six components of the learner-centered method of education, illustrating the many parallels with the patient-centered clinical method. Key points include the following.

- The way teachers relate to their learners will influence the way in which learners interact with their patients.
- It is important to incorporate learners' ideas and aspirations about what they wish to learn into all educational planning.
- There are two dimensions of understanding the student as a whole person: the student's life history, and personal and cognitive development; and the learning environment.
- There are three key elements in finding common ground in the learner-centered approach: establishing priorities; choosing appropriate teaching/learning methods; determining the roles of both teacher and learner.
- Previous knowledge of learners' strengths, weaknesses and special interests accelerates the learning process and increases the potential intensity and complexity of the knowledge, skills and attitudes that can be mastered.
- Above all else, the relationship between teachers and learners is the single most important variable affecting the outcomes of learning.
- Teachers need to role-model a realistic approach to their many responsibilities, demonstrate exemplary teamwork, and portray a balanced lifestyle.

12

Challenges in learning and teaching the patient-centered clinical method

W Wayne Weston and Judith Belle Brown

In the previous chapter, describing the learner-centered method of education, we outlined a framework for teachers enacting this approach to teaching. In this chapter we present some of the common challenges faced by those who strive to learn, or to teach, the patient-centered clinical method and then provide practical, hands-on teaching tips to assist teachers at all levels of training. Teaching and learning the patient-centered clinical method is demanding for many reasons.

The nature of medical practice

Medical practice often seems arduous enough when limited to the diagnosis and treatment of disease; suggesting to doctors that they must also consider patients' perspectives of the illness experience and the social context in which patients live their lives may seem overwhelming. This is especially true for young doctors who are struggling to learn their craft. Several characteristics of practice pose difficulties for learning. Hippocrates (1982) commented on this 2000 years ago in his aphorism: 'Life is short; art is long; opportunity fugitive; experience delusive; judgment difficult.' The long hours, lack of sleep, and the personally draining nature of patient-care often leave students and practitioners exhausted and emotionally spent. Physicians, in this state, may have little energy to invest in learning to be patient-centered. In the long run, we argue, patient-centered care is more rewarding for both doctors and patients. But, when doctors are harried, they are tempted to focus narrowly on the patient's presenting complaint alone and to end the visit as quickly as possible by ignoring any other concerns the patient may have. When doctors appear rushed, patients may collude in this approach by keeping their worries to themselves. This reinforces some physicians' beliefs that most patients are primarily interested in quick solutions (Brown *et al.*, 2002a).

Although there are undeniable time pressures in practice, sometimes doctors are caught up in 'busy work' to avoid the emotional demands of practice. Without a commitment to continuing personal growth and self awareness, physicians may evade confronting the reasons for their avoidance. The following case serves as an example.

Case example

> Michael Wong, a first year internal medicine resident, described his discomfort with the recent death of his patient. He found the experience painful because, in spending time with the patient, he had developed a relationship. Unlike the deaths of other patients who had remained strangers, this patient's death touched him deeply. Michael almost wished he had not become attached and was ambivalent about allowing himself to become vulnerable again. This experience was a turning point in his education – the opportunity to discuss his feelings with his peers and teachers helped him to accept his pain as a necessary part of his learning and growth. Michael realized that protecting himself from further painful experiences, by avoiding getting to know his patients, would rob him of one of the most valued aspects of practice. He also recognized that his relationship with the patient was the most helpful element of his care.

Discomfort with relinquishing power to patients

In disease-centered interviews, doctors simplify their patients' problems by reducing them to disease categories. The focus is on the problem, not the person; the personal, social and cultural contexts are not relevant to the physician's central mission of diagnosis and cure. Another way in which the interview is simplified is for both doctor and patient to agree that the doctor is in charge. The roles of doctor and patient are clear and distinct; the doctor's task is to make a diagnosis and to tell the patient what to do to recover and the patient's job is to comply with the 'doctor's orders'. Patient-centered interviews may be more complicated. Not only are doctors looking for disease but also actively seeking to comprehend their patients' suffering; in addition, doctors are striving to determine the extent to which patients wish to be involved in the decisions about what should be done. Many physicians are reluctant to inquire about their patients' expectations for fear they will ask for something that the doctor disagrees with; they are uncomfortable with confrontation and saying no. And if they acquiesce to the patient's wishes and a poor outcome ensues, they worry about the threat of lawsuits. Doctors tend to see such disagreements as win-lose situations, where one opinion must prevail, rather than potential win-win situations where the ideas of both may lead to a more creative solution. In this approach, the textbook answer may not be the best response under the special circumstances of the individual patient. It may be particularly difficult for young physicians, still struggling to develop their self-confidence as professionals, to share power with their patients. The following example illustrates some of the issues that lead to power struggles between doctors and patients and the resultant failure to find common ground.

Case example

Jill Kline, aged 48, presented to the clinic complaining of a cough and shortness of breath. This was her second episode in the past three months. The third year resident, Christopher Torrance, who was new to the clinic, quickly scanned Mrs Kline's chart, observing that there were reports from two walk-in clinics and the Emergency Department, also in the past three months, where she had been treated for symptoms of wheezing and shortness of breath. After gathering a history of her symptoms and conducting a physical examination he inquired: 'Are you a smoker?'

Jill hesitated, and reluctantly replied: 'Well, yes, sort of . . .' Her voice trailed off and her head fell forward in embarrassment.

Recalling the strategies for helping patients to quit smoking, which he had learned in medical school, Dr Torrance's first reaction was to apply these principles to Mrs Kline. He assailed her with facts and figures in order to convince the patient to quit smoking. The more enthusiastic and adamant he became the more Jill became entrenched in her position that she 'only smoked a bit' and remained unconvinced that it was worth the effort to quit. Finally, exasperated, Dr Torrance wrote out a prescription for antibiotics urging Mrs Kline to return to see him if her symptoms did not improve. He concluded the visit with a warning that he would not be responsible if she experienced any serious respiratory problems as a result of her failure to comply with his advice to quit smoking.

Jill Kline left the office feeling misunderstood and chastised. Christopher Torrance also felt misunderstood and frustrated by the patient's 'non-compliance' and shared his concerns with his supervisor. They quickly agreed that the doctor and patient were not on the same wavelength regarding the importance of smoking cessation and began to explore how Christopher and his patient could find common ground on this issue. In the discussion with his supervisor Christopher recognized that, in his eagerness to apply the principles of smoking cessation, he had failed to ascertain some key information. What was the relationship between her ongoing health problems, her smoking behavior and her current life situation?

Four weeks later Jill returned to the clinic because her symptoms persisted and she was continuing to smoke 'but just a little bit'. Recalling his discussion with his supervisor, Dr Torrance decided to alter his approach and inquired about what was currently happening in Mrs Kline's life. Instead of admonishing her, he decided to try to understand her reluctance to quit smoking in spite of her health problems.

Jill told him that she had been a single mother for ten years because her husband had left her after the birth of their Down's Syndrome child. The child had been one year of age at the time and her husband could not accept the fact that she would never be 'normal'. Jill had cared for her daughter for the past 11 years but had had to place her in an institution one year previously because of medical complications. This represented a tremendous loss and sense of failure. Then six months ago her 17-year-old son had been caught downloading pornography from the Internet for sale. She was humiliated by this event and felt great dismay, and again failure as a mother.

While Jill had smoked sporadically during her teenage years she had only started smoking regularly four months ago. Jill speculated that this had been in response to the multiple losses and disappointments she had endured over the past 16 months. Feeling ashamed and embarrassed she had not told anyone about starting to smoke again, except the resident.

Dr Torrance validated her feelings and empathized with the difficult events she had recently faced. Together they agreed that the optimal goal for restoring her health was to quit smoking. But, they also appreciated that this was perhaps not a priority in Jill's life at the present time. While he wanted to apply his knowledge of smoking cessation, he also acknowledged that this skill was dependent on the patient's life circumstances. Jill Kline had many difficult issues to confront and resolve. Quitting smoking would come later and be a potential success for both the patient and the doctor.

Need for self-awareness

Doctors who explore patients' cues to personal problems quickly find themselves discussing intensely intimate issues. When confronted with having a serious illness, patients often wonder about its meaning for them and their families. For example, it may raise fundamental questions such as: 'Why me?' or 'What will happen to my children if I die?' Other patients may present with symptoms that reflect their concerns about their marriage or employment. These situations may trigger questions and feelings in physicians' minds related to their own current relationships or to unresolved issues from their families of origin. As a result, young physicians, with little life experience, may be overwhelmed by their feelings and retreat into the conventional medical model for self-protection. Additionally, physicians may form relationships with some patients which unconsciously replicate troubled relationships from their past; without insight the physician is likely to become entangled in the same difficulties.

Because the patient–doctor relationship is so intensely personal, such difficulties are inevitable at times. Students and physicians need opportunities to develop self-awareness. These issues must be addressed with sensitivity by the teacher, taking into consideration the students' level of comfort in discussing their feelings. Often this can be done in a small group so that all students learn from each other's insights; but sometimes this may be too threatening or overwhelming. Opportunities for one-to-one discussion also need to be available. Self-awareness is an important aspect of what Epstein (1999) describes as mindful practice. He outlines five forms of self-awareness:

> Intrapersonal self-awareness helps the physician be conscious of his or her strengths, limitations, and sources of professional satisfaction ... Interpersonal self-awareness ... allows physicians to see themselves as they are seen by others and helps to establish satisfactory interpersonal relationships with colleagues, patients and students ... Self-awareness of learning needs allows physicians to recognize areas of unconscious incompetence and to develop a means to achieving their learning goals. Ethical self-awareness is the moment-to-moment cognizance of values that are shaping medical encounters. Technical self-awareness is necessary for self-correction during procedures such as the physical examination, surgery, computer operations, and communication. (1999: 836)

He goes on to discuss the implications for teachers: 'The teacher's task is to invoke a state of mindfulness in the learner, and, thus, the teacher can only act as a guide, not a transmitter of knowledge' (Epstein, 1999: 838). Kern and colleagues (2001) describe the importance of powerful experiences, which evoke strong feelings, as a stimulus for personal growth particularly if they are accompanied by introspection, a helping relationship, or both. 'Powerful experiences occur commonly in medicine but may lack optimal conditions for personal growth. To promote practitioner personal growth, medical faculties may wish to explore methods to promote introspection, helping relationships, and the acknowledgment of powerful experiences when they occur' (Kern *et al.*, 2001: 97).

The following example describes a teaching intervention that promoted self-awareness.

Case example

> In a teaching practice, Sarah Valiquet, a first year family medicine resident, stepped out of an interview to consult with her supervisor. This was the second time she had seen the patient for tension-type headaches. Toni Sanatani, a 45-year-old executive, was not improving and initiated this visit in order to be referred for a CAT scan. The resident was frustrated and angry with what she described as an 'abuse of the system'. Her attempt to persuade Mr Sanatani that the test was unnecessary terminated in a heated disagreement. Dr Valiquet felt her medical knowledge had been rejected and her professional credibility undermined. She needed to win this argument!
>
> While the resident was describing her frustration and the stand-off with her patient, the supervisor recognized Dr Valiquet's vulnerability and need for support. But, from previous knowledge of Mr Sanatani, the supervisor understood his request probably stemmed from the death of his uncle from a brain tumor six months ago. The teacher's task was to help the resident air her feelings and then to help her explore why she had fallen into a win-lose relationship with the patient. Dr Valiquet needed to understand how both she and her patient had contributed to this impasse. Then she had to find a way to convert the struggle into a win-win outcome. The resident recognized that her recurrent conflict with authority figures led her to experience Mr Sanatani's request for reassurance as a demand for an unnecessary test and a challenge of her medical competence. Instead of exploring his fears, she reacted by defending herself. Dr Valiquet dismissed the patient's request as unwarranted and the fight was on. After realizing what had happened, Dr Valiquet was able to return to the patient, acknowledge that they had reached an impasse and ask if they could begin again. This culminated in an exploration of the patient's concerns and fears about the headaches. Following a careful neurological examination and discussion about why a brain tumor was highly unlikely, the patient was prepared to consider other causes for his headaches.
>
> Later, Dr Valiquet sat down with her supervisor to discuss options for exploring her problem with authority figures. The supervisor's recognition of Dr Valiquet's vulnerability had prevented him from criticizing her error and engaging in a parallel struggle which would have replicated the student's difficulties with authority. Instead, his non-judgmental stance encouraged the development of her self-awareness.

For the most part, as physicians mature in personal and clinical wisdom, they become more comfortable with the uncertainties of medicine and the complexities of their patients' problems; ongoing self-reflection promotes a deepening understanding of the patient–physician relationship.

In an inspiring paper, Michael E McLeod, a gastroenterologist, reflects on his struggle toward self-awareness:

> I worked to keep my emotions and intuitions from influencing medical decisions because they were subjective and not measurable. I became adept at hiding the feelings of vulnerability and helplessness that I felt when my patients died, and those of anger and frustration with 'hateful' patients … As a result I became increasingly isolated from my own emotions and needs: I shared less with my colleagues at work. I evolved a workaholic lifestyle with the subconscious expectation that others would figure out my needs and satisfy them because I was 'doing so much'. I did not take the risk of identifying and asking for what I needed. I hid behind a mask of pseudocompetence and efficiency. I let power, money, and position take the place of empowerment, love, and meaning. But because they were substitutes for my primary needs, they were never enough. (1998: 678)

Overemphasis on the conventional medical model

There are several features of medical education and professional socialization that may interfere with learning an effective clinical approach to the familiar problems presented by patients. Medical training indoctrinates students to see patients' problems as derangements of the 'body-machine' and to be concerned about missing some rare but deadly disease. As a result, most students and many physicians attempt to find a disease to explain each of their patients' complaints. This may result in over-investigation, unnecessary referral and over-prescribing. Also, patients' personal concerns may receive little attention because physicians are concentrating all of their thought and energy on ferreting out pathology. This is not surprising since the majority of medical students' clinical experience is in large tertiary care hospitals where they are exposed to very seriously ill patients. They are often overworked and may have little time to do anything but tend to the grave physical needs of their patients.

In the absence of an alternative model, it is understandable that young physicians will use the framework they are most familiar with – the conventional medical model. Physicians, when stressed or overwhelmed by the problems of a patient, will often revert to a simplistic focus on conventional medical diagnosis even if they have learned and have used a more sophisticated and comprehensive patient-centered approach.

One of our students, in describing her struggle to use the patient-centered clinical method, expressed her fears that she would be mandated to relinquish the conventional medical model altogether:

I want to remember that stuff (textbook information), you know?! Not only did I work hard to learn it and to remember it for a short while, and it has helped me to fend off staffmen in the past, but even without the quizzing, it is a form of security, a teddy bear of sorts. Beyond that, sometimes it's a source of pride, of excitement, of fun, of conversation with colleagues, a worldly treasure. Yeah, I know it's a treasure moths will soon destroy (to coin a phrase), but meanwhile I am trying to live in a world that demands these things!

The conventional medical model has a long history of success, it is highly respected in our culture and it allows physicians to remain comfortably distant from patients and their problems. Also, if doctors do their best (biomedically speaking), and their patients do not improve, the physicians need feel no blame. If the patient did not 'comply' with the doctor's 'orders' then the lack of improvement can be blamed on the patient.

Students and physicians need to learn a more appropriate clinical method, one which incorporates the power of the conventional medical model but which is not constrained by its narrow focus on disease. Such a clinical method cannot be learned all at once. Students may need to learn each component of the patient-centered clinical method separately and they will also require opportunities to practice integrating their clinical skills into a unified whole.

Concentration on history-taking rather than listening to the patient

Students in first year medical school have little difficulty learning how to inquire about patients' ideas and expectations concerning their illnesses but, as they progress through medical school, they become consumed by the task of making the right diagnosis and their interviews become less patient-centered (Barbee and Feldman, 1970; Cohen, 1985; Helfer, 1970; Preven *et al.*, 1986). This may be a consequence of the emphasis on taking a thorough history of each disease and completing a comprehensive functional inquiry. Much less attention is given to open-ended exploration of the patient's feelings and ideas. Without practice, most young doctors feel uncomfortable inquiring about patients' personal lives. Often there is concern that patients will become emotional and perhaps cry or show anger; they worry that they will open up a 'can of worms' which they will not be able to handle. Physicians' training tends to make them cautious about trying new approaches with patients where they feel uncertain about the outcome; they are also reluctant to try unfamiliar techniques if they feel uncomfortable or awkward. The commonest excuse given to avoid asking about patients' personal concerns is lack of time. But it is not efficient use of time to search for a disease that is not present or to ignore a major source of patients' distress such as their fear or concern about the possible cause and implications of their symptoms.

Alternatively, when physicians are learning the patient-centered clinical method, they mistakenly equate it with a 'psychosocial functional inquiry'. The following example typifies this common misunderstanding.

When a patient presented with concerns about her severe sore throat and about how long she was going to be off school the resident interrupted her story with: 'Wait, I need to get to know more about your personal situation. Where did you grow up? What was your childhood like? Was there much conflict in your family?' These questions would be very useful in the appropriate context, but in this case they seemed unconnected from the patient's practical concerns about receiving effective treatment and getting back to school as soon as possible. The physician needed to be sensitive to any cues about how this patient's home and school situation were related to her illness but was not being patient-centered by imposing a psychosocial inquiry.

Teacher inexperience

It takes considerable experience, first as a doctor and then as a clinical teacher, before a physician is able to integrate secondhand information about patients in order to make good decisions. To make the task even more complex, teachers are trying to assess not only the patients' problems but also the learners' problems. To achieve this, teachers must consider many different factors at the same time. First, there are several questions about students: Did they establish a comfortable relationship with patients that allowed the patients to mention everything they had in mind? Did the students pick up on all the important cues the patients gave? Did the students mention to the teacher all of their concerns about the patient, or did they avoid those topics that might have disclosed their own ignorance? What are the students' blind spots? Unless the teacher has prior knowledge of the students or has witnessed their conduct in actual interviews with patients, it may be difficult to answer many of these questions. It is important to establish a climate of acceptance, where students are not punished for admitting ignorance. Students need to know that the teacher is depending on the information they gather to make important management decisions; hence they must state where they are confused or uncertain so that the teacher will explore or double-check these areas.

Second, there are questions to be considered about the patients: What more information does the physician need to make a reasonable diagnosis? Why did the patient present now? What are the patient's feelings, ideas and expectations about the problem? Here, too, prior knowledge is invaluable. But unless teachers have seen the patient–student interactions, they must depend on obtaining secondhand information from students. Here is where a patient-centered case presentation, described in Chapter 14, is an invaluable tool for both the learner and the teacher.

Finally, inexperienced teachers may be concerned about their reputation among their students and may feel a need to prove themselves by demonstrating their excellence as clinicians. The dilemma for physicians who are teaching a patient-centered approach is that the value system of the medical school is often at odds with this approach. Excellence may be defined in terms of one's technical prowess and diagnostic acumen but rarely in terms of one's ability to relate to patients. In teaching at the bedside, the discussion may focus on the latest drug for the patient's problem rather than exploring the patient's experience of their illness. For young students, desperate for unambiguous answers in the chaotic and messy domain of clinical medicine, knowing the latest drugs for various diseases is highly valued. They have not yet learned how to deal with uncertainty. Students may reward teachers who can provide black and white answers and discount teachers who urge them to address not only the patients' diseases but their illness experiences in the context of their life setting. Young students may feel overwhelmed by the complexity of clinical medicine and resent the teacher who appears to make their task more difficult. Thus, student's needs for certainty and simplicity coupled with the teacher's need for acceptance by peers can have a powerful influence on novice teachers.

Competing demands on teachers

Teachers are pulled in many different directions at once: they are expected to be exemplary role models and to see enough patients to earn a living; they must prove themselves credible among their academic colleagues by engaging in research and publishing papers; they must add their fair share of teaching of both undergraduate and postgraduate students; and they must serve on the many committees and working groups of the university and professional associations that depend on their involvement. Faculty members are increasingly finding themselves stretched thin and forced to set priorities. Too often it is time for teaching that is cut back, since there are fewer institutional rewards for these activities than for research or clinical care. Teaching the patient-centered approach may be time-consuming considering that teachers would want to observe student–patient interactions, to provide constructive feedback and to adequately explore students' personal issues that may be evoked by the discussion.

Teacher over-protectiveness

Including students in patient-care changes the patient–doctor relationship and creates several dilemmas for teachers. Clinical teaching makes the doctor's job more complicated – the teacher, in this context, is responsible not only for the quality of patient-care but also for the quality of the student's learning experience. Sometimes the two responsibilities seem to be at odds. Physician discomfort in these situations may interfere with student learning. Doctors may be more hesitant to allow students to practice on their patients than the patients are themselves. For example, physicians may falsely assume that their patients would not want to discuss their feelings about being ill with a student. This may be more of a reflection the physician's discomfort than the patient's uneasiness. Most patients are willing to cooperate to benefit the students' learning, provided the students are appropriately supervised and not trying to do something for which they are ill-prepared. It is essential that teachers not undermine the student's position with patients. Whenever possible, teachers should function as consultant to the student and point out their agreement with his or her approach. However, if the student has made an error, the fact needs to be addressed honestly. One approach is for the teacher and student to excuse themselves from the examining room to allow for frank discussion. When they both return, the student discusses with the patient the error and the new plans for treatment. With postgraduate students, the patient may have already gone home before the error is noted. In this situation, it is essential that the patient be contacted to correct the mistake as quickly as possible. Not everyone will support the use of such candor in this age of litigation. But such honesty reassures patients that the monitoring system works, and that a teaching practice offers the advantage of at least two opinions on their problems.

Teachers as role models

The most important teaching method used by clinical teachers is role-modeling. Whether they are conscious of it or not, clinical teachers act as models of the profession for students and house staff. Whatever is taught in the preclinical years of medical school is either accepted or rejected depending on whether they see 'real doctors' doing it. For example, exhortations to 'listen to the patient' will be scoffed at if most clinicians routinely conduct disease-centered interviews and cut off patients' attempts to express their concerns.

In a case-control study of the attributes of excellent attending-physician role models in internal medicine, conducted in four teaching hospitals in Montreal and Baltimore, Wright and colleagues (1998) found five attributes independently associated with being named as an excellent role model: spending more than 25% of one's time teaching (odds ratio 5.12); spending 25 or more hours a week teaching and conducting rounds when serving as an attending physician (odds ratio 2.48); stressing the importance of the patient–doctor relationship in one's teaching (odds ratio 2.58); teaching the psychosocial aspects of medicine (odds ratio 2.31); and having served as a chief resident (odds ratio 2.07). In addition, excellent attending physicians were more likely to engage in activities that build relationships with residents such as organizing an end-of-month dinner with residents, sharing personal experiences, talking about their personal lives, and trying to learn about the lives of the house staff (Wright *et al.*, 1998).

In an accompanying editorial, Skeff and Mutha (1998: 2016) point out that: 'Teachers, even those who are motivated and highly skilled, cannot accomplish these goals without institutional support.' In order to develop and nurture excellent teachers, the institution must reward those who spend time with house staff and in workshops and faculty development activities honing their skills.

In another study of clinical teachers in three medical schools in Quebec, Beaudoin and colleagues (1998) surveyed all senior clerks and second year residents about their perceptions of the qualities of their teachers. Almost half of the clerks and one-third of the residents perceived that most of their teachers did not display the humanistic characteristics that were examined in connection with their roles as caregivers and teachers (e.g. valuing contact with patients as an important part of patient care, concern about the overall well-being of patients and not just their presenting complaints, spending time educating patients about their health problems); 75% of clerks agreed that their teachers seemed unconcerned about how their patients adapted psychologically to their illnesses; 78% felt their teachers did not try to understand students' difficulties; and 77% felt their teachers did not try to support students who were having difficulties. Residents were somewhat less critical suggesting that perhaps they were being socialized to accept these deficiencies in patient care and teaching. The authors speculate: 'Perhaps their perceptions show how difficult it becomes to attain high standards of humanistic care when healthcare personnel must deal with increasing strains, constraints and uncertainties. Under these circumstances, perhaps there are limits to one's caring' (Beaudoin *et al.*, 1998: 769).

Students can have mixed experiences in learning the patient-centered clinical method as opportunities for learning from their role models may vary. In focus group interviews with clinical clerks at The University of Western Ontario, students described their observations of their role models and the conflict they experienced in the transition from theory to practice. As one student said, 'I think we have been trained well but putting it into practice is another story.'

The following comments highlight students' awareness that the patient-centered clinical method is applicable to all physicians and not just family doctors. 'I think that any specialist can be just as patient-centered as the family doctor. It's just how you approach it.' Furthermore, a paucity of role models in the specialties was a concern. 'We don't have the role models in the specialties to reinforce it. I think that time is just an excuse. In an extra minute you can do so much more. Being patient-centered affects everything from helping you with your diagnosis to helping with your treatment plan and management.' As one student observed, 'It's hard to be optimistic about the way we're going to practice patient-centered medicine when we have no role models.' The following comment illustrates the negative effect a role model can have on students when they are attempting to apply patient-centered concepts to clinical practice: 'If you're laughed at by physicians for using this, and they say, "Don't bother with those questions," you stop doing it. Your residents will be directing a lot of your learning along the next two years and when they say, "You don't want to piss off your Attending. He hates those patient-centered questions." So you're not going to ask patients, "What are your ideas about your illness?" ' When role-modeling was effective, it provided a powerful and memorable learning experience. 'One orthopedic surgeon I had for clinical methods, I still remember this, I was FIFEing the patient and I found out that the patient had diabetes and was worried about their upcoming surgery, and possible complications. When I told the surgeon that, he didn't laugh at me; he didn't think it was ridiculous. He then went in to see the patient and said, "So do you have any concerns about the upcoming surgery?" And they talked about it. It only took a few minutes.'

Conclusion

In this chapter we have described some of the challenges experienced by both teachers and learners as they endeavor to practice, learn and teach the patient-centered clinical method. These challenges include personal, professional and systemic aspects. Each one affects the others. Thus solutions are not simple and must include tackling the educational challenges in concert. It is particularly important to recognize the impact of the dominance of the medical model and the powerful influence of role models on the socialization of medical students. Learning to be patient-centered cannot happen in isolation but must be respected and reinforced at all levels of medical education.

Teaching the patient-centered clinical method: practical tips

W Wayne Weston and Judith Belle Brown

In previous chapters we addressed a number of theoretical issues and explored general principles of teaching communication skills; in this chapter we concentrate on the practical application of these principles to the day-to-day challenges of teaching patient-centered medicine in a clinical setting.

The context of learning: the setting and the participants

The learning environment determines what will be reinforced and what will be very difficult to teach or learn. For example, students are unlikely to learn patient-centered medicine in a setting where it is not practiced or from teachers who do not value the principles underlying the method. On the other hand, effective teaching is more apt to occur in a setting that supports and rewards it.

Several issues about teachers need to be considered:

- *Interest and skill in teaching*: Not all faculty members have a talent for teaching; some are more interested in clinical care, research or administration. Academic units need to be set up so that faculty members can focus on what they most value and not be forced to spend too much time on activities for which they have no aptitude.
- *Faculty 'reward system'*: Faculty should be promoted on the basis of excellence in one or two areas of academic work and not be expected to be all things to all people. In many universities, teaching and patient care are undervalued; faculty who devote most of their energies to these areas may

jeopardize their careers. This creates a conflict of interest – spend more time with their patients and students or commit more time to academic areas, such as research, which are rewarded by promotion and tenure. Teaching and practice must be seen as scholarly activities in their own right (Boyer, 1990; Glassick *et al.*, 1997; Hansen and Roberts, 1992; Richlin, 1993). Fortunately, academic culture is changing and, in many schools, faculty are being promoted for their contributions to teaching and education.

- *Opportunities for faculty development*: Teachers are made not born. Without training in teaching, medical faculty tend to emulate previous medical school teachers. Often this means copying less effective approaches. Many faculty members are interested in teaching but find it difficult or frustrating because they have had no preparation for the job. All faculties of medicine need a well-planned program of faculty development with a special emphasis on helping new faculty members learn their academic craft. Faculty members are often selected for their skills in research, administration or teaching. Their reputation as clinicians is considered but their clinical skills are rarely assessed in a rigorous manner. As a result, some faculty members will need additional training to improve their skills in using a patient-centered approach. Even faculty who are intuitively patient-centered will need opportunities to learn the theoretical basis of the model and to master the techniques to pass these skills on to their students. It is very difficult to teach the patient-centered clinical method in an environment that does not enthusiastically embrace the approach or which fails to acknowledge the need for ongoing development and renewal.
- *Time*: A central challenge for academe is to find a way to restore the 'sacred idleness' so necessary for reflection and creativity. Without time for contemplation, teachers end up going through the motions, following algorithms or recipes that are often unproven. Good teaching takes time – to establish intimate relationships, to challenge the status quo and to search the literature for better answers. Teaching the patient-centered clinical method also requires time for observation and feedback.

There are also several important aspects of the practice setting which need to be considered:

- *Setting*: Tertiary care teaching hospitals are becoming less and less appropriate sites for learning about relationships and communication with patients. Patients are either being admitted for day surgery or are so sick that they can barely converse with the doctor. It is next to impossible to develop meaningful relationships with these patients. Alternative settings, which are more conducive to learning the patient-centered clinical method include: physicians' offices in the community, patients' homes, chronic care facilities, and palliative care settings.

Clinicians are busy and not always available when students are scheduled to arrive. Consequently, effective teamwork is needed. Much of the teaching falls on the shoulders of the residents, nurses and other members of the team who are usually given no preparation for the task. They may be unaware of the objectives for the students, and may be asked to evaluate them without being provided with any guidelines. They are rarely given any advice about how to teach. As a minimum, all members of the practice team should be aware of the following:

- when students are going to arrive
- the objectives for the students' experience
- how the students are assessed
- the role of the students on the team and level of responsibility expected of them
- any special tasks or assignments expected to be completed by the students
- in particular, they need to be thoroughly familiar with the patient-centered approach and the various methods used to teach it in that setting.

- *Patients*: Students and physicians learning patient-centered medicine, need opportunities to work with patients of both sexes, all ages, different cultures and with a vast range of problems. Patients also need to be given adequate preparation for, and explanation of, the students' roles and responsibilities. It is helpful to post a sign in the reception area or waiting room proudly announcing the involvement of the practice in the teaching of medical students. Including the current student's name on the sign adds a valuable personal touch.
- *Physical plant*: There must be adequate space for students to be integrated into the setting – they need a place to put their personal belongings as well as a comfortable work space. In ambulatory settings there need to be sufficient examining rooms for students to see patients on their own without interfering with patient flow. Space for debriefing about patients, for feedback about student performance, or for private discussions about students' concerns is essential.

It is impossible to teach the patient-centered clinical method without providing constructive feedback to students. Effective feedback requires repeated direct observation of the student interacting with patients. Opportunities for observation, either with one-way mirrors or videotape, are invaluable. Videotape review, in particular, provides a powerful opportunity for enhancing self-awareness. *See* Appendix 1 for additional information about the use of videotape in teaching the patient-centered clinical method. But, even without such equipment, it is possible to observe student–patient interactions directly by sitting quietly in a corner of the examining room. However, it is often difficult for the teacher to avoid being drawn into the interaction and quickly taking over. Sitting behind the patient may reduce this challenge.

Common teaching methods

There are several commonly used teaching methods – some are very effective but others can be destructive to student learning. (*See* Table 13.1 below.) Great teachers over the ages have used parables – stories with a message – to instruct and inspire their students. 'War stories' may be entertaining and even instructive, but often they are told to enhance the reputation of the teller. A crucial distinction rests in the purpose of the narrative – whether to brag or teach. Using a one-to-one interaction with a student to give a lecture misses out on the major advantages of clinical teaching. Learning is directly proportional to the learner's degree of involvement.

A common distortion of the Socratic method is: 'Guess what I'm thinking!' Rather than probing and questioning learners to help them deepen their own understanding, the teacher asks leading questions or gives hints to help students guess the 'right' answer. One hazard of this approach is that students stop thinking for themselves and, instead, start second-guessing the teacher. Some teachers think that being Socratic means never answering students' questions. Often teachers like this will turn every student question back on the student: 'What do you think about that?' or 'Why don't you look that up tonight and tell me tomorrow what you learned?' Used appropriately, these techniques are invaluable but sometimes students are so confused or overwhelmed that they need more help. Sometimes the answers they seek are not in the books; sometimes, especially in an ambulatory care setting, the student needs immediate advice to help a waiting patient. Sometimes, when teachers never answer students' questions, students begin to think they do not know any of the answers and their credibility and effectiveness as teachers are lost. On the other hand, answering students' questions too often may foster dependence and might convey the message that students are not capable of learning for themselves.

Table 13.1   Comparing common teaching methods

Less effective	More effective
'War stories'	Parables
Mini-lectures	Dialog
'Guess what I'm thinking!'	Guided discovery
'Put down'	Critique the behavior, not the person
Never answering the question	Sometimes answering the question
Grilling	Challenging
Dictating	Coaching

One of the most destructive acts a teacher can commit is to 'put down' a student; students rarely forgive such behavior and will not respect a teacher who does not show respect for them. Students may learn facts from teachers they do not like but they will not heed the teacher's principles or values. It is especially dangerous for teachers to put down one student in front of others; they then lose the respect and credibility of the whole group of students.

While drill may be appropriate for memorizing the dosages of emergency drugs, grilling – putting a student 'in the hot seat' – is usually inappropriate. Those who advocate its use argue that it helps toughen up students and prepares them to keep cool in the stressful situations of clinical practice where they must think and act quickly. In its typical form, grilling involves repeated questioning of one student until he or she gives a wrong answer or 'gives up' by confessing that he or she does not know the answer. The teacher moves on to other students and continues the process until all have been shown inferior to the teacher. This approach is said to motivate students to try harder but usually ends up in a game of clinical one-upmanship and the focus is often on esoteric or trivial information. This approach may encourage competition rather than teamwork, teaches that not knowing is 'bad' and may leave students feeling put down. It is difficult for students to develop comfortable relationships with teachers who utilize this approach excessively. The vast majority of students in medicine are motivated to work hard. Excessive pressure from the teacher is not only unnecessary but may also be counterproductive. An over-anxious student does not learn well. In a supportive environment where teachers demonstrate a genuine interest in the people they teach, students generally blossom and put forth their best efforts. In such a setting, teachers can challenge students' conclusions or even their basic assumptions without provoking so much defensiveness that they cannot learn. An effective challenge preserves, and may even enhance, the learner's self-esteem.

Another important teaching strategy is coaching. The teacher, as coach, works with students to identify skills to be learned and, together, they decide on how best to learn them. For example, a student has difficulty finding common ground with diabetic patients who seem uneasy taking responsibility for self-care. The student has already discovered that providing lots of advice and cajoling patients is ineffective and is looking for more effective strategies. The teacher can direct the student to try specific interviewing methods and perhaps replicate the ineffective strategies the student had tried with patients. Alternatively, the teacher can collaborate as a coach. The coach will assist the student to clarify his or her learning needs and identify specific skills to practice either by using role-play or observing the student with real patients and providing constructive feedback. While teachers who act as directors dictate the learning agenda, coaches support and encourage self-directed learning.

Each of these teaching methods illustrates the distinction between teacher-directed and learner-centered approaches to education as described in Chapter

11. The more effective methods which we have seen in Table 13.1 all focus on the needs of the learner more than the interests of the teacher and are rooted in a fundamental respect for the learner.

Characteristics of constructive feedback

Many of these effective strategies require the teacher to provide constructive feedback as outlined below. This description is based on work adapted by John Casbergue (1978).

'Tell it like it is' is a popular saying. It is based on the assumption that complete honesty is a highly desirable human condition, but it might better be said, 'Don't tell it like it isn't.' Leveling or responding with absolute openness is sometimes inappropriate and may be harmful. This is particularly true in working with people in learning situations in which human beings interact. In learning situations where constructive feedback is essential, what should be avoided is deceiving other people about what you see or what you feel. This brief commentary focuses on characteristics that a physician-educator might consider in giving constructive feedback to learners at all levels as well as to colleagues. The intent is to suggest specific ways for genuine communication to occur between teachers and learners while preventing the learner–teacher relationship from being destroyed by insensitivity or lack of recognition that learners, at all levels, must receive ongoing, constructive and systematic feedback.

The following are among the characteristics of constructive feedback that faculty and students can use in giving feedback. These points can assist faculty in recognizing the role and importance of feedback and to aid them in establishing effective relationships with learners.

1   Feedback should be descriptive rather than judgmental. Descriptions are limited to what was said and done, or how it was accomplished (e.g. 'You presented a very clear outline of the microbiology of pneumonia but you did not mention the role of host defenses.' Another example: 'You started the interview with two excellent open-ended questions but then almost all of your questions were closed-ended and did not give the patient much chance to open up new areas for discussion'). Avoid assumptions about motive or intent (why you think someone did 'that'). By avoiding judgmental language, we avoid having the recipient react defensively (e.g. 'I didn't do that!' whether stated verbally or in their mind).

2   Feedback should be specific rather than general. To be told that one is 'domineering' is not as useful as being told that, 'In the discussion that just took place, you did not appear to be listening to what others were

saying, and I felt forced to accept your arguments.' Or, in providing feedback about a student's interview, rather than saying, 'You aren't interested in the patient's social situation,' it is more helpful to say, 'When the patient indicated he could not afford the medication, you did not respond.' Of course, in order to provide such specific feedback, the teacher must have observed the student firsthand. Secondhand feedback (passing on comments from another teacher) is, at best, of little use and, at worst, misguided and possibly harmful.

3   Feedback should focus on behavior rather than on personality. It is important to focus on what persons do rather than on what we think or imagine they are. Thus, we might say that a person 'talked more than anyone else in this meeting' rather than that he or she is a 'loud-mouth'. The former allows for the possibility of change; the latter implies a fixed behavioral trait. Another example: 'Didn't you see how upset the patient was? How could you be so uncaring as to ignore her feelings by changing the subject and focusing on the functional inquiry?' Such a criticism will upset most students (and any other students within earshot). It would be more helpful to comment: 'I noticed that, when the patient became tearful, you changed the subject. What were you feeling at that moment in the interview?' Chances are, the student was upset too and didn't know what to do and so reverted to the old standby, the functional inquiry. This second approach will facilitate the student disclosing personal feelings and bewilderment that the teacher can help the student to understand and then consider other approaches in the interview.

4   Feedback involves sharing of information, rather than giving advice. Feedback is a gift – it should help the recipients gain a better understanding of themselves; it provides insights into the students' blind spots. By sharing information, we leave individuals free to decide for themselves in accordance with their own goals and needs. When we give advice, we often tell another what to do (we take away some of their freedom to decide for themselves), or we 'put them down' (the perception might be that they aren't bright enough to come up with their own solution). Admittedly, there is a fine line in working with students, but the intent is to move away from advice-giving as a primary form of feedback.

5   Feedback should be well timed. In general, feedback should be given at the earliest opportunity. The sooner it is done, the more details the teacher and learner can remember so that the feedback can be very specific. A chart record or a videotape of the interview can be used to stimulate the student's recall of the interaction and thus make the feedback more valuable. This suggestion depends, of course, on the recipient's readiness to hear it; feedback presented at an inappropriate time may do more harm than good (e.g. 'I see that you just punctured his eardrum.')

6   We should limit the amount of information to how much the recipient can use rather than the amount we would like to give. To overload individuals with feedback is to reduce the probability that they will be able to use any that they receive. When we give more than can be used, we are more often than not satisfying some need of our own (e.g. to control, to direct) rather than helping the other person. Feedback can be destructive when it serves only our own needs and fails to consider the needs of the person on the receiving end. Too often we give feedback because it makes us feel better or gives us a psychological advantage.

7   Feedback should be directed toward behavior which the receiver can do something about. Frustration is only increased when a person is reminded of some shortcoming that he or she cannot easily remedy (e.g. nervous mannerisms, stuttering).

8   Feedback should be solicited rather than imposed. It is helpful to think of the teacher as a coach – someone who is trying to help the students to be the very best that they can be. No one would ever dream of hiring a high-priced coach to give them only compliments about how well they are doing – they expect feedback about their weaknesses so that they can get better. Feedback is most useful (and more easily heard) when the recipients actively seek feedback or have asked observers to answer specific questions for them. Even in a teaching situation, it is helpful to offer the feedback rather than automatically present the feedback. One helpful approach is for the teacher and learner to agree in advance on how and when feedback is to be given/received. Such 'contracting' eliminates misunderstanding or avoidance of very useful and helpful feedback. 'Pendleton's Rules' provide an excellent framework for structuring a feedback session (Pendleton *et al.*, 1984; 68–71). (The learner provides feedback first about what was done well, then the teacher comments on what went well. Next the learner comments on what could be improved and the teacher does the same. Finally, the learner summarizes the feedback, comments on what was learned and what he or she will do to continue to improve.)

9   Feedback can be verified or checked by the recipient. What is heard is very often not what was intended. The recipients should try to rephrase the feedback they are receiving to see if it corresponds to what the sender has in mind (e.g. 'What I hear you saying is . . . '). No matter what the intent, feedback is often threatening and thus subject to considerable distortion or misinterpretation. It is also helpful, when wrapping up a feedback session, to ask the students to summarize what they will take from the discussion and what they plan to do about it, e.g. learning plans.

10 Feedback can be verified or checked to determine degree of agreement with others. Others may not share one person's reaction to a situation. When an action is noted or feedback is given in the presence of other people, both giver and receiver have an opportunity to check with others in the group

about the accuracy of the observed action or feedback. Do others share one person's impression? Such 'consensual validation' is of value to both sender and receiver. It should be recognized that private feedback may be very acceptable to a receiver, whereas it may be very threatening or embarrassing if others are around.

11 Avoid collusion. Collusion is characterized by an unwillingness on the teacher's or the learner's part to take the risk of giving and/or receiving feedback regarding the performance or actions of the other person. This might be characterized by the following. Suppose we have a less than open teacher talking with a learner after observing a rather mediocre performance. Teacher: 'That was okay,' (while really being concerned about the quality of the action). Learner: stays silent, while really thinking, 'That really wasn't too good – I wonder what he or she really thinks?' In this situation, the teacher and learner are colluding by remaining silent or indirect at a time when both (but particularly the learner) could benefit by open communication.

12 Feedback skills can be improved by paying attention to the consequences of the feedback. The person giving feedback should be acutely aware of the effects (verbal and non-verbal) of the feedback. It is often helpful to check out the recipient's reaction, i.e. to receive feedback on feedback. This is most effective when there is trust in the relationship.

13 Constructive feedback is an important step toward authenticity. It opens the way to a relationship which is built on trust, honesty and genuine concern. Through such a relationship, we will have achieved one of the most rewarding experiences that a person can achieve and will have opened a very important door to personal learning and growth.

A compendium of teaching strategies

There are a great many ways to help students learn the patient-centered clinical method at all levels of education. Many of these learning methods involve practice followed by feedback. In the structured environment of the preclinical curriculum, it is relatively easy to teach the basic skills of patient-centered care, e.g. in clinical skills courses. But, in the hurly-burly of clinical education, these skills may be easily ignored. Table 13.2 outlines several practical methods to incorporate the teaching of patient-centered medicine into day-to-day clinical education.

The roles of patient, student and teacher

Teaching in the ambulatory setting involves a complex triadic relationship between teacher, learner and patient. The teacher in this context is responsible

Table 13.2 A compendium of teaching strategies

Method	Indications	How
Demonstrations of skills by faculty	To help a novice learner understand what they are trying to learn. To demonstrate to an experienced learner that there is still more to be learned	Prepare the learner for the observation – discuss with them what to watch for in the demonstration. A 'debriefing' afterward is helpful to consolidate the learning and to respond to questions
Role-plays	To provide an opportunity to 'try out' a new skill in a safe situation and receive immediate feedback about how to improve before trying the skill on a patient	Teachers need to be aware of the common 'first time' skills of students at different stages in their learning and have examples of role plays to practice, e.g. exploring the illness experience with a patient who has chronic relapsing disease
Standardized patient interviews	To practice more complex skills which are difficult for amateurs to role-play, e.g. an angry or depressed patient	Lay out the 'ground rules' carefully first. Allow 'time-out' if the student-doctor is stuck. Provide constructive feedback allowing the 'doctor' to go first. Some standardized patients are trained to provide constructive feedback
Patients playing a role, e.g. a recovered alcoholic playing the role of an alcoholic in denial	To practice complex skills with a real patient and get feedback from the patient. All of these role-playing approaches can be used to provide experiences with important but uncommon situations which the student might otherwise not experience	These patients are carefully prepared in the same way as standardized patients. But they are playing 'themselves' at an earlier phase in their illness when they were still having problems coming to terms with their diagnosis. Because of their personal experiences they are able to create more depth to the role and provide invaluable insights about the impact of interviewing methods on patients with similar problems
Extended discussions with patients	To help students understand the impact of illness on the lives of patients	Set aside 45–60 minutes for the student to have an extended conversation with a patient (or group of patients with the same problem). The focus should not be on the diagnosis but on the patient's unique illness experience. Seeing more than one patient with the same disease will highlight the distinct impact of the same disease on different individuals

Table 13.2 (*continued*)

Method	Indications	How
The student presenting the patient by role-playing the patient	To help the student experience the patient's situation and to give the other team members an opportunity to practice interacting with the patient's 'proxy'	The student is instructed to interview the patient in sufficient detail and depth to be able to role-play the patient for the team. Other team members interview the student who is in the role of the patient. The focus can be on the interview or on the diagnosis or both (information about physical examination and lab findings are provided when requested)
Presenting a short video clip of an interview with a patient	To provide feedback on patient-centered skills and to demonstrate them to the other members of the team. It is helpful if the faculty members also show segments of their own interviews	This requires a setting in which video cameras are mounted on the wall of the interviewing room. Students are encouraged to view the tape themselves first and to select a short segment or segments to show to the team. The segments can be as short as one or two minutes to illustrate a particular skill or can be 20 to 30 minutes long if there is time. The other team members provide constructive feedback
Using the 'Patient-centered case presentation' (*see* Chapter 14)	To practice 'seeing' patients in a broad context which includes the humanistic aspects of illness. This is a powerful way to reinforce the other teaching strategies listed here	This approach adds to the traditional case presentation of the disease. It incorporates a description of the patient's experience of illness and the family and community context. Developmental and relationship issues and finding common ground about management are also included
Screening exercise with real patients	To provide practice using screening methods with real patients	Assign the student to approach two patients on the ward and screen them for (e.g.) alcohol problems. Ask them to describe the screening technique used and the results obtained. Ask how they might apply what they learned to other patients. Option: the interview could be audiotaped and constructive feedback provided

Table 13.2 *(continued)*

Method	Indications	How
Observed interviews with real patients followed by constructive feedback	'Real' patients are often more challenging and unpredictable than standardized or role-played patients. It is important to consolidate skills learned in simulated situations by using them in the 'real' world	Faculty can observe directly or by videotape or monitor. Alternatively they can hear about the interaction from the student describing what happened
Self-reflection and reading	To enhance self-awareness and to consolidate learning from the other methods. New ideas from the literature can also be learned this way. It is important to begin self-directed learning during medical school in preparation for a lifetime of learning after graduation	Provide time for thinking and reading. Annotated reading lists are invaluable for helping students quickly find readings that match their needs. Convenient access to Medline searching is also invaluable. Include discussion of articles about communication at journal clubs. Model self-reflection
Evidence-based discussion	To help learners realize that patient-centered care is a science as well as an art	Refer to the increasing volume of research in patient–physician communication

not only for the quality of the learning experience but also the quality of patient care. It is important to patients for the teacher to be clearly involved in their care. Teacher and student may take on a variety of roles depending on the situation and the educational goals.

Observation: The teacher acts as a role model and provides the patient care. The student observes. This is especially useful to help clarify objectives by demonstration. New students benefit from this but so also do seasoned learners who are trying to learn from teachers a skill that is difficult to describe in words.

Partial care: The student provides a portion of patient care, e.g. taking a history and performing part of the physical examination. This is especially suited to inexperienced students who need help with management decisions. It is also a useful format for practicing a newly learned skill.

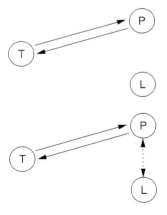

Collaborative care: Teacher and learner together provide care, e.g. discussing management options and finding common ground with a patient. This allows the student to see how it is done and to be actively involved at the same time. The teacher may gradually withdraw and give more responsibility to the student. The roles of teacher and learner need to be clearly understood and their relationship should be secure before attempting this approach.

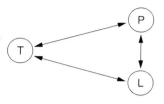

Supervised care: The teacher provides 'back-up' and may double-check portions of the history and physical examination, but the student provides the majority of care. This is appropriate for situations where the patient problem is within the competence of the learner. The teacher monitors the care for a variety of reasons – to respond to learner's questions, to provide feedback to the learner or to reassure the patient about the quality of care.

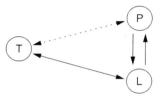

Facilitator: The teacher functions as a facilitator of learning rather than as a physician. The learner provides full care to the patient. This situation is appropriate where the patient problem is well within the competence of the learner. The teacher observes in order to provide constructive feedback.

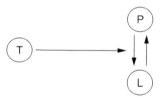

Tips on clinical supervision

When a student is seeing a patient in the hospital and/or clinic setting and comes to the supervisor, the following process is suggested.

- First clarify the patient's situation and the major problems to be addressed. Guide students to present the case in an organized fashion without unnecessary detail. Students should also learn to recognize their specific learning needs and to address these at the start of a case presentation so that the teacher can focus on them.
- Ask the patient's name. In settings where patients are well known, the teacher will have a vast store of knowledge about previous illnesses, life experiences and typical responses to stress. Knowing which patient the student is discussing will often generate key hypotheses about the current

situation. This process models the importance of continuity of care and the value of the patient–physician relationship.

- Avoid premature conclusions. One of the hazards of familiarity is the danger of drawing conclusions before fully exploring all possibilities of the current situation. It is often useful to brainstorm – considering all options without the constraints of what is probable or practical.
- Refrain from being the fountain of all knowledge. It is important for students to take ownership of their own learning and to relate the current clinical situation to their own experiences.
- Ask students to 'think out loud'. This will often reveal to them where they are stuck.
- Provide a conceptual framework. Decision trees and diagrams are helpful to organize masses of data or to uncover gaps in information. Use the chalk board for clarification. When students are confused or unclear about a patient's problem, it is often useful to depict the situation as shown in Figure 13.1. In these situations it is common to have a large mass of data about the patient's diseases and even some ideas about the patient's illness experience. But often, the sections on 'Person' and 'Context' are sparse. This visual representation assists the student to recognize the deficiencies in their understanding of the patient and suggests areas for further inquiry. The diagram can also be used to document the accumulating knowledge about the patient. When a student is having difficulty working with a patient, the source of trouble is often related to finding common ground. Box 13.1 illustrates a useful grid for identifying disagreements between patient and physician regarding management. In our experience, difficult interactions are reflected by differences of opinion about the nature of the problem, the goals of treatment and/or management and the respective roles of the patient and doctor. Filling in the grid makes the conflict obvious and leads naturally into a discussion about how to deal with their differences.

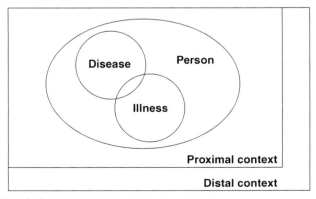

Figure 13.1 The whole person.

Box 13.1   Finding common ground

Issue	Patient	Doctor
Problems		
Goals		
Roles		

- When students reach the limits of their knowledge, ask how they are going to seek more understanding of the issues. Schedule a definite time to follow up on what they learn. When the decision cannot wait, you may need to offer a suggestion. If possible, offer options and encourage students to choose from them and to explain their choices. Use questions to clarify what students are saying rather than to probe their ignorance.
- Chart review is particularly helpful for assessing the strength of the evidence for the student's diagnostic conclusions and proposed investigation and management. The traditional record needs to be modified to fit the patient-centered clinical method. For example, students should include information about the patient's 'illness experience' (feelings, ideas, effects on function, and expectations).
- Videotape review is vital for helping students examine their own reasoning process. Videotaping the consultation has the special advantage of allowing students to monitor their own performance, with the teacher acting as a facilitator. It also enables the teaching occasion to be postponed until more time for the analysis of the tape is available. The videotape stimulates recall of the student's thought processes during the interview and can be used to challenge them about why they asked certain questions, why they ignored others and why they did not ask questions which were on their minds. *See* Appendix 1 for a detailed discussion of the use of videotape review in teaching and learning the patient-centered clinical method.
- Role playing with simulated patients offers students the possibility to practice in a safe situation and to try several different approaches to the same situation. The opportunity to stop for a 'time out' is valuable for reflecting

on the interaction and to receive feedback from the 'patient', teacher and other observers. This technique is also helpful to learn how to manage clinical situations that are uncommon and may not present themselves to every student.

- Learning from role models should not be a passive activity. Students must be prepared, by their teachers, to focus on specific behaviors and then have an opportunity to discuss their observations. For example, before the teacher and student enter the examining room, it is helpful to explain what the teacher will be attempting. For example, if the student has already seen the patient but been unable to determine the patient's experience of illness, the teacher may remind the student about the four dimensions which need to be explored and briefly outline the kinds of questions which could be asked. Following the encounter, they will discuss the student's observations and the teacher's reasons for certain actions.

Conclusion

In this chapter we have highlighted a number of practical guidelines for teaching the patient-centered clinical method. Effective teaching and learning require an environment which provides the necessary resources – patients, time and space. It must also reward faculty for contributing their energies to becoming exemplary role models and clinical supervisors. It may be possible to teach some of the elements of the patient-centered clinical method in the absence of this infrastructure, but without it, success is limited.

14

The case report as a teaching tool for patient-centered care

Thomas R Freeman

This chapter presents a potentially powerful tool for teaching patient-centered concepts: the patient-centered case presentation. The chapter begins with a review of the evolution of case presentation approaches, next presents the patient-centered case presentation with an example and concludes with an assessment of the advantages of such an approach.

Review of case presentation approaches

The traditional format of the case presentation which evolved during the time of Sir William Osler was recognized very early as a valuable tool in the teaching of medicine (Cannon, 1990). It generally begins with a brief description of the patient, followed by the history of the present illness. Next comes past history, family history, patient profile and examination findings. Investigative results such as laboratory work, x-rays, pathology reports, a problem list and management plan usually round out the presentation. This form of presentation accurately reflects the conventional clinical method which is based on the biomedical model (McWhinney, 1988).

The written medical record was greatly improved by the method described by LL Weed (1969), and his Problem Oriented Medical Record has been widely accepted. This method made problems the organizing principle of the record and separated subjective and objective elements. This form of written record has had a great influence on the format of oral case presentations, as well.

The bio-psychosocial model proposed by Engel (1977) was an attempt to apply systems theory to clinical problems. This model, along with the recognition that psychological and social factors play a role in illness events, has led to the inclusion of these topics in many case presentations.

The conventional case history or report has been criticized for being heavily dependent on scientific language which, although seemingly precise, leaves much of reality aside (Schwartz and Wiggins, 1985). Abstract scientific language excludes the human, lived experience of patients and obscures the fact that where illnesses are unique, disease labels are classificatory terms only (McCullough, 1989). This problem is as true of chronic illness as it is of acute illness (Gerhardt, 1990). By minimizing the importance of the patient's story and subjective experience, the conventional case history separates biological processes from the person (depersonalization) and minimizes the physician's role in producing findings or observations (Donnelly, 1986). This form of presentation is primarily doctor and disease-centered. 'The message is clear, disease counts; the human experience of illness does not' (Donnelly 1986: 88).

Hawkins (1986) advocates a method she calls the clinical biography in which the scientific and humanistic are complementary, each representing different attitudes to the human experience. She points out that case history and biography are similar in that they involve a lot of interpretation and are to be understood in the 'context' of the narrative.

From a phenomenological perspective, the clinical encounter can be viewed as a hermeneutical exercise involving the interpretation of multiple 'texts'. Such a hermeneutic model poses a number of questions, the most important being: 'How can the ill person, both as text and co-interpreter, be restored to centrality in the clinical encounter?' (Leder, 1990).

Efforts to change the focus of case histories to include more accurate descriptions of patients as persons, range from the elegant literary work of Luria (Hawkins, 1986) and Sacks (1986) to the innovative and pragmatic teaching methods of Donnelly (1989) and Charon (1986).

Donnelly (1989) suggests that the human aspects of medicine can be addressed by teaching stories (which pay attention to what has happened in the interior world) instead of chronicles (which stick simply to a recitation of events). He asked house staff to include, in the history, one or two sentences about what the patients ' understanding of the illness was and how it affects their lives in an effort to help the physician empathize more accurately.

Charon (1986) states that the physician's effectiveness increases with empathy and teaches the 'empathic stance' by asking medical students to write stories about their patients. These stories are considered as adjuncts to the hospital chart and do not replace the traditional case write-ups. Charon has suggested that the students are molded into the kind of doctor their teachers want by becoming the kind of writer their teachers want (Charon, 1989). Narrative medicine has developed a literature in its own right (Charon, 2001; Greenhalgh and Hurwitz, 1998), and has helped inform our understanding of how we seek meaning in the events of our lives. For the most part, however, the narrative format lacks the structure desirable in transmitting important knowledge quickly in clinical settings. There remains the need for a bridge between the thin description of the traditional case presentation and the thick description of the narrative approach especially in the teaching of students and house staff. Basic changes have to occur in the way that medicine is taught.

Anspach (1988) points out that the presentation of case histories is an important part of the medical training of students, interns and residents. Usually presented before an audience of peers and senior medical people, these presentations are important for both their content and as part of the socialization process. They are a powerful way of teaching and reinforcing a particular worldview. With the evolution of the clinical method, it is an appropriate time for a change in the way that case histories are presented to reflect more accurately and reinforce the patient-centered clinical method and the worldview on which it is based.

Description of the patient-centered case presentation

In a sharp departure from the conventional case report, which focuses on the organic pathology of the patient, the patient-centered case presentation (PCCP) gives primacy to the patient and the total experience of the illness and associated pathology. Unlike the conventional method, in which 'the objective truths of medicine are recorded in the "language of abstraction"' and are not 'related to the existence of the individual patient' (Wulff *et al.*, 1986: 132), the PCCP regards objective truth as of less interest when it is not related to the individual.

The PCCP focuses on an 'acquaintance with particulars' (McWhinney, 1989a). It begins with a description of the particulars of the case under study and then proceeds to a discussion of the general, i.e. other cases or studies that may share similar features. There may be a discussion of a single case or several cases that seem to express a common theme.

The PCCP, by going from the particular to the general and from the subjective to objective and back again, performs a cycle that ultimately informs the presenter with a greater understanding of the patient.

Table 14.1 compares the conventional case presentation and the patient-centered case presentation and highlights how the items of information of the conventional approach are incorporated into the PCCP.

1   *The patient's chief concern or request*: This consists of a brief statement of the symptomatology as well as the illness behavior (McWhinney, 1972) that brought the patient to the encounter. It should address the patient's actual reason for coming.

Table 14.1   Comparison of conventional and patient-centered case presentation

	Conventional case presentation	*Patient-centered case presentation*
1	Chief complaint	Patient's chief concern or request
2	History of present illness	Patient's illness experience; quotes from the patient; feelings, ideas, effects on function, expectations, meaning of illness
3	Past medical history: medications, allergies; observations	Disease: • history of present illness • past medical history • review of systems • physical exam • laboratory etc.
4	Family history	Person: • patient profile • individual life cycle phase
5	Patient profile	Context: • proximal (e.g.): – family history – genogram • distal (e.g.): – culture – ecosystem
6	Review of systems	Patient–doctor relationship (the clinical encounter); the dyad itself; transference/counter-transference issues; finding common ground: problems, goals, roles
7	Physical exam	Assessment (problem list)
8	Laboratory database	General discussion; illness experience; literature (pathographies, poetry); medical literature (clinical epidemiology, pathophysiology, other case reports, medical anthropology)
9	Problem list	Proposed management plan
10	General assessment	
11	Proposed plan	

2   *The patient's illness experience*: A description of the experience of the illness should include some quotations from the patient which particularly illustrate the subjective quality of the illness. For example, when discussing an individual for whom pain is a predominant feature, it would be appropriate

to include the pain descriptors that the patient used in communicating the discomfort. Metaphors are particularly helpful here as they are linguistic structures that bear epistemological weight (Carter, 1989; Donnelly, 1989). Knowing the metaphors that patients use to describe their illness gives the clinician greater insight, understanding and empathy. The language for the metaphoric landscape is 'not found in traditional textbooks of medicine, but in articulate memoirs of illness, insightful fiction, poetry, drama and the examined experience of our own illnesses and those of our family and friends' (Donnelly, 1989: 134–5). As in the patient-centered clinical method, the patient's feelings, ideas, effects on function and expectations are mentioned here including the meaning of the symptoms to the patient.

3   *Observations*: The observation portion of the presentation involves the Disease, Person and Context dimensions shown in the diagram which presented an overview of the patient-centered clinical model (Figure 1.1 in Chapter 1). This section is subdivided into observations about the disease, including the standard elements of the medical history (history of present illness, past medical history, review of systems, physical exam and relevant laboratory work), issues related to the person (patient profile, life cycle phase), and context, both proximal (e.g. family, employment) and distal (e.g. culture, ecosystem).

4   *The patient–doctor relationship (The clinical encounter)*: This involves a discussion of not only the technical management issues (e.g. drug and non-drug therapies), but also a discussion of how the patient–doctor dyad can be developed into a healing relationship (Cassell, 1985b). Issues of self-awareness, feelings about the patient and struggles to make effective connections are appropriate, as are any issues related to finding common ground between the doctor and the patient. *See* Chapter 6 for a detailed description of finding common ground and Chapter 8 for more on enhancing the relationship.

5   *Assessment (Problem list)*: This section summarizes the issues that need further assessment or intervention in any of the four areas of disease, illness, person or context.

6   *General discussion*: Having discussed the particulars of the case, the presentation then turns to the general issues raised by the case. The issues selected for discussion are chosen by the presenter from elements of the case which he or she found most interesting or puzzling. In this way the case helps to instruct the presenter. General issues can be subdivided into those that relate to the experience of the illness and those issues related to pathophysiology, epidemiology, sociology and medical anthropology.

First person accounts of the experience of illnesses are becoming more common. Literature and poetry provide many examples of individuals who have written in a lucid and illuminating way of their personal experience of an illness (Broyard, 1992; Cousins, 1979; Frank, 1991; Mukand, 1990;

Styron 1990). Indeed, this type of writing has recently undergone a resurgence and an acquaintance with it will provide the presenter with improved insights into the way in which the illness is affecting their patient. It will be necessary for faculty to accumulate a usable bibliography of such material as it appears not only in journals but also in newspapers, magazines and books (Baker, 1985). In addition, the movie industry has focused on this area and occasionally a short video can very effectively communicate the trials of a particular sickness.

This section of the PCCP includes a discussion of any relevant medical literature pertaining to the case. It should incorporate the current understanding of any pathology or clinical epidemiology (i.e. prevalence, natural history, the sensitivity and specificity and predictive value of any tests, effects of intervention).

This section also demonstrates a knowledge of the published scientific literature concerning the disturbed psychological and social functions that have been observed in other individuals with similar problems.

7 *Proposed management plan*: This is an opportunity to use the information gleaned from the discussion of the general issues and to integrate this knowledge into a management plan.

An example

The following example of a PCCP is derived from the author's practice. The presentation begins with a description of the particulars of this case. This is followed by an outline of some of the general issues raised by the case. Many of these issues have been identified by residents when this case has been presented to them. In a full case presentation it is expected that the presenter will choose one or more of the issues to discuss in detail. The general issues chosen should be decided by the presenter and reflect that person's learning needs. I have emboldened keywords in the patient's discourse that he used repeatedly to describe his understanding of the situation.

1 *Patient's chief concern/request*: Brian (a pseudonym) was a 26-year-old man attending the office because he had become more interested in doing something about his **lifestyle**. This was precipitated by recent laser surgery for treatment of diabetic retinopathy. As a result of the laser treatment, his vision had become more blurry, leading to some difficulty reading and causing him to rethink what was going on with his life.

2 *The patient's illness experience*: To a great extent, Brian's illness experience revolved around his feelings and ideas about diabetes and the meaning, to him, of this label.

When asked about the personal meaning of diabetes he replied: '... a change in lifestyle ... your life has to be more routine ... eating ... exercise ... you have to **control** eating, **control** your insulin. At one point it [diabetes] was running my life; I wavered from letting it run my life to wanting to make it a very minimal part; now, I'm trying to find a **balance** between a routine and not letting it run my life.'

His greatest fear developed after receiving laser treatments, when his vision became blurred. 'Oh, my God, I'm going to go blind.' Some of this blurring had resolved. He had since learned that, to a certain extent, this was to be expected after laser treatments. He expressed some anger at not being warned of the side effect of the procedure. He understood that the blurring may also have been related to **control** of his blood sugar. Even though some of the blurring had cleared, it forced him to consider some of the long-term consequences of diabetes. 'My vision could become bad enough that I couldn't read.' This fear took on even greater dimensions in view of his recent decision to become a teacher. The consequences of his recent treatments made it necessary that he sit at the front of the classroom. He denied that this change was a concern, but one sensed that this denial was wearing thin as evidenced by the fact of his attendance to the office at this time.

3   *Observations (Disease)*:

a   *History of present illness*: He was diagnosed with insulin dependent diabetes mellitus at age 11. He had been on varying doses of insulin since that time. In his early adolescence, there were several episodes of hypoglycemia.

His experience with visual difficulties was the most recent reminder of diabetes. When this first developed, he was new to the city and attended a walk-in clinic and was subsequently referred to an ophthalmologist.

b   *Past medical history*: Aside from his diabetes, his past medical history was without significant events. There had been no surgery. There were no known drug allergies.

Current medications: Insulin Lente 15 units, Crystalline 15 units in a.m.; Lente 20 units, Crystalline 15 units in p.m. He only occasionally checked his blood sugars with a glucometer at home when he felt that it was particularly high (he associated this with feeling 'sluggish', e.g. 'in my mind I visualize my *blood getting thicker*.'). He was evasive when pressed about what levels of glucose he was finding at these times but finally recalled numbers in the 300s or 400s on the 'old scale'.

c   *Review of systems*: Aside from some persistent blurred vision, ROS revealed only occasional intestinal gas every three to four months.

d   *Physical exam*: Brian presented himself in a detached manner. Even when talking about his fear of blindness, he talked in a monotone. He was clearly articulate and intelligent, but left you with the impression that he distanced himself from his feelings as much as possible. He declined being weighed but appeared to be 10 to 15 pounds overweight. BP 126/ 82. Examination of the optic fundi revealed numerous microaneurysms but no hemorrhages. He declined any further examination at that time.

4 *Person*: Over the past 15 years Brian's experience and understanding of the disease had undergone some changes. As a child his mother was deeply involved with the treatment of his diabetes. This was not without its problems. He stated that when it was time for him to leave home and go to university, one of the best parts was that his mother would not be there to **control** his diabetes.

He came to this city to start his university education and was involved in a program that emphasized tight control and careful monitoring of diet and exercise. Brian felt that this approach was consistent with other parts of his life at the time, in that he could keep fairly consistent hours. However, when he had finished his undergraduate education his life became less controlled and predictable and so did his diabetic control. He found that close control interfered with his **lifestyle** and he felt at that point in his life that he needed more spontaneity and that routine was not consistent with this. This coincided with frequent moves and an uncertainty about where he was going in his career. He 'let go' of routine and his lifestyle became scattered. He did the minimum required to manage his diabetic condition – took his insulin and watched his diet – but exercise and rest were ignored.

Brian described himself as an optimistic person. He said that he bored easily and this was why he had gone through a period of frequent changes, although he thought that presently he was fairly settled. Recently he had married a woman who was a social worker and had taken a job with a local social agency. Brian felt more settled in terms of his career and his personal life. He felt that things were 'on track'. Being married provided more routine. He had started teacher's college this past fall.

Brian viewed himself as a lot like both of his parents. 'I want to deny that I'm like my father but . . . ' He felt that he shared with his father the orientation that 'my motivation comes from inside me. I know that I should look at external factors, but I don't. He's organized and so am I.' Like his father, Brian sometimes liked to be alone.

5 *Context*: His family of origin consisted of his parents and two sisters. His older sister developed hydrocephalus and epilepsy, both of which were under control. She currently worked for the Board of Education in a neighboring city. His younger sister was alive and well. His father was 56 years old and had been diagnosed as having hypertension and circulatory problems. He had 'several times been close to a heart attack'. Brian attributed this to his father's 'self-imposed stress . . . he isn't very social and he doesn't get much exercise. I think that's contributing to his problem.' His mother was 55 years old and basically healthy although she used to be overweight.

6 *The patient–doctor relationship*: 'I don't like people helping me. I'm really strong about that.' He was unable to think of any way that his doctor could be of help to him except for 'routine medical problems'. This clearly excluded helping to manage his diabetes as he made clear that that would be too much like his mother and he refused to let that type of relationship develop again. This suggested some developmental and some transference issues.

He did not comply with a request to have some basic blood work done although he took a laboratory requisition with him. He was invited several times to return for a complete physical assessment or simply to talk but, so far, has not done so, continuing to attend for minor episodic problems. To date, common ground has not been found and agreement on the goals and priorities has not been reached.

7 *Assessment (Problem list)*:
   a insulin dependent diabetes mellitus
   b diabetic retinopathy/threatened visual loss
   c unresolved family of origin issues
   d questionable compliance with diabetic regimen
   e failure to find common ground about management.

8 *General discussion*: In an oral case presentation, it is expected that the pre-senter would fully discuss at least one of the issues raised in this section. The others may be outlined.
   a *The experience of the illness*: Two prominent issues that are suggested by this case with respect to the experience of the illness are: the issue of control and the fear of visual loss.

   The potential or actual loss of control is a characteristic of most illnesses whether acute or chronic. It is essential that physicians recognize the centrality of loss of control to any state of illness. Part of the physician's role as a healer is to restore a sense of control to the patient (Cassell, 1985b).

   Compelling accounts of what it means to be blind or to face the imminent loss of vision are common in literature and poetry (Longhurst and Grant, 1989). Occasionally there appear, in the lay press, eloquent first person descriptions of individuals struggling with the fall-out of diabetes (Fields, 1990).

   A familiarity with such material will serve to inform the physician tending to Brian and to deepen his or her understanding of the subjective aspects of this man's illness. It may help the physician to provide advice on the day to day coping with the problems caused by the illness.

   b *The observations*: From the standpoint of the biomedical model some of the issues that this case raises are: euglycemia and diabetic retinopathy, the use of laser technology in treating such retinopathy and the common sequelae of this procedure.

Under the heading of contextual issues could be considered the family and the child with chronic disease (Battle, 1975; Leichtman, 1975).

Many of the life phase issues which Brian is facing are related to late adolescence. Consideration of the adolescent coping with chronic illness would therefore be appropriate here (Wolfish and McLean, 1974). The developmental tasks of identity and the capacity to form intimate relationships may be thwarted by an excessive pre-occupation with illness and the sick role.

c *The patient–doctor relationship*: Stein (1985b) argues convincingly for physician awareness of the unconscious communications taking place between the patient and the doctor which influence the illness/disease process. One of the cases he reports ('The Contest for Control: a case of diabetes mellitus in multiple contexts') is an excellent introduction to consideration of the relationship issues with patients such as Brian.

9 *Proposed management*: In a situation such as has developed with Brian, it is clear that common ground has not yet been defined. It becomes necessary for the physician to go back and find common ground with the patient on each of the three areas: problem definition, goal setting, and roles.

As Brian enters the early adulthood phase of his life it will be particularly important that his physician develop a congenial relationship and avoid an authoritarian one which would echo the type of relationship he experienced with his mother and which he has spent at least six years trying to escape. The management can be summarized in Box 14.1.

In a formal case presentation, therefore, a presenter could choose to expand on any one of the identified topics (the issue of control in illness experience, fear of

Box 14.1 Finding common ground with Brian about management

Issue	Patient	Doctor
Problems	Diabetes mellitus Interference with lifestyle	Diabetes mellitus Poor adherence Complications
Goals	Fewer symptoms Less interference with lifestyle	Better glucose control
Roles	Independence Self-control	Provide information Gentle challenge but avoid paternalism

visual loss, euglycemia and diabetic retinopathy, laser treatment of diabetic retinopathy and sequelae of treatment, the family and child with chronic disease, adolescence and chronic disease and transference/counter-transference issues). A review of such topics will help to inform more fully the development of a management plan.

In using this method of case presentation with residents my experience has been that there is a tendency to avoid topics pertaining to the experience. This avoidance is best dealt with by stating the issue in the beginning, when the method is first presented and by meeting with the learner/presenter at least a week before the presentation to go over the proposed case and direct him or her to the appropriate resources.

Advantages of the patient-centered case presentation

Case presentations can be viewed as 'highly conventionalized linguistic rituals' which serve to socialize physicians in training to a particular worldview (Anspach, 1988). The PCCP, by placing the patient at the core of the presentation, reinforces the primacy of the person rather than the disease, without excluding the process of clinical decision making. In this way it can serve to inculcate a more humane form of medicine and reinforce the basic values inherent in the patient-centered clinical method. It does this without sacrificing the more conventional type of information found in the standard case presentation.

In most medical schools, learning is largely passive (i.e. lectures) in the initial years. This gradually gives way to the less structured format experienced in clinical rotations and residency training in which the learner is expected to take a more active part in learning. It is not an unusual experience after starting into practice, to feel somewhat at a loss as to how to continue to be well informed. The rapid expansion of medical knowledge makes it impossible for any individual to always be completely up-to-date. Therefore, it is necessary that the practicing physician have a method for continuing medical education which takes into account one's individual learning needs. Most experienced physicians acknowledge that their most demanding teachers are ultimately their patients. The PCCP offers a format that can serve as a bridge between the passive learning of medical school and the active learning of medical practice. It recognizes the role of the patient in teaching us what we most need to know.

The usual reasons for making a case report are: a unique case; a case of unexpected association; or a case of unexpected events (Morris, 1991). The philosophy of the PCCP is that every case is unique and may, and often will, involve the unexpected. The only necessary motivation for undertaking a PCCP is a desire to come to a deeper understanding of the patient.

Teaching experience with the patient-centered case presentation

The patient-centered case presentation is a regular part of the teaching program for senior residents in family medicine at The University of Western Ontario. Residents have appreciated this component of their structured teaching because of the variety of topics covered and the fact that they themselves control the topics based on their own clinical experience and self-perceived learning needs.

Residents in their second and final year of training are introduced to this method of case presentation making clear how it differs from the usual case presentations they have done elsewhere in their training. A case is presented to them using the PCCP format and they are each assigned a date to make their own case presentation. They are asked to reflect on a case that they have encountered in their training that caught their interest or is memorable in some way. Then they are asked to consider what aspect of the case stimulated their interest and from that derive a learning issue that they then research and present to their peers. They are explicitly asked to ensure that the case is presented in such a way that the audience appreciates the patient involved as a person, rather than simply a disease label.

Due to time constraints, each presentation is given 15–20 minutes including time for questions. In many cases, more time is desirable to discuss a case fully, but one advantage of the shorter presentation time is that many more topics are covered. Depth of material is sacrificed for breadth. If more time is made available, it is reasonable to expect that the material covered would be more comprehensive.

The following summary is based on 73 such presentations made by residents in family medicine. Some cases involved more than one diagnosis. There are a number of ways to classify learning topics (Northrup *et al.*, 1983). One method is by identifying the organ system involved, another way is to categorize by whether the question raised involves assessment/diagnosis or treatment/management. Of the 73 presentations, 41 dealt with assessment/diagnosis issues and 48 with treatment/management issues.

The classification by system involved uses the categories of the International Classification of Primary Care (ICPC) as this provided a diagnostic vocabulary most suitable for the setting of the participants. The two most common categories were: psychological and neurological (*see* Table 14.2). In addition to the problems listed below, nine of the cases also dealt with what can best be described as issues of process and ethical issues. Examples were:

- continuity of care in a 70-year-old man with bursitis
- how aggressively to pursue investigations of vague complaints in an 84-year-old with advanced Alzheimer's disease

Table 14.2   Residents ' case presentations by category (ICPC)

ICPC system	No. (%)
Psychological (P)	17 (21)
Neurological (N)	12 (15)
General* (A)	8 (10)
Pregnancy (W)	8 (10)
Digestive (D)	5 (6.25)
Respiratory (R)	5 (6.25)
Musculoskeletal (L)	4 (5)
Endocrine/metabolism (T)	4 (5)
Female genital (X)	4 (5)
Social (Z)	4 (5)
Blood/blood organs (B)	3 (3.75)
Cardiovascular (K)	3 (3.75)
Male genital (Y)	2 (2.5)
Urinary (U)	1 (1.25)
Total:	80 (100.0)

* 6 of the 8 problems in this category were adverse events of medical interventions such as drug reactions.

- organ donation in a 48-year-old woman dying of astrocytoma
- naturopathy in a 72-year-old man with cancer of the colon.

A few residents addressed issues that related to physician discomfort or the patient–doctor relationship. Examples of this were:

- the physician's discomfort with domestic violence issues
- how intrusive a physician should be with a 23-year-old woman with an unwanted pregnancy and a history of sexual abuse
- learning to use one's intuition when uncertain of diagnosis
- how to cope with patients complaints against the physician when he/she feels that everything has been done correctly.

It is clear that while some cases presented by these groups of learners were very similar in content to the traditional case reports, many more focused on patient-care issues that revealed a more patient-centered focus. Learners' needs vary and teaching techniques need to be flexible enough to take this into account. The PCCP allows a learner to choose from a broad range of topics as well as depth of inquiry. By providing a structure consistent with patient-centered medicine, PCCP ensures that the principles of this approach are reinforced.

Conclusion

The patient-centered case presentation suggests a way of presenting case material in medicine that is consistent with new clinical methods. It recognizes that case presentations are an important part of the socialization of training physicians. By giving primacy to the subjective aspects of illness, this form of presentation reinforces an attitude of 'patient-centeredness'.

This way of presenting a case forms a useful 'bridge' between the passive and detached learning characteristic of much of undergraduate medical training and the active, personal learning required of a practicing physician.

Acknowledgments

Parts of this chapter have been previously published in *Family Practice: An International Journal* (1994) 11(2).

15

Developing a patient-centered curriculum

W Wayne Weston and Judith Belle Brown

Patient-centered medicine is not simply an 'add on' to the curriculum; it can be its very core. In fact, unless the underlying values of the curriculum reflect commitment to the patient as the center of medicine's professional work, all efforts to produce a different kind of doctor, one sensitive to the needs and concerns of patients, will fail. Patient-centered values are often incorporated into courses on communication but are rarely integrated with other pre-clinical courses. During clerkship, students are often exposed to role models who demonstrate a traditional disease-centered method of care. These role models may even put students down for 'wasting time' on patients' ideas and concerns. The curriculum must be of-a-piece, presenting a unified and consistent message about the importance of a patient-centered approach to care. In this chapter we will outline the principles of curriculum development and will illustrate the theoretical principles with a case study of the curriculum renewal in the Faculty of Medicine and Dentistry of The University of Western Ontario. We will present our failures as well as our successes in the hopes that our experiences of both will be instructive.

Curriculum derives from the Latin verb 'to run', as in a race – an apt description of the experience. The word is used in various ways by different authors at different times and may refer to a collection of courses or to the entire course of study over the years of medical school. The broader definition can also include the methods of teaching and assessment as well as the underlying philosophy on which the curriculum is founded. Stenhouse defined curriculum as 'everything that is happening in the classroom, department, Faculty or School, or the University as a whole' (Stenhouse, 2001: 338). We will use the term 'curriculum' in this broad sense.

A patient-centered curriculum

How can an entire curriculum be patient-centered? Isn't there a risk of watering down the basic sciences or ignoring traditional subjects when more time is devoted to teaching students to be patient-centered? When is enough enough? Isn't there a risk of turning students off by spending too much time on this topic and leaving out organic medicine? These are all valid concerns. Sometimes it seems that there is so much to learn about human biology and pathology that there is no time left for anything else. Being patient-centered does not mean giving up traditional biomedical studies. Patients expect physicians to be experts in the pathophysiology of disease. But, as explained throughout this book, they expect physicians also to be experts in the experience of illness. Therefore, curriculum planners must find ways to integrate the study of biomedicine with a study of the human condition and the responses to illness and suffering. Lowenstein describes how he addressed similar concerns:

> Physicians today, in their roles as teachers, complain that they feel overburdened by their responsibilities for the care of patients whose illnesses are complex and often require the expertise of teams of specialists. Many physicians are intimidated by the very large body of knowledge they must master and transmit to students and house officers. One way of coping with these very understandable feelings is to narrow one's focus, to deal with only that part of the disease one knows best and leave the rest to others with different areas of expertise. This does not work well in the care of patients, nor does it make for good teaching or role modeling. To focus on a specific problem, no matter how important or interesting, it is usually necessary to direct attention away from the patient where all problems intersect. (Lowenstein, 2002: 24–5)

He goes on to describe how he altered his ward teaching to include at least some small reference to the patient as a person:

> I remember vividly the first morning when I interrupted an intern in the middle of his opening sentence, 'This is the first admission of this thirty-five-year-old IVDA . . .' I asked, 'Would our thinking or care be different if you began your history by telling us that this is a thirty-five-year-old Marine veteran who has been addicted to drugs since he served, with valor, in Vietnam?' There was an embarrassed hush. As I left the ward later that morning, I reflected that the few minutes taken up by my question might have been my most important contribution of the day, possibly more instructive than my comments about pneumocystis pneumonia, arterial oxygen saturation, or respiratory alkalosis. I have continued to insist that patients be 'personalized' in case presentations and find that I have been able to integrate details about

patients' perceptions, responses, and needs without sacrificing attention to other aspects of clinical medicine. (Lowenstein, 2002: 26)

Most medical schools teach interviewing in the first two years in clinical skills courses and provide opportunities to hone these skills in the clerkship. Other courses that may focus on related skills and concepts include: medical humanities, behavioral sciences, and courses focusing on self-awareness. Usually there is little connection between these courses and the big courses on physiology, anatomy, pathology, pharmacology and the courses related to the major clinical disciplines. Problem-based learning provides a method of learning which has the potential to integrate these subjects but often the students focus most of their attention on biomedical topics.

Why do students concentrate on biomedicine and tend to disregard everything else? Where do they get the message that interviewing, medical humanities and behavioral science are less important than traditional courses? Even in curricula that espouse a patient-centered mission, students do not take these subjects as seriously as the big biological courses. A key to understanding this puzzle is the environment for learning in medical school. One of the key features of the learning environment is the hidden curriculum which reflects beliefs and values that may support or criticize the official curriculum or bring an alternative perspective to the learners (Hafferty, 1998). The same phenomenon is found in all professional schools. Writing from the perspective of nursing, Bevis and Watson describe the hidden curriculum in these terms:

> It is the curriculum in which we are unaware of the messages given by the way we teach, the priorities we set, the type of methods we use, and the way we interact with students. This is the curriculum of subtle socialization, of teaching initiates how to think and feel like nurses. It is the curriculum that covertly communicates priorities, relationships, and values. It colors perceptions, independence, initiative, caring, colleagueship, and the mores and folkways of being a nurse. It is taught by subtle, out-of-awareness things that pervade the whole educational environment: when classes are scheduled, how much time is given a subject in relationship to other subjects, how many test items are assigned a topic or whether or not a term paper is given to the area, who addresses whom in what way, how the teacher responds to students who openly differ in opinion from the teacher, how students are or are not encouraged to work together, and how teachers interact with students. All of these give the value messages to students that shape their learning in this curriculum. (Bevis and Watson, 2000: 75–6)

In medical school, the central concept that permeates the deep structure of the hidden curriculum is the notion of disease – ferreting out and 'fixing' the patient's disease becomes the pre-eminent focus of the physician's purpose

(Armstrong, 1977). The importance of the human connection between doctor and patient, emphasized in the official statements of curriculum committees, is easily lost during the commotion of clinical education. When the focal point is disease, students learn to see the world as a dichotomy between those who have a disease and those who do not. The dilemma they face is that they have no categories to describe people who are ill but have no disease – why would such a person seek assistance from a physician? It makes no sense from a purely biomedical perspective. The teachers' challenge is to confront the hidden curriculum by making it explicit so that students will consider alternative conceptual frameworks.

Principles of course design

In this next section we outline the various domains of learning the patient-centered clinical method. There are knowledge, skills and attitudes to be acquired and each demands specific and unique conditions to facilitate learning (Haney, 1971; Gagne *et al.*, 1992; Gagne and Medsker, 1996). For example, learning a new concept, such as the distinction between disease and illness, requires a much different educational experience than learning a skill, such as responding with empathy. Thus, it is important for teachers and learners to recognize these differences between the types of learning in planning any instructional event. Because a learner-centered approach requires collaboration between teacher and student, it is important for both teachers and students to be conversant with these distinctions.

Verbal information

These are ideas, propositions, 'facts' – the basic alphabet of knowledge. Without knowing the names of things, it is difficult to communicate with others in the field or to learn more complex knowledge. For example, the terminology used in the patient-centered clinical method of practice provides teachers and learners with a common vocabulary for discussion. Much of this material can be effectively learned from lectures and reading and benefits from repetition.

Intellectual skills

These are discriminations, concepts and rules – the ability to interact with the environment using symbols. Individuals possessing intellectual skills have a sufficient understanding of a body of knowledge that they can elucidate principles and identify novel examples of concepts. For example, the student will be able to discuss the four dimensions of patients' illness experience – feelings, ideas, effects on function, and expectations – and be able to recognize each element in their encounters with patients.

This type of learning is facilitated by stimulating recall of previous related knowledge and guiding the new learning by a statement, question or cue. Concepts 'discovered' in this manner, as compared with being learned in a lecture, are more accessible to learners when they need to retrieve the concept in a new clinical situation. Providing occasions for learners to perform their just-learned skill in connection with a new example is invaluable. For example, after a student has learned the concept of finding common ground, it is invaluable to provide opportunities to practice applying the concept with several patients. Forgetting to apply the newly learned skill is often stimulated by their discomfort with feeling awkward or incompetent. It is useful to remind students, just before seeing a patient, about the concepts they will be trying out.

Problem-solving skills

These are the abilities to use verbal information and intellectual skills to deal with a situation which is novel to the learner at that point in time. Problem-solving is a complex process that includes the capability to recognize the problem, skill in generating alternative solutions and judgment in selecting an appropriate option. Attitudes relating to the content of the problem, self-confidence and comfort with uncertainty will all greatly influence the learner's ability to deal with a specific problem at a specific time (Haney, 1971). Prerequisite intellectual skills and verbal information are needed to solve specific problems. For example, when students are learning to reach mutual agreement with patients regarding treatment, it is useful for teachers to remind them about the three aspects of finding common ground – problems, goals and roles. This will be of particular importance when learners find themselves disagreeing with their patients about one or more of these aspects. Learners will need the skills to recognize when these prerequisites are missing and should be able to seek them out appropriately. There is no substitute for practice, using problem-solving skills in a variety of novel situations.

Psychomotor skills

This is the ability to coordinate muscle movements in a smooth, regular and precisely timed fashion, e.g. using body language and communication skills. Students need to know what the skill looks like. Written educational objectives or a description of the skill may help but a demonstration is even more helpful, especially for novices. Students need to learn each of the 'part' skills and also the order in which each part is performed. Learning is facilitated by repeated practice in a situation that provides feedback. Feedback is absolutely essential to effective learning of psychomotor skills. The nature of the feedback should be varied, depending on the level of skill of the learner. Novices will need fairly detailed and specific feedback about their performance – what was done well and what needs more practice or additional skills. As learners improve and develop a clearer idea of what a good performance looks like they will be more aware of their own shortcomings. At this stage they need guidance to improve specific, discrete skills and practice putting them all together. It is important to distinguish between application and acquisition practice. Acquisition practice occurs when a student is first learning a skill. It is useful at this stage of learning to practice one component of a skill at a time and to do it over and over again. Simulated patients are useful for this type of practice, but even real patients can be used. Students can be asked to concentrate on a specific part of the patient-centered clinical method, e.g. determining patients ideas and expectations about the visit. Application practice is done to consolidate learning of 'part' skills in a coordinated and integrated manner similar to the manner in which the skills will be used in the application setting. It is important to recognize students' levels of skill. They should not be expected to perform a complex communication skill on a real patient, e.g. breaking bad news, if they have not had an opportunity to practice the essential 'part' skills first, e.g. empathy and support. Coaching is also vital; learners need someone to provide continuing feedback and moral support in the setting in which they will apply their new skills.

Attitudes

These are internal states that influence the choices of personal action made by individuals – predispositions to approach or avoid a situation. A number of attitudes have been identified as important for effective practice, e.g. a willingness to become involved in the full range of difficulties which patients bring to their doctors and not just their physical problems. Attitudes may be learned from an emotionally toned experience following a course of action. For example, while a doctor was conducting a routine cervical smear he uncovered a history of brutal childhood sexual abuse. Following self-disclosure of her story the patient began to weep and then sobbed uncontrollably for some time. The doctor was overwhelmed by the patient's story and felt anguished and helpless. From that point on he was extremely reluctant to inquire about the sexual histories of his female patients. Another example is the satisfaction and sense of connectedness experienced by physicians when patients gain insight into the relationship between their physical symptoms and prior traumatic events thus freeing them from years of suffering. *See* Chapter 12 for a discussion of the importance of role models in learning attitudes.

The principles of course design may be summarized as follows. The needs of the learner and the tasks of the teacher will vary with the desired learning outcome (Gagne *et al.*, 1992; Gagne and Medsker, 1996). Facts are effectively learned from books and lectures; principles are learned by struggling with the material and applying it to new examples; problem-solving is best learned by trying to solve problems in a variety of situations; psychomotor skills are learned by practice in situations which provide feedback; attitudes are usually learned by interacting with respected models. Hence teachers must be prepared to fill many roles – resource person, facilitator of learning, manager of learning resources, provider of feedback, and role model.

Example: curriculum renewal at The University of Western Ontario

Shifting focus from general principles to an actual example of curriculum renewal at The University of Western Ontario Medical School, we will examine the history and context in which the changes occurred and briefly describe the mission of the curriculum. Then we will outline the role of new courses in reinforcing the patient-centered philosophy.

> A curriculum that is static gradually declines and dies. A successful curriculum is continually developing. It must respond to evaluation results and feedback, to changes in the knowledge base and the material requiring mastery, to changes in resources (including faculty), to changes in its targeted learners, and to changes in institutional and societal values and needs. A successful curriculum requires understanding, sustenance, and management of change to maintain its strengths and to promote further improvement. Related activities, such as development of the environment in which the curriculum occurs, faculty development, networking with colleagues at other institutions, and scholarly activity, can also strengthen a curriculum (Kern *et al.*, 1998: 99).

The history and context

The Medical School at The University of Western Ontario (Western) is an old school by Canadian standards, having been established in 1881. The curriculum was the traditional 'two plus two' falsely attributed to Flexner (Flexner,

1910; Jonas, 1978) – two years of basic science followed by two years of clinical learning. Although Western had a reputation as a fairly conservative school, it was the first Canadian school to establish a division of family medicine within the Department of Epidemiology under the leadership of Ian R McWhinney in 1968. In 1999, Western became the first Canadian school to have a woman family physician, Carol Herbert, as its Dean. Thus, Western represents a unique mosaic of conventional traditions and forward-thinking approaches. A 'new' curriculum in the 1970s moved the clerkship from the fourth year to third year and introduced a 'back to basics' block in the fourth year. The next curriculum change, in the early 1990s, introduced Problem-Based Learning (PBL) one day a week in the first and second years but faced the difficulties common to many schools that developed a 'hybrid' curriculum that combined PBL with traditional teaching methods. Partly because of poor integration of PBL with the rest of the curriculum, the accreditation team demanded significant changes in the curriculum and this served as the impetus to change once again in the late 1990s. A new Assistant Dean was appointed to lead the process. He was the first to admit that he knew little about curriculum but he was an expert in leading diverse groups to a consensus, having been involved as a leader in the difficult changes associated with hospital restructuring. He created a process that included over 200 faculty members as well as many students and lay persons. He had also been the coordinator for the clinical methods course in the first and second years and had been responsible for incorporating the patient-centered clinical method as a new framework for that course. He wanted to use the patient-centered clinical method as a framework for the whole curriculum.

There were several factors that influenced Western to make the patient-centered clinical method a core principle in the undergraduate curriculum. First, there was an accumulation of evidence supporting the importance of patient-centered practice. Second, society had changed – patients were expecting to have more involvement in decisions about their care. Third, and perhaps most importantly, the patient-centered clinical model proved to be a clear model that all participants could support. It was the 'common ground' on which the Faculty developed a common vision. At the time Western was developing its new curriculum, all five Ontario medical schools were collaborating in the EFPO (Educating Future Physicians for Ontario Project) – one of the largest and most ambitious educational projects ever conceived (Maudsley et al., 2000; Neufeld et al., 1998). The goal of this well-funded ten-year project was to change medical education in Ontario, making it more responsive to the needs of Ontarians. The project provided funding for educators at each school to devote time to curriculum development and to meet and learn from one another. The needs of the people were articulated in terms of eight physician roles (expert, communicator, advocate, collaborator, gatekeeper, scholar, scientist and person) which formed the focus for curriculum innovation, faculty development and student assessment. The project spawned the CanMEDS 2000 Project (CanMEDS, 2000) which redefined the competencies of specialists in Canada in terms of similar physician roles. This was an exciting time of renewal in medical education in Ontario which provided a supportive climate for the type of change Western was planning. Both projects, rooted in the recognized needs of the people, legitimized the primacy of the patient in medical care and education.

Curriculum renewal at Western involved making changes in several aspects of the curriculum: changing the process of selecting students for admission to the school; restructuring content into system blocks; adding a 'case of the week' as a focus for small group discussions of illness issues related to the disease topics of the week; synchronizing the skills learned in the clinical methods course with the topics covered in the rest of the curriculum; adding a new course on 'Health, Illness and Society' into the first and second years and a new elective course on 'Ecosystem Health' in the fourth year; including teaching of the patient-centered method in the clerkship in addition to Years 1 and 2.

Mission of the curriculum

The mission of curriculum renewal at Western was to create an integrated curriculum that was patient-centered in content, student-centered in delivery, and accountable to the community.

Mission statement of the Western curriculum

Medicine is a calling, a call to service. The patient-centered curriculum reflects this noble tradition of commitment to individual patients, their families and community. The physician's covenant is a promise to be fully present to patients in their time of need – to 'be there', even when the physician can offer no cure, to provide relief whenever possible, and always to offer comfort and compassion.

The patient is the center of our clinical work and, consequently, the center of our learning. Patient-centered care requires a relationship in which patients will feel that their concerns have been acknowledged and that the physician has understood their plight from each patient's own unique perspective. Patients and physicians must work together to find common ground regarding management – reaching a mutual understanding of their problems, goals of treatment and respective roles of patient and physician. Patient-centered care also incorporates the concept of ecosystem health which studies human health within the interrelations between economic activity, social organization and the ecological integrity of natural systems.

Our curriculum is a reflection of our responsibility to attend to our patients' suffering in the broadest and deepest sense. Our graduates must have a thorough understanding of the biological, behavioral and population sciences basic to medicine. They will apply their medical learning within the integrated context of patient's lives, families and communities and they must also begin a lifelong quest to understand the human condition, especially the unique responses of patients to their illnesses (The University of Western Ontario Medical School Calendar, 2002).

Admissions

The admission process gradually changed at Western to reflect a growing awareness of the importance of the humanistic qualities of our students. Instead of relying primarily on grade point average, we placed more emphasis on the student interview and a student essay. As a result, the average age of our incoming classes increased and they were more diverse. In addition, for a variety of reasons, the proportion of women in the class increased to approximately 50%.

The patient-centered clinical methods course: Year 1

The clinical skills course was revised and based on the patient-centered model. A standardized patient program was developed and cases were written to illustrate the components of the patient-centered clinical method. The course was divided into three segments. First was five weeks of classroom instruction – lectures providing an overview of the patient-centered clinical method and included video demonstrations and role plays. This was followed by four weeks of small groups composed of four students each where the students had an opportunity to role-play a patient. Students were prepared for these role play experiences by the coordinator of the standardized patient program. The cases played by the students needed to be common enough problems that the students would require minimal instruction or knowledge about the disease but could be familiar with the illness experience. The case content of the student role plays included problems such as upper respiratory infection, chest wall pain, headache and problems sleeping. As a result, they were often able to get 'under the skin' of the patients they were playing and experience their dilemmas first hand

and also, when being interviewed by their classmates, feel what it is like to be interviewed by skilled or not so skilled students. Finally, there were eight weeks of small group teaching with 16 standardized patient role plays. The objectives of the course were to provide students with advanced skills in communication particularly with emphasis on the first two components of the patient-centered clinical method – exploring disease and illness and understanding the whole person. Key to the success of this course was the development of cases that would reflect a wide range of problems both acute and chronic. The standardized patient role plays were much more complex including drug seeking, 'non-compliance', woman abuse, Alzheimer's disease, sexual abuse, an angry patient, a seductive patient, breaking bad news, and obtaining informed consent for patient's wishes regarding resuscitation.

The format of the eight weeks of small-group teaching consisted of groups of eight first year medical students, with two instructors per group, meeting three hours a week over an eight-week period. During each session, two standardized patients would be interviewed. At the end of each interview, the student would experience constructive feedback, beginning with the students' own observations, followed by group and instructor feedback and concluding with feedback from the standardized patient. Approximately 90 course instructors were recruited from family medicine, internal medicine, psychiatry, pediatrics, emergency medicine and anesthesia. As much as possible, co-facilitators included both male and female teachers in each group, each from a different discipline. Inexperienced teachers were paired with experienced teachers. All the instructors participated in a day-long faculty development workshop which included a review of relevant research relating patient-centered medicine with patient outcomes (similar to Chapter 17), an overview of the patient-centered clinical method and a videotape demonstration. The session also included working with several of the standardized patient cases that would be used in the course. During the workshop, participants had an experience that paralleled what the students were exposed to at the outset of the course and what they would be teaching in the upcoming course.

The eight-week advanced communications course has been highly rated by both faculty and students. They view the role plays as very effective and the use of standardized patients as important. In addition, they find the standardized patient feedback very useful. Students feel that they have gained knowledge about component 1, 'Exploring both the disease and the illness', but feel less confident in their skills in 'Finding common ground' (component 3). This is not surprising given that they are just concluding their first year of medical school and have not had adequate knowledge and/or exposure to therapeutics. Faculty viewed the use of small groups as appropriate and perceived having a co-facilitator to be an important advantage. Over 80% of the instructors reported a desire to teach the course again in the future.

'Case of the week' and 'Patient-Centered Learning'

Each week during first year begins with a case, usually a real or standardized patient, who is interviewed by the teacher or one of the students in front of the whole class. The interview focuses on the patient's medical history and also on their illness experience. After the interview, the class, guided by the teacher, outlines a number of key objectives for personal study in preparation for small group discussion at mid-week and a wrap-up discussion at the end of the week. These small group discussions, labeled Patient-Centered Learning (PCL), replaced the Problem-Based Learning (PBL) tutorials of the previous curriculum and some of the old PBL cases are still used. One principal objective of these sessions is to explore the common experiences of illness related to the diseases being discussed each week. In addition, these sessions provide opportunities to explore broader social and ethical issues related to the case of the week. These sessions work well when the case is well-developed and the teacher is familiar with the purpose of the PCL discussions. But, with faculty turnover and increased workloads, this is not always true and sometimes the case of the week is focused primarily on disease. This is a good example of the need for continuing faculty development and careful monitoring of any new curriculum innovation. There is a tendency to slip back into the old familiar patterns.

'Health, Illness and Society' course

This course, modeled after the 'Health, Illness and Community' course developed at the University of Toronto (Wasylenki *et al.*, 1997), provides students with opportunities to learn about the social determinants of health through longitudinal exposure to patients in the community and placement with community agencies. These experiences help students to learn about component 2 of the patient-centered clinical method – understanding the whole person.

'Ecosystem Health' course

This course expands the context of the patient to include the ecosystem and challenges students to ask, 'What can I do to prevent others from getting my patient's disease?' The course builds on the patient-centered clinical method by adding additional rectangles to the whole person figure to include both proximal (i.e. employment, social support) and distal (i.e. community, culture, ecosystem) factors of the patient's context.

The clerkship

We still face the challenge of incorporating the patient-centered clinical method into all services in the clerkship for all the reasons already described in earlier chapters: entrancement with the medical model; false perception that being patient-centered would take too long; and lack of understanding or skill in using the method. The key is the resident group who do the bulk of clerkship education. We have begun the process of providing workshops to faculty and residents about how to teach the patient-centered clinical method in the clinics and on the wards. Students have begun to criticize services that do not provide good role models of patient-centered care and this may be a potent force for change. Patients are more vocal about their expectations and complain more often when they are dissatisfied. More articles on communication are being published in mainstream journals and the evidence is irrefutable that good communication results in better outcomes. All of these forces should help to bring about changes in the next decade.

Lessons learned

Curriculum renewal requires more time, energy, and commitment than most of us imagine. It is a huge undertaking that taxes even the most idealistic faculty member. Mutual support and encouragement are essential to sustain the effort. Faculty members will play various roles – innovators, sponsors, champions, and key opinion holders. Each group will assume a unique and important role. It is also important to recognize that some faculty will never change. Pay attention to the skeptics – they often have important questions that need to be answered. But do not waste time and effort on the cynics who only want to subvert the process. Nurture the leaders who are essential to the change process, rather than trying to satisfy everyone.

Strong support from the Dean is essential. Without it, strong department chairs opposed to the changes may block curricular reform. For a patient-centered curriculum to flourish, the curriculum as a whole must present a congruent message across disciplines and throughout all years. Several forces were present at Western that posed challenges to this principle. There was a vocal minority of faculty, in both basic science and clinical departments, who cast doubt or openly disagreed with the patient-centered approach. The clerk-ship posed the greatest challenge in part because a large number of faculty and resident teachers had not been exposed to the concepts of patient-centered medicine.

Students play a pivotal role as partners and ambassadors. They have the most to gain or lose in a new curriculum; consequently they are deeply committed to making the reforms effective. Also, they are still full of energy and idealism and can sustain the momentum when faculty members are starting to fade. Their role as ambassadors is particularly important when students make the transition from the classroom to the clerkship; they can carry the message about patient-centered care to the residents on each service. Also, they can use the official curriculum, which pledges to be patient-centered, as a standard to be achieved when they evaluate each service.

It is helpful to involve lay persons on key curriculum committees. They remind the faculty of the importance of sticking to the mission and reduce the bickering that sometimes takes over committee deliberations.

It is well known that student assessment drives the curriculum – students focus their time and energy on those topics that are evaluated most thoroughly. This posed our greatest challenge. The knowledge, skills, attitudes and values taught in the clinical methods course or in the other courses mentioned above do not lend themselves to multiple choice or short answer exams. Students quickly realized that they could coast through these courses while they concentrated on what they considered to be the hard biomedical courses. It is ironic that what students considered to be the softer subjects are in reality so much harder to learn and assess. While Objective Structured Clinical Examinations (OSCEs) offer a rigorous approach to assessing communication skills, they are very labor intensive and expensive, thus reducing the frequency with which they can be used.

A strong, well supported program of faculty development is essential for the ongoing success of any curriculum innovation. Faculty members need to have opportunities to learn the new skills needed for the new teaching methods. Even more important, faculty development helps to bring about the needed changes in the academic environment of the medical school. D'Eon and colleagues present a strong case for viewing faculty development as a social practice:

Faculty development should not be an isolated event in the lives of teachers (as is currently often the case because of limited understanding of the nature of the practice). It would be an ongoing matter of groups of teachers spending time questioning and clarifying the purpose of the teaching that they do, and explaining, criticizing and justifying activities in the light of a renewed understanding of purpose and context. One teacher's performance would improve, not only because she had learned a new strategy, but as a result of her critical and collegial examination and understanding of a wider range of norms that influence what she does in the classroom. Teaching practice would improve but not as a result of prescriptive rules being invoked to mandate certain actions. Teaching would improve because teachers better understand their purpose and the activities that achieve it and are able to reform the normative standards of the practice. To reiterate, rules and norms, as social constructions, can be changed, but only when they become subject to collective criticism and redevelopment. (D'Eon *et al.*, 2000: 160)

Conclusion

This chapter has outlined some core principles of curriculum development and how to create a patient-centered curriculum. Using the experience of curriculum renewal at the Faculty of Medicine and Dentistry at The University of Western Ontario we have explored some of the successes in implementing a patient-centered curriculum as well as the challenges and lessons learned.

PART FOUR

Research on patient-centered care

Introduction

Moira Stewart

The following section summarizes the research relevant to the patient-centered clinical method. Researchers from a variety of research backgrounds have asked questions about the nature and impact of the kind of medical practice that we call patient-centered.

Oversimplifying somewhat, one can argue that there are two broad analytic perspectives that need to be present in a doctor's mind to support patient-centered practice. To gain an integrated understanding of the patient's problem, the doctor needs to seek information from the patient about both the disease and the illness experience, weaving the conversation back and forth between these two broad areas of inquiry. (*See* Figure 3.1 on page 41.) Analogous to this distinction between disease and illness experience is the distinction between the perspective of doctors as they participate in patient-centered visits, i.e. the perspective of analytic thinking about the disease and the perspective of empathetic listening about the illness experience. *See* Figure A, overleaf. Doctors will have to weave back and forth between these perspectives during any patient encounter. Similarly, the evidence base needed by medicine to attain high quality patient-centered care will have to provide relevant research findings from epidemiologic and basic sciences to support the analytic thinking about the disease, as well as from qualitative research (including narratives) to support empathetic listening to the patients' illness experience. *See* Figure B overleaf. A research program aimed at enhancing patient-centered practice, therefore, ought to include both epidemiologic and qualitative methodologies weaving back and forth between these two broad research traditions as the research questions dictate.

Hence, this section will first summarize the evidence from qualitative studies which illuminate patient-centered principles in practice and next turn to a summary of evidence from the epidemiologic tradition on the impact of patient-centered communication on a variety of important outcomes. Our hope is that these two current reviews will help clinicians first learn about the distinctive

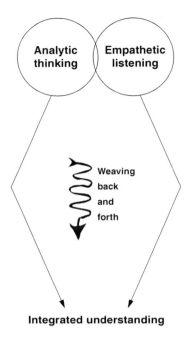

Figure A   Perspectives of physicians.

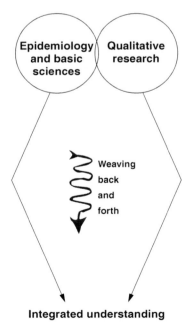

Figure B   Evidence base for patient-centered care.

contributions from both these traditions before creating their own integrated understanding which underpins quality patient-centered practice.

Next, this section presents updates on the research measures which we have developed, tested and used in a variety of medical settings.

Finally, this section provides a summary of results from our research program leading to the research questions which we believe need to be addressed in the future.

16

Using qualitative methodologies to illuminate patient-centered care

Carol L McWilliam and Judith Belle Brown

In the past decade, professionals from all health and social service disciplines have made tremendous progress in advancing knowledge through application of qualitative research approaches. This chapter presents an overview of the current state of the art in using qualitative methodologies to illuminate and develop the theory and practice of patient-centered medicine.

Of the three paradigmatic options available to researchers wanting to apply qualitative research methods, perhaps the easiest option for those living and pursuing their careers in the Western world is to apply descriptive qualitative research methods within the post-positivist, or Western Scientific paradigm. As the following sections reveal, researchers have taken fairly extensive advantage of this option for investigating patient-centered care in recent years. But human inquiry invites the adoption of two less familiar paradigms as well, specifically the interpretive paradigm and the critical paradigm. These options have seen more limited application in medical fields.

Parallels between the patient-centered method and humanistic inquiry invite the application of qualitative methods in investigating patient-centered care in all three of these paradigmatic options. The patient-centered method is a process of acquiring qualitative knowledge and understanding of a fellow human being. Patient-centered care focuses on the patient's disease and illness, and the patient as a whole person. In interpretive humanistic inquiry, the researcher and research participant together strive to capture the needs, motives, and expectations of the participant to construct the interpretation of their experience. The patient-centered processes of finding common ground and building a relationship have similarities to the process of interpretive inquiry. In both interpretive research methodologies and clinical practice of the patient-centered method, interpretive or hermeneutic analysis is a central component (Good *et al.*, 1985) of achieving the desired outcome, be it good research or good care. The 'high context' nature of patient–doctor communication invites research in both the interpretive and the critical paradigms, as in all patient–professional communication, much is influenced by the hidden, invisible dimensions of 'external' and 'internal' context.

Those whose practice affords more prolonged and/or more intensely patient-centered contact have begun to make much more use of methodologies in these research paradigms. Interpretive research methodologies aim to promote understanding of subjective, intuitive, dynamic, interrelated, context-dependent experiences of human life. The patient–doctor encounter constitutes one such experience. Researchers have used interpretive research to elicit particulars about human nature and experience, extracting meaning and understanding from words, behaviors, actions and practices of people (Zyzanski *et al.*, 1992).

The critical paradigm presents researchers with the opportunity to achieve both qualitative understanding and quantified generalizable results about human experiences of social injustices, particularly unconscious or hidden exercise of power and control contained in social relationships. Undertaking research in this paradigm would enable researchers to uncover understandings of the potential for power imbalances in the patient–doctor relationship. The potential of research conducted in this paradigm challenges researchers and practitioners alike to illuminate the importance of patient-centered practice as a means of preventing or overcoming human experience of social injustice in the process of seeking and receiving healthcare. However, to date, there has been very limited application of this paradigm in research in the field of patient-centered care (Waitzkin, 1984), notwithstanding the powerful syntheses provided by Candib (1995) and Malterud (1994).

The following sections illustrate how the application of qualitative research methods has begun to advance the theory and practice of patient-centered medicine. As well, the examples presented illuminate new directions for qualitative research to further our understanding of patient-centered care.

Capturing the needs, motives and expectations of patients as individuals

Qualitative methodologies are helpful in gaining a greater understanding of the needs, motives, and expectations of patients and, to date, have proven to be particularly helpful in identifying the specific needs of patients whose care may present particular challenges for physicians. Four examples in the current literature illustrate the utility and applicability of qualitative investigation with this emphasis.

Peremans *et al.* (2000) used focus groups and basic content analysis to identify the needs and expectations of adolescent girls concerning contraceptive use. Findings revealed that knowledge concerning the daily use and side effects of contraceptives was insufficient. Much more pressing needs articulated in the focus groups were: assurance of confidentiality; adequate time for consultation; guidance and support for overcoming fears about the gynecological examination; and anxieties associated with waiting to be seen. Findings describe the important priority that this patient population places on their needs for patient-centered care.

Insights gained in another focus group study of pregnant women's needs, motives and expectations related to maternal serum screening similarly add to physicians' understanding of the uniqueness of their experience (Carroll *et al.*, 2000). Researchers uncovered three factors influencing women's motives for undergoing or declining prenatal genetic screening: personal values, attitudes, beliefs and experiences; social support from family and friends; and the quality of the information provided by their physicians. In addition to the desire for quality information, the expectations of this patient population encompassed the right to make an informed choice, and the sensitivity of physicians to their individual needs. As in the previous example, both the expectation of patient-centered care and what constitutes a patient-centered sensitivity to unique needs, motives, and expectations are readily apparent.

A third example (Boon *et al.*, 1999) illustrates how grounded theory method can be used to illuminate the social processes of cancer patients' enactment of effort to meet their own needs, motives and expectations for care. Findings more peripherally showed how patient-centered physicians may engage these patients as partners in achieving their own priorities for care, exposing the intricate details of decision making to use or not use complementary/alternative medicine (CAM). Furthermore, the findings revealed helpful and non-helpful responses of healthcare practitioners to what participants experienced as their personal responsibility or desire for control in managing their own care. Patients' need for guidance when making decisions about using specific CAM therapies was particularly apparent, highlighting the importance of health professionals' willingness and preparedness to meet this need in a patient-centered way.

Finally, in a substudy of a multimethod comparative case study of community-based family practices, researchers (Smucker *et al.*, 2001) used the hermeneutic interpretive analysis strategy of immersion and crystallization to explore and characterize patient–physician encounters with frequent attenders in family practice. Findings revealed that the nature of these visits could be differentiated on three dimensions: biomedical complexity; psychosocial complexity; and the degree of dissonance between patient and physician. Six typologies of visits were identified including: simple medical; ritual visit; complicated medical; the tango; simple frustration; psychosocial disconnect; medical disharmony; and the heartsink visit. While not generalizable, these interpretive findings afford many insights into what elements of patient need may enter into the patient–physician relationship, and how these elements may unfold in the office encounter with frequent attenders. The interpretation provides a framework that may help physicians to sort out the needs, motives and expectations of frequent attenders and to develop patterns of and parameters for communication to achieve their goals for patient-centered care.

Understanding the patient as a whole person

Understanding the patient as a whole person invites the application of qualitative research methodologies to elicit a more in-depth picture of the larger life context than is immediately apparent. Insights acquired through qualitative investigations not only add to the practitioner's understanding of the specific individuals who have participated in the study, but also have the potential to be applicable in achieving a greater holistic understanding of other patients who may share similar life contexts.

Three studies illustrate the applicability of qualitative research for enhancing understanding of the patient as a whole person. A focus group study (Brown et al., 1997a) conducted with seniors and informal and formal caregivers explicated the barriers and facilitators of seniors' independence in obtaining appropriate medical, home-based and public healthcare. The study findings described four main themes characterizing the barriers and facilitators to seniors' independence: personal attitudes and attributes; service access issues; challenges in communication and coordination; and continuity of care. Findings from the basic content analysis conducted in this post-positivist study typify the utility of this approach to qualitative research for understanding the patient as a whole person. The comprehensive overview of barriers and facilitators obtained in the study may guide physicians' explorations of the experiences of their older patients, thereby enabling them to focus and individualize their care in ways that optimize their patients' independence in seeking out and following up on appropriate heathcare.

In another substudy of the previously mentioned multimethod comparative case study, Main et al. (2001) used participant observation of encounters in community-based family physicians' offices to elicit findings that enhance understanding of the patient as a whole person. Team analysis of field notes uncovered the contextual involvement of patients' families in facilitating healthcare. Findings revealed how physicians may use the patient's family as social context: to illuminate the patient's disease, illness and health; to discover the source of an illness; to manage and coordinate the patient's health and illness; and to address the family's concerns, health and illness, thereby achieving not only patient-centered, but cost-effective family-centered care. Here, too the applicability of findings to enhancing both the theory and practice of patient-centered care is readily apparent.

A third example illustrates how very intersubjective hermeneutic interpretive investigation may be used to advance patient-centered practice. In their analysis of health promotion through critical reflection, McWilliam *et al.* (1997) illuminated the contextual factors that underlie patient behaviors, presenting challenges to all care providers, including their physicians. Findings enable professionals to understand how life context priorities and goals (such as a life of hardy independence followed by an illness which threatened the patient's ability to live at home with her beloved adult son) serve as important motivators of patient behaviors that appear on the surface to constitute unreasonable resistance to medical advice (such as the advice to move to a nursing home). The findings also provide insights into how professionals might refine care approaches to promote the health of older persons with chronic conditions.

These three examples typify the application of qualitative methods ranging from more objective, post-positivist investigation to more subjective, interpretive investigation. While we could find no examples of critical research to investigate understanding of the whole person, this range within the post-positivist and interpretive paradigms illustrates the opportunities for variety, and invites researchers to creatively apply qualitative methods to understanding the whole person in context.

Finding common ground

Finding common ground with patients presents many challenges and opportunities. Coming to a mutual agreement about diagnoses and treatment plans is critical to ensuring patient adherence, but can readily overtax the patience and time of physicians, particularly when relationships are new or have had inadequate time to develop. Qualitative research may elicit insights into factors that achieve or impede finding common ground, and may facilitate the development of the social interaction processes required.

Two qualitative studies describe key elements of the process of finding common ground, illustrating the potential of these methodologies. In one study, researchers (Scott *et al.*, 2001) used a multimethod comparative case study and basic content analysis with a quasi-statistical approach to identify the nature and incidence of patient pressure tactics that countered physician efforts to find common ground regarding the use of antibiotics to treat acute respiratory tract infections. Findings illuminate the complex connection between physician prescribing practices and patient expectations, revealing the significance of the nature and content of patient–physician communication. The study also addresses some of the challenges in finding common ground when patients and physicians may not agree.

In a second investigation, researchers applied grounded theory research methods to illuminate how the physician's and the patient's experiences together constitute the elements essential to finding common ground (Tudiver *et al.*, 2001). Using constant comparative analysis, researchers described how a number of patient factors (i.e. expectations, anxiety) and physician factors (i.e. clinical practice experience, influence of colleagues) interacted in the process of finding common ground in making cancer screening decisions. Findings also illustrate how a strong patient–physician relationship is central to finding common ground when cancer screening guidelines are unclear or conflicting.

Incorporating prevention and promotion

Incorporating health promotion and disease prevention to achieve patient-centered care presents many unique challenges. The patient's own knowledge, attitudes and beliefs, often subconscious, very much affect whether he or she is receptive to a proactive approach to healthcare. Furthermore, the physician needs to have a tremendous depth and breadth of understanding of the patient's stage of readiness and self-efficacy related to promoting health or preventing disease in order to determine the appropriate approach to any intervention. As well, it is essential for the physician to know what health and/or the prevention of disease means to the patient so that approaches to incorporating prevention and health promotion can be aligned to his/her needs, motives and expectations, with a view to optimizing positive outcomes. The physician needs to understand strategies for achieving outcomes that are neither readily nor quickly apparent. Above all, as quantitative research captures the linkages between the broader determinants of health and health outcomes, qualitative methodologies provide the opportunity to capture in-depth descriptions of the experience of health, indirectly informing health promotion and disease prevention.

Seven studies illustrate a variety of qualitative methodological applications that inform the incorporation of health promotion and disease prevention in patient-centered care. In two of these studies, researchers have used basic content analysis to identify patients' knowledge, attitudes and beliefs about primary and secondary disease prevention. To inform interventions for increased colorectal cancer screening in men and women aged 50 and older, Beeker *et al.* (2000) used focus groups. The purpose was to identify knowledge, attitudes, and beliefs about coloretal cancer screening, perceived barriers to screening, and strategies for motivating and supporting behavior change. Findings revealed that participants were poorly informed about but receptive to this topic, suggesting the appropriateness of public education campaigns, decision aids and targeted interventions to increase awareness of the prevention and early detection benefits of screening.

In another study (McMichael *et al.*, 2000), interviews, case studies and focus groups were conducted with Aboriginal women and service providers in rural and remote areas of Queensland, Australia. The purpose of this study was to identify social, structural and personal factors associated with the detection of breast cancer, as well as the treatment and post-treatment care and support of cancer patients. The study findings revealed that personal history of health services, information about mammography, the cost of treatment and care, the availability of personal support and relationships with practitioners all influenced women's willingness to access services and maintain treatment. Findings suggested the importance of patient-centered efforts to increase women's awareness of breast cancer and the benefits of preventative health efforts.

In a third interpretive study to explore decision making by menopausal women initiating or remaining on hormone replacement therapy (HRT), Marmoreo *et al.* (1998) used focus groups to examine women's thoughts, feelings, attitudes and behaviors regarding HRT. Researchers identified four spheres of influence on the participants' decisions (internal perceptions and feelings; interpersonal relationships; external societal pressures; and anticipated consequences, as informed by research evidence), weighted by the intensity of the influence on the decision-making process. These more interpretive findings underscored the importance of considering the context of patients' decisions regarding elective preventive care, the dynamic interplay among the spheres of influence upon decision making, and the various strategies that women therefore employ in deciding their participation in preventive care.

In a fourth study, Backett-Milburn *et al.* (2000) used interpretive analysis of women's wider accounts of their lives, health, lifecourse and experience of menopause to make sense of their disinterest in the prevention of osteoporosis. Adding further insights to those gleaned by Marmoreo *et al.* (1998), findings revealed the tremendous challenge of undertaking preventive care for these women, who poignantly conveyed their inclination to 'worry about that when it comes along' (1998: 153).

Similarly, in a hermeneutic phenomenological investigation, McWilliam *et al.* (1996) exposed the essence of the human experience of health amongst older persons with chronic illness as 'being able to do the things one wants to do'. Older participants described numerous personal strategies used for health promotion. These two studies by Backett-Milburn *et al.* (2000) and McWilliam *et al.* (1996), in particular pinpoint the importance of understanding the patient's perspective on, valuing of, and action toward health and health promotion before deciding to provide proactive care.

How health professionals might go about incorporating disease prevention and health promotion has also begun to be illuminated by qualitative investigation. Working in the post-positivist paradigm, Jaen *et al.* (2001) used cross-sectional direct observation of outpatient visits by cigarette smokers to determine the patterns and quality of tobacco counseling. They discovered that only one-third of eligible visits included tobacco cessation counseling, a pattern that was related to competing priorities and physicians' non-adoption of the recommended practice approach of asking, advising, assessing, assisting and arranging preventative healthcare.

In a phenomenological investigation of a critical reflection approach to promoting health as a resource for everyday living, McWilliam *et al.* (1997) uncovered essential aspects of practice focused on promoting the individual's health. These included relationship-building, and increasing conscious awareness of the individual's life and health goals, priorities, resources, actions toward those goals, and experience of outcomes. Findings from McWilliam *et al.* (1997) and Jaen *et al.* (2001) not only inform practice, but invite further investigation to refine intervention strategies.

Enhancing the patient–physician relationship

As described in Chapter 8, the patient–physician relationship constitutes the primal exchange within which all medical care transpires. For this reason, research that uncovers the essence of the complex interactions that occur between patient and physician is foundational to building the theory and practice of patient-centered care. Greater in-depth understanding of the attributes of therapeutic relationships, how power is expressed in patient–physician relationships, how caring and healing transpire, and ways of being in relationships with patients may do much to enhance the self-awareness and practice expertise of professionals, thereby enhancing patient-centered care.

Four studies exemplify how the findings of qualitative investigation may enhance the patient–physician relationship. Two studies used focus groups and basic content analyses to obtain patient perspectives on important elements of the patient–physician relationship. At the individual relationship level, Thom and Campbell (1997) delineated nine categories of physician behavior that patients described as promoting their trust in the physician: thoroughness in evaluation; providing appropriate and effective treatment; understanding the patient's individual experience; expressing caring; communicating clearly and completely; building partnership/sharing power; honesty/respect for the patients; predisposing factors; and structural/staffing factors. On a macro level, Brown *et al.* (1997b) delineated four primary factors contributing to long-term attendance at a family practice teaching unit: the relationship context; the team concept; professional responsibility and attitudes; and comprehensive and convenient care. These complementary findings convey the attributes of the practice setting that patients perceive as foundational to good patient–physician relationships.

Another study offers a non-partisan perspective on the physician's role in the patient–physician relationship. Applying grounded theory methods, Robinson *et al.* (2001) used field researchers' direct observations and field notes to investigate 379 outpatient encounters of 13 family physicians, ultimately developing a typology of physicians' responses to patients presenting with emotional distress. Findings categorized physicians' responses by their philosophy and management skills: biomedical and basic ('the technician'); biopsychosocial and basic ('the friend'); biomedical and advanced ('the detective'); or biopsychosocial and advanced ('the healer'), as well as by their degree of response: 'actively ignore[d]'; 'postponed or triaged'; or 'actively manage[d]'. These findings entice physicians to examine and refine their own responses to emotionally distressed patients, with due consideration of their own natural proclivity and skills, their patients' needs, motives and expectations, and the contextual barriers and facilitators.

The experiences of patient–physician encounters of women with breast cancer have been studied using phenomenological methodology (McWilliam *et al.*, 2000). This investigation elicited in-depth insights into the important elements of relationship-building for these patients, whose symptoms and diagnosis often trigger challenging feelings, such as vulnerability. Findings revealed that physicians who work at relationship-building along with information-sharing ultimately contribute positively to their patient's experience of control and mastery, and, in turn, their learning to live with cancer. By contrast, when patients experienced physicians to be paternalistic, negative, non-accepting, angry, falsely reassuring, giving poorly timed information and no hope, the patients were left feeling vulnerable and out-of-control. Patients who failed to have a connection with their physician experienced a continued search for meaningful patient–physician communication. Findings not only underscore the importance of creating a working relationship built upon a patient-centered approach, but also illuminate key efforts that might contribute to success in this process.

Being realistic

In the current context of healthcare, being realistic presents an ever-increasing challenge. The complexity of patient problems, available resources and treatments, the time pressures associated with diminished resources and increased demands for care, and the escalating pressure for cost-effective services all must be confronted. Qualitative research helps to uncover the multifaceted issues that arise in the real-life practice context, affording insights and understandings that may help to evolve the theory and practice of realistic patient-centered care.

Four studies illustrate the potential of qualitative research for guiding the evolution of realistic patient-centered practice. Using a post-positivist paradigm and basic content analysis of 106 transcripts of consultations provided to 50 patients with complex chronic conditions by 14 Australian general practitioners, Martin *et al.* (1999) discovered the topics addressed in short (less than ten minutes), standard (between ten and 19 minutes) and longer (20 minutes or longer) consultations. Findings revealed the physician's review of treatment was the most common element, and physician's review of illness the second most common element, the two together dominating the dialog of short and medium-length consultations. The physician's providing of information was the third most common element, while patient-initiated discussion of illness occurred much less frequently (14% of the content in shorter consultations, 12% in those of standard length, and 23% in long consultations). In longer consultations, these four most prominent elements each occurred in approximately 25% of consultations. Emotional support was not offered very frequently, but occurred more frequently in longer consultations. Qualitative findings from this investigation illuminate the opportunity for improving patient-centeredness and invite more qualitative exploration of the challenge of providing patient-centered care within realistic time frames.

A hermeneutic phenomenological study by Brown *et al.* (1998) illuminated the importance of the physician's own personal and professional life context and philosophy in being realistic about practice orientation. This study uncovered the interactivity of past influences (the physician's education, professional, and personal experiences) and current system factors (inadequate remuneration, time, personal support and knowledge of resources) entering into physicians' approaches to providing palliative care.

In a focus group study, Brown *et al.* (2002a) explored the evolution of walk-in clinics describing patients' expectations for immediate and convenient healthcare and a lack of family physician availability; thereby illuminating the challenges of being realistic. In another study, Brown *et al.* (2002b) used in-depth interviews with physicians to identify their experiences in caring for patients with serious mental illness in a shared mental healthcare model. Several challenges to being realistic were described: poor communication; lack of access to services; fragmentation of care; and lack of accountability. All of these problems undermined realistic evolution of the collaborative relationships required for shared care. The importance of all of these multiple factors to realistic expectations for physician involvement in providing patient-centered care was made readily apparent by these investigators.

Conclusion

Much progress has been made through the use of qualitative research to investigate patient-centered care. However, many opportunities to further advance the theory and practice of patient-centered care exist. While some of the studies to date were conceived to directly address patient-centered practice, many have been undertaken for other purposes. Nevertheless, by virtue of the nature of qualitative inquiry, these studies too illuminate components of the patient-centered clinical method. These studies are important in as much as they spontaneously document the clinical validity of the patient-centered clinical method. As well, they illustrate the many opportunities for researchers committed to the evolution of the theory and practice of evidence-based patient-centered care.

To date, research primarily has explored either the physicians' or the patients' perspectives, rather than the perspective of both partners in care on any one experience or component of patient-centeredness. More direct observation and more interpretive analysis of the two-way communication that transpires to create patient-centered care will be important. As well the absence of work in the critical paradigm invites initiatives in this area of qualitative research.

17

Questions about patient-centered care: answers from quantitative research

Moira Stewart

In the past decade new studies and meta-analyses of previous studies have provided insights into the dimensions of patient-centered medicine which positively influence a variety of physician and patient outcomes. The quality of the quantitative evidence varies by the design of the study, and includes A-level evidence from rigorously designed randomized controlled clinical trials (as defined by the Canadian Task Force, 1994). A key precursor to such studies was the development of the measures to transform the interactive process between a patient and a doctor into a category or a score. Examples of such measures are described in Chapters 18 and 19.

The studies reviewed in this chapter will be presented by outcome. The physician outcomes include: malpractice claims, time, and physician satisfaction. Patient outcomes include: patient satisfaction, patient adherence, and patient health outcomes. At the end of the chapter, we will present a summary of the elements of patient-centered communication which were repeatedly found to be positively associated with outcomes. The evidence included in this chapter has been summarized in two published systematic reviews (Brown *et al.*, forthcoming; Stewart *et al.*, 1999). For each outcome, the chapter first presents the studies, then gives an example of the magnitude of the impact, and finally, presents the kind of communication that has made a difference to the outcome.

Malpractice claims

There were eight studies that related patient–physician communication with malpractice complaints/claims against the physician. These eight included

Table 17.1 Magnitude of the relationship between patient–physician communication and malpractice claims*

	% Poor patient–physician communication
No claims	8.2
All others	17.7
High frequency	27.6
High pay	24.7

* Based on Hickson *et al.*, 1994.

randomized controlled trials as well as other designs (Beckman *et al.*, 1994; Hickson *et al.*, 1992; Hickson *et al.*, 1994; Lester and Smith, 1993; Levinson *et al.*, 1997; Penchansky and Macnee, 1994; Shapiro *et al.*, 1989; Vincent *et al.*, 1994).

Table 17.1 illustrates the magnitude of the relationship between patient–physician communication and malpractice using one study as an example. Hickson *et al.* (1994) found the presence of poor patient–physician communication to be quite low in the group of patients whose doctors had no complaints (8.2% in the no claims group). The high-frequency claims and the high-payout groups had more than three times the percentage of poor communication (approximately 25% in these latter groups).

Taking all eight studies, one can summarize the kind of communication that is problematic. Five important issues emerged:

1 *Time*: Patients who complained about their physicians felt rushed or had shorter visits than other patients.
2 *Inadequate explanation*: Physicians provided minimal information and there were fewer orienting statements by the physician.
3 *Connection*: The patients felt ignored, felt no acknowledgment of their statements, no reflection of their affect, no eye contact, no friendly physical contact and no humor.
4 *Facilitation*: The physician did not facilitate an explanation to arrive at an understanding of patient and family perspectives.
5 *Support*: Patients felt that their own and their family's views were devalued by the physician.

Time

The relationship between patient–physician communication and time has been widely studied and is also discussed in Chapter 9. As well, the most frequently asked question, when our team leads workshops with physicians, is whether patient-centered communication will take more time. Nineteen studies were found on this topic and some were randomized controlled trials, as well as other designs. The conclusions of these studies are conflicting with regard to time. Six studies demonstrated no differences between patient-centered visits of physicians and non-patient-centered visits in terms of time (Arborelius and Bremberg, 1992; Greenfield *et al.*, 1988; Henbest and Fehrsen, 1992; Marvel *et al.*, 1998; Roland *et al.*, 1986; Wilson, 1991). In other words, in the same amount of time physicians who were rated by their patients or rated by experts as patient-centered explored psychosocial issues, engaged in collaboration with patients, explored the patients' ideas and concerns, and listened more to the patients who showed higher frequencies of speaking. However, ten other studies found differences, not in patient-centered communication directly, but in other relevant outcomes, for visits which were of longer duration; these tended to be studies where there was a random allocation of patients into a time slot that was longer (≥ 15 minutes) or one that was shorter (Ferris, 1998; Hornberger *et al.*, 1997; Howie *et al.*, 1991; Hull and Hull, 1984; Jacobson *et al.*, 1994; Marvel, 1993; Ridsdale *et al.*, 1992; Verby *et al.*, 1979; Westcott, 1977; Williams and Neal, 1998). For example, in longer visits Zyzanski *et al.* (1998), found that more counseling was undertaken, more preventive activities including vaccinations occurred, a larger portion of patients' needs were recognized, patients indicated higher satisfaction, more discussion occurred about follow-up and guidelines were more often implemented.

In situations where time was limited, two factors were found to be related to patient satisfaction: a brief period of time to chat about non-medical topics; and providing patients with feedback on clinical findings (Gross *et al.*, 1998; Stange *et al.*, 1998).

Physician satisfaction

The third physician outcome covered in this review is physician satisfaction. We found only one cohort study that related physician satisfaction to a communication rating of the visit (Roter *et al.*, 1997). Such findings, if replicated in randomized trials, imply that there may be direct benefits to physician morale if patient-centered practice becomes more widely practiced.

Patient satisfaction

There are many studies of patient–physician communication in relation to subsequent patient satisfaction. None of the studies reviewed was a randomized trial. As well, three review papers have summarized the findings on patient satisfaction (Hall and Dornan, 1988b; Dietrich and Marton, 1982; Linn *et al.*, 1982). These concluded that there was a significant relationship between patient-centered communication and patient satisfaction. Five aspects of communication were related to patient satisfaction:

1 a warm and caring demeanor
2 the patient's assessment of medical competence
3 a balanced communication of both psychosocial and biomedical concerns
4 continuity of the relationship
5 the facilitation of the patient's expression of their expectations.

Patient adherence

Sixteen studies (none of which were randomized controlled trials) and several review papers showed clear evidence of the importance of communication in determining patient adherence (Anderson *et al.*, 1982; Blackwell, 1996; Coe *et al.*, 1984; Garrity, 1981; Garrity and Leaviss, 1989; Golin *et al.*, 1996; Kjellgren *et al.*, 1995; Ley, 1982; McLane *et al.*, 1995; Roter, 1989; Sanson-Fisher *et al.*, 1995; Salzman, 1995; Sbarbaro, 1990; Squier, 1990; Svarstad, 1985; Wilson, 1995). A study of our own found that if the visit was rated as being low on patient-centeredness, the patient adherence was the usual 55%, whereas if the visit was rated as being high on patient-centeredness, the patient adherence was 73%, almost a 20% difference in patient adherence (Stewart, 1984). The kinds of communication that were associated with better patient adherence in the 16 studies reviewed were:

1 information exchange and patient education
2 finding common ground regarding expectations
3 an active role for the patient
4 positive affect, empathy and encouragement.

Patient health outcomes

There are many in the medical field who think this to be the most important outcome. The tasks of medicine are variously defined, but many would agree that improving the health of the patient is the most important task of medicine. To what extent has the literature shown that patient-centered communication actually has an important effect on the patient's health? Twenty-four studies have been reviewed (Brown *et al.*, forthcoming; Stewart, 1995; Stewart *et al.*, 1999); 12 of these were randomized controlled trials and, of these, 11 demonstrated significant, positive relationships between communication (or interventions to improve communication) and better patient health outcomes (Egbert *et al.*, 1964; Evans *et al.*, 1987; Greenfield *et al.*, 1985; Greenfield *et al.*, 1988; Johnson *et al.*, 1988; Kaplan *et al.*, 1989a, b; Roter and Hall, 1991; Savage and Armstrong, 1990; Thomas, 1978, 1987; Thompson *et al.*, 1990). One of the most famous of these studies was conducted by Kaplan *et al.* (1989a, b). In this instance, the study was conducted with chronically ill patients who were being seen by their primary care internist in the USA. Table 17.2 shows that the experimental group (patients were encouraged to change their communication style towards a more participatory style) and the control group patients were quite similar in terms of their blood pressure before the intervention. After the intervention the experimental group showed a drop of 12 points in diastolic blood pressure while the control group dropped only 2 points in diastolic blood pressure, a clinically significant improvement in the chronic disease physiologic outcome. A classic study in the surgical field published in the *New England Journal of Medicine* in 1964 showed the important effects of an education strategy conducted by anesthesiologists before and immediately after surgery in terms of a decrease in the patients' pain, a marked decrease in the use of narcotics by the patients, as well as earlier discharge from hospital (Egbert *et al.*, 1964).

The kinds of health outcome that have been studied range from patient anxiety, psychologic distress, symptom resolution, functional status, self-reported health status, to physiologic status (for example the HA1 and blood pressure). In our view, if a new product was shown to be as effective in rigorous studies as patient-centered communication, industry would aggressively market this product. From these health outcome studies, the patient-centered product would be defined as: during history-taking ask about the patient's feelings and show support; ask many questions about the patient's ideas and expectations; during the discussion of the management plan, encourage patients to ask questions

Table 17.2 Magnitude of the relationship between patient–physician communication and patient physiologic health outcome*

	Diastolic blood pressure in mmHg	
	Experimental	*Control*
Pre	95	93
Post	83	91

* Based on Kaplan *et al.*, 1989a.

and get information, provide information packages to patients, share decisions with patients; and finally, come to an agreement on the nature of the problem and the follow-up plan.

Conclusion

In summary, what is the answer to the question, 'Does patient-centered communication matter?' Yes, patient-centered communication matters to physicians in terms of: the malpractice claims that they might have to endure; the time that it takes them to do their job; and physician satisfaction itself. Yes, patient-centered communication matters to the patient in terms of: patient satisfaction; patient adherence to medication regimens; and patient health outcomes. Based on the literature reviewed for this chapter, the definition of patient-centered communication can be summarized in four principles shown in Box 17.1: clear information provided to the patient; mutually agreed-upon goals between the doctor and the patient; an active role for the patient in asking questions, having them answered and decision making about treatment; and positive affect, empathy and support from the physician to the patient. We therefore recommend these four evidence-based guidelines for patient–physician communication.

These principles are congruent with the definition of the patient-centered clinical method contained in this book, particularly emphasizing component 3, 'Finding common ground'. The research measures used in these studies were not, for the most part, based on a patient-centered conceptual framework. Most were atheoretical, as were many of the interventions evaluated in these studies. In the future, interventions and measures should build on both empirical findings to date and conceptual development which arises out of clinical practice.

Box 17.1   Evidence-based guidelines for patient–physician communication

- Clear information provided to the patient.
- Mutually agreed upon goals.
- An active role for the patient.
- Positive affect, empathy and support from the physician.

18

Measuring patient-centeredness

Judith Belle Brown, Moira Stewart and Bridget L Ryan

Concurrent with the theoretical development of the patient-centered clinical method and subsequent educational programs was a research initiative to support the empirical basis of the method. Central to the research program was the creation of tools to measure patient-centered care. Many methods of measuring communication have been developed since Bales first introduced the Bales Interaction Analysis in 1950 (Bales, 1950; Kaplan *et al.*, 1989a; Roter, 1977; Roter *et al.*, 1990; Stewart, 1984).

Advances in assessing the patient–physician interaction have led several authors to provide comparisons of various coding schemes. In a special issue of *Health Communication* (2001) six research teams coded the same dataset using their respective measures (McNeilis, 2001; Meredith *et al.*, 2001; Roter and Larson, 2001; Shaikh *et al.*, 2001; Street and Millay, 2001; von Friederichs-Fitzwater and Gilgun, 2001). Commentaries on the results highlight what certain coding schemes can and cannot measure (Rimal, 2001; Frankel, 2001). In addition, Mead and Bower (2000) have assessed the reliability and validity of various observation-based measures of patient-centered behaviors, including an earlier version of the Measure of Patient-Centered Communication described in this chapter.

Many of these measures, while effective in assessing patient–physician interaction, are not specific to the patient-centered clinical method as we envision it. Thus, rather than import parts of measures relevant to patient-centered care, a new research measure was created – the Measure of Patient-Centered Communication (MPCC). This chapter describes this measure.

The measure of patient-centered communication (MPCC)

Development

Based on the patient-centered clinical method described in this book, a method of assessing and scoring patient–physician encounters, either audiotaped or videotaped, was developed. The MPCC has evolved significantly since its inception in the early 1980s. The development of the MPCC is detailed below. The MPCC has several advantages over other methods (Bales, 1950; Kaplan *et al.*, 1989a; Roter, 1977; Roter *et al.*, 1990; Stewart, 1984): first, it does not require that the taped interview between the patient and the physician be transcribed; and second, it is theory-based, that is, it was developed specifically to assess the behaviors of patients and physicians ascribed by the patient-centered clinical method as detailed in this book.

The initial version of the coding and scoring of the MPCC was published in 1986 and used in a study of family practice residents (Brown *et al.*, 1986). At that time the measure only captured component 1, 'Exploring both the disease and the illness experience'. As a result the measure underwent significant expansion including component 2, 'Understanding the whole person' and component 3, 'Finding common ground', and provided more detailed process categories as well as coding and scoring instructions (Brown *et al.*, 1995). This 1995 version of the measure was used in a number of subsequent studies in family practice (Kinnersley *et al.*, 1999; R Epstein, personal communication), emergency medicine (W McCauley, personal communication), and surgery (K Leslie, personal communication). The 2001 version arose in response to patients' expressed needs regarding communication (McWilliam *et al.*, 2000) and is detailed in the MPCC manual (Brown *et al.*, 2001). This latest version has been used in a number of funded studies with family physicians, surgeons and oncologists (Stewart *et al.*, submitted), family physicians (R Epstein, personal communication; D Post, personal communication), and adapted for use in a USA randomized clinical trial (M Kemp White, personal communication). These USA and Canadian projects have obtained adequate reliability after two-day workshops and follow-up telephone advice.

The current measure incorporates coding and scoring of component 1, 'Exploring both the disease and the illness experience', component 2, 'Understanding the whole person', and component 3, 'Finding common ground'.

Components 4 through 6 represent aspects of the patient–physician relationship that either evolve over time or may not be measured in each encounter. Many activities inherent to components 4, 5 and 6 will not be verbalized by the physician (i.e. issues about time management, touch as an expression of warmth and concern). While always an important part of the patient-centered method, these components have not been measured in our previous studies.

Application of the MPCC: who and where

The MPCC can be used in a variety of patient–physician settings. In previous studies, it has been successfully used during office visits when patients are presenting with acute and/or chronic illnesses, routine physical examinations or check-ups, office procedures such as mole removal and follow-up visits for previous problems. It has also been used in the Emergency Department where real-time coding was conducted. As well as being used with actual patients, the MPCC has been employed in office visits with standardized patients.

This latter application offers the advantage of standardization but presents specific challenges because coders may work with a preset template of patient statements and expected behaviors (i.e. specific feelings, ideas, effects on function and expectations) on the part of the standardized patient. In reality, these behaviors may not be elicited by the physician or the encounter may proceed in a manner that does not provide the standardized patient with an opportunity to articulate programmed statements, either at all, or at an appropriate time. For example, a standardized patient may be directed to provide the physician with a statement about the effect of a sore back on his/her ability to work. If the physician moves quickly to the treatment of the problem, and it is only then that the standardized patient has an opportunity to raise this issue, the coder would normally place the statement in component 3, coding it as part of the mutual discussion surrounding the treatment. With standardized patients, coders must decide how to handle these situations, balancing the goal of consistency afforded by standardized patients with the goal of accurately capturing the interaction. In the case of the effect of the sore back on work, the coders might decide to move back to component 1 so as to ensure that this statement was captured in a consistent way for all standardized patient visits.

Occasionally, an additional person such as another healthcare professional will be present during an interview. If the healthcare professional is not an integral part of the visit, this person should not be considered as part of the interview to be coded. However, if the visit does involve two healthcare professionals, such as a medical student and a staff physician, who are taking equal part in the interview, these two people, depending on the research question, may be seen as one physician and the interview will be coded as if these two people speak as one physician.

The other situation where an additional person may be present is when another person accompanies a patient. In this case, the coder must decide with whom the interview is being conducted. If, for example, a mother accompanies her child who does not speak for herself, then the interview will be coded between the mother and the physician. If however, the child is older and is an active participant in the discussion, the interview will be coded between the child and the physician. In the case of an adult patient, the interview will usually be coded between the patient and the physician unless the adult patient is unable to speak independently. This can happen, for example, in the case of a patient who is severely mentally challenged or is cognitively impaired.

Reliability and validity of the MPCC

Interrater reliability of the scoring of the initial version of the MPCC was established among three raters at $r = 0.69$, 0.84, and 0.80 (Brown *et al.*, 1986). Using the 1995 version (Brown *et al.*, 1995), Stewart *et al.* (2000) established an interrater reliability of 0.83 and an intrarater reliability of 0.73. A recent study using the current version (Brown *et al.*, 2001) established an interrater reliability of 0.80.

The validity of the scoring procedure of the 1995 version was established by a high correlation (0.85) with global scores of experienced communication researchers (Stewart *et al.*, 2000).

Coding the MPCC

Coding takes place while listening to an audiotape/videotape/CD (either in segments or in full) of a patient's visit to the physician. It is often necessary to listen to all or parts of the recording a second time in order to fill in gaps in coding that were not captured on the first pass.

Coders listen for statements from the patient and the physician that are pertinent to the patient-centered clinical method and list only those pertinent statements. Not every statement the patient or physician makes will be coded. Coders must place statements under the most appropriate component. Components 1, 2 and 3 of the patient-centered clinical method are coded. *See* Figure 18.1 for the coding template of the MPCC.

Coding under appropriate headings

Once the appropriate component is identified, the coder will list the patient or physician statement under the most appropriate heading. In components 1

Component 1. Exploring both the disease and the illness experience

Symptoms and/or reason for visit	Preliminary exploration	Further exploration	Validation	Cut-off	SCORE
1 _____	Y N	Y N	Y N	Y N	_____
2 _____	Y N	Y N	Y N	Y N	_____
3 _____	Y N	Y N	Y N	Y N	_____
4 _____	Y N	Y N	Y N	Y N	_____
5 _____	Y N	Y N	Y N	Y N	_____
				ST**	

Prompts

1 _____	Y N	Y N	Y N	Y N	_____
2 _____	Y N	Y N	Y N	Y N	_____
3 _____	Y N	Y N	Y N	Y N	_____
4 _____	Y N	Y N	Y N	Y N	_____
5 _____	Y N	Y N	Y N	Y N	_____
				ST**	

Feelings

1 _____	Y N	Y N	Y N	Y N	_____
2 _____	Y N	Y N	Y N	Y N	_____
3 _____	Y N	Y N	Y N	Y N	_____
4 _____	Y N	Y N	Y N	Y N	_____
5 _____	Y N	Y N	Y N	Y N	_____
				ST**	

Ideas

1 _____	Y N	Y N	Y N	Y N	_____
2 _____	Y N	Y N	Y N	Y N	_____
3 _____	Y N	Y N	Y N	Y N	_____
4 _____	Y N	Y N	Y N	Y N	_____
5 _____	Y N	Y N	Y N	Y N	_____
				ST**	

Effect on function

1 _____	Y N	Y N	Y N	Y N	_____
2 _____	Y N	Y N	Y N	Y N	_____
3 _____	Y N	Y N	Y N	Y N	_____
4 _____	Y N	Y N	Y N	Y N	_____
5 _____	Y N	Y N	Y N	Y N	_____
				ST**	

Expectations

1 _____	Y N	Y N	Y N	Y N	_____
2 _____	Y N	Y N	Y N	Y N	_____
3 _____	Y N	Y N	Y N	Y N	_____
4 _____	Y N	Y N	Y N	Y N	_____
5 _____	Y N	Y N	Y N	Y N	_____
				ST**	

** Sub-total
*** Grand total

GT*** _____ ÷ =

Figure 18.1 Coding template of the MPCC.

Component 2. Understanding the whole person

Any statements relevant to FAMILY, LIFE CYCLE, SOCIAL SUPPORT, PERSONALITY, and CONTEXT are to be listed below:

		Preliminary exploration	Further exploration	Validation	Cut-off	SCORE
1	_____	Y N	Y N	Y N	Y N	_____
2	_____	Y N	Y N	Y N	Y N	_____
3	_____	Y N	Y N	Y N	Y N	_____
4	_____	Y N	Y N	Y N	Y N	_____
5	_____	Y N	Y N	Y N	Y N	_____
6	_____	Y N	Y N	Y N	Y N	_____
7	_____	Y N	Y N	Y N	Y N	_____
8	_____	Y N	Y N	Y N	Y N	_____
9	_____	Y N	Y N	Y N	Y N	_____
10	_____	Y N	Y N	Y N	Y N	_____

** Sub-total

*** Grand total

ST**

GT***   ÷ 5 =

Figure 18.1   (*continued*)

and 3, there is a choice of headings. In component 2, there is only one heading. The headings for each of these components are described below.

Component 1: Exploring both the disease and the illness experience

Symptoms and/or reason for visit

Patients' symptoms are listed using the patients' words in the upper-left portion of the component 1 coding form (*see* Figure 18.1). Patients' symptoms are the stated conscious expression of their physical, emotional, or social problem, usually representing their reason for the visit. While a statement of symptoms normally initiates an office visit, it may occur at any stage of the interaction. For example, a patient may say at the end of the visit, 'By the way, doctor, I've also got a pain in my knee.'

Symptom and/or reasons for visit fall generally into six categories as follows:

1   The patient initiates the description. ('I've been having a lot of chest pain.')
2   The patient responds positively to a physician inquiry about a sign or symptom. (The physician asks: 'Have you been having any allergy problems this spring?' The patient responds, 'No, they seem to be under control.')

Component 3. Finding common ground

Problem definition:	Clearly expressed	Opportunity to ask questions	Mutual discussion	Clarification of agreement	SCORE
1 _____	Y N	Y N	Y N	Y N	_____
2 _____	Y N	Y N	Y N	Y N	_____
3 _____	Y N	Y N	Y N	Y N	_____
4 _____	Y N	Y N	Y N	Y N	_____
5 _____	Y N	Y N	Y N	Y N	_____
6 _____	Y N	Y N	Y N	Y N	_____
7 _____	Y N	Y N	Y N	Y N	_____
8 _____	Y N	Y N	Y N	Y N	_____
9 _____	Y N	Y N	Y N	Y N	_____
10 _____	Y N	Y N	Y N	Y N	_____
				ST**	

Goals of treatment/management

	Clearly expressed	Opportunity to ask questions	Mutual discussion	Clarification of agreement	SCORE
1 _____	Y N	Y N	Y N	Y N	_____
2 _____	Y N	Y N	Y N	Y N	_____
3 _____	Y N	Y N	Y N	Y N	_____
4 _____	Y N	Y N	Y N	Y N	_____
5 _____	Y N	Y N	Y N	Y N	_____
6 _____	Y N	Y N	Y N	Y N	_____
7 _____	Y N	Y N	Y N	Y N	_____
8 _____	Y N	Y N	Y N	Y N	_____
9 _____	Y N	Y N	Y N	Y N	_____
10 _____	Y N	Y N	Y N	Y N	_____
				ST**	

Responded appropriately to disagreement with flexibility and understanding

1 _____	Y N	N/A			_____
2 _____	Y N	N/A			_____
				ST**	

** Sub-total   GT***   ÷   =

*** Grand total   _____   _____

Figure 18.1 *(continued)*

3 The patient responds either positively or negatively to a physician inquiry regarding a known problem that the patient has not presented at the current visit. (The physician asks, 'So how has it been since your bowel surgery?' The patient responds, 'It's been going well, actually.')

4 The patient raises a problem or management issue from a previous visit. ('That antacid you gave me last time didn't help at all.')

5   The physician elicits the patient's personal and/or family history or con-
    ducts a check-up as part of the visit. (The physician asks, 'Any history of
    heart disease in your family?' or 'Do you smoke?' or 'Any hospitalizations?')
6   The patient is present to have a procedure. In this case, there may be very
    little conversation but it is appropriate to code the physician's conversation
    with the patient both before and during the procedure. This is where the
    physician would be scored on how he/she handles the issue of informing
    the patient about the procedure and the issue of patient consent. (The
    patient begins, 'I'm here to have this mole removed.' The physician
    responds, 'Okay, now did I explain to you what is going to happen?' The
    patient indicates, 'Yes, we discussed that last time.')

Prompts

Prompts are listed in the patients' words in the second left-hand section of the
component 1 coding form. Prompts are signals from patients that their feelings,
ideas or expectations have not yet been explored. Prompts may be verbal, behavioral or arise from the context of the consultation. Prompts are defined as either
statements that are out of context or restatements of a problem that has already
been mentioned.

Feelings

Feelings are listed in the patients' words in the third left-hand section of the
component 1 coding form. Feelings reflect the emotional content of the patient's
illness. They may be the predominant aspect of the illness, as in a grief reaction,
or be a contributory factor, as in the anxiety of a discovery about a breast lump.
They may arise directly out of the stated symptoms and/or reason for visit,
prompts, ideas, effect on function, or expectations, as when a patient who has
requested a check-up discloses during the course of the interview that she is
anxious (feeling) about the effects of dyspareunia (symptom and/or reason for
visit) on her sexual function. Words commonly used by patients to express their
feelings are: troublesome, concerned, preoccupied, afraid, fearful, worried, sad,
depressed, anxious.

Ideas

Ideas are listed in the patients' words, in the fourth left-hand section of the
component 1 coding form. Patients form ideas about their illness in their
attempts to make some meaning or sense of their experience, that is, they develop

an explanatory model of their illness. Patients' health beliefs, values, and life experiences can inform this explanatory model. These ideas may be based on prior experiences or influenced by present events such as a recent death of a friend.

Effect on function

Effects on function are listed in the patients' words in the fifth left-hand section of the component 1 coding form. The illness may have an effect on the patient's daily function including the patient's capacity to fulfill certain roles and responsibilities such as a worker, spouse or parent. Questions by the physician may include: how the illness limits daily activities, impairs family roles, requires a change in lifestyle. Specific activities relevant to the heading 'Effect on function' are: physical mobility, eating, dressing, sleeping, toileting, working and socializing.

Expectations

Expectations are listed in the patients' words in the lower left-hand section of the component 1 coding form. Every patient who visits a physician has some expectations of the visit. The patient's expectations often relate to a symptom or a concern about which the patient anticipates exploration or response from the physician. The presentation of the patient's expectations may take many forms, including a question, a request for service or a statement of the purpose of the visit. Expectations are also reasons for the visit other than symptoms (i.e. annual health visit, request for service, request for completion of a disability form, request for a prescription refill).

Component 2: Understanding the whole person

There are five topics specific to component 2 and patient statements relevant to these five topics are to be listed (*see* Figure 18.1, second section, for the component 2 coding form). The five are: family; life cycle; social support; personality; and context (i.e. employment/schooling, culture, environment, healthcare system). Often, statements relevant to one topic may also be relevant to another. However, we do not consider it important for these topics to be mutually exclusive and, consequently, we have not separated them by sub-headings. This is a difference from the coding for component 1 with its sub-headings.

Component 3: Finding common ground

There are two areas specific to component 3 (Finding common ground) – problem definition, and goals of treatment and management – which represent establishing the nature of the problems and priorities and the goals of the treatment and management (*see* Figure 18.1, third section, for the component 3 coding form).

Problem definition

Problem definition is the physician's statement of the nature of the problem(s). These statements are listed in the top left-hand section of the component 3 coding form. This statement is not necessarily a restatement of the patient's initial presentation but is the physician's formulation after the patient's presentation has been explored. It may be that on certain occasions the physician does not know what the problem is but may offer a number of possible definitions of the problem. In this instance, each separate hypothesis/problem definition is to be documented under problem definition.

Goals of treatment and management

Goals of treatment and management are the present treatment plan. These are listed in the second left-hand section of the component 3 coding form. These goals are sometimes future-oriented but reasonable and attainable. Both the physician's stated goals for treatment and management as well as any patient expressions of goals or patient comments on the physician goals are listed. Goals of treatment and management include such things as ordering a test, suggesting an examination, prescribing a medication, or suggesting a treatment. Typically, these are instrumental suggestions on the part of the physician.

Coding of appropriate process categories

After writing the statement in the appropriate place, the coder must assign process categories to each statement. These process categories describe the physician's response or lack of response to the patient's statements. The following two sections describe the process categories for components 1 and 2 and for components 3 respectively.

Component 1 and Component 2 process categories

The process categories include: Preliminary exploration (yes/no); Further exploration (yes/no); Validation (yes/no); Cut-off (yes/no); and Return (®).

Preliminary exploration

Preliminary exploration is the immediate response of the physician to the patient's expression of symptoms and/or reason for visit, prompts, feelings, ideas, effect on function, and expectations. A code of 'yes' is any acknowledgment that the physician heard and accepts the patient's symptoms and/or reason for visit, prompts, feelings, ideas, effect on function, expectations. Alternatively, when the physician cuts off the patient, the categorization would be 'no' to preliminary exploration and 'yes' to cut-off. Premature reassurance by the physician does not count as preliminary exploration.

Further exploration

Further exploration is the second and subsequent responses of the physician. Further exploration means that the physician's response facilitated the patient's further expression either with verbal facilitation or by silence allowing the patient to amplify and/or redirect the conversation.

Validation

Validation is an empathetic response by the physician to the patient's expression. A code of 'yes' means that the physician has acknowledged the patient's expression in an empathetic way. Validation would include phrases such as, 'I understand that ...'; 'This must be a difficult time ...'; 'These are difficult decisions to make ...'.

Cut-off

A cut-off is defined as the physician blocking the patient's further expression of symptoms and/or reason for visit, prompts, feelings, ideas, effect on function, or expectations, for example, by changing the subject, excessive focus on disease, jargon or premature reassurance.

Return

The final process category is a specific physician behavior called a return. The return will be indicated by an ⓡ in the margin. This occurs where a physician has cut off a patient but subsequently in the interview returns to the patient's symptoms and/or reason for visit, prompts, feelings, ideas, effect on function, or expectations. With a return, the physician is considered to have initiated preliminary exploration of the patient's problem and this nullifies the cut-off.

Component 3 process categories

The process categories include: Clearly expressed, (yes/no); Opportunity to ask questions (yes/no); Mutual discussion (yes/no); and Clarification of agreement (yes/no).

Clearly expressed

'Clearly expressed' requires that the physician clearly states in language the patient can understand what he/she believes is the problem or what the management should be. Statements are not clearly expressed if the statement is garbled, incomplete or contradictory; or the statement is not comprehensive enough for the patient to understand the reasoning behind the statement.

Provided an opportunity to ask questions

Providing an opportunity to ask questions includes the explicit request from the physician, 'Do you have any questions about this?' It can also be the patient asking a question or the patient making a comment on the problem definition or goal.

Mutual discussion

Mutual discussion is not achieved when the physician describes the problem definition or goal without any evidence of the patient participating in a discussion either by asking questions or stating opinions. The patient also has to provide verbal content for there to be a discussion.

Clarification of agreement

Clarification of agreement can take two forms. The first form is where the physician explicitly asks 'Do you agree with this?' and the patient responds to the question. The second form is where the physician encourages, through silence or the implicit tone of the interaction, the patient to express agreement or disagreement.

Responded appropriately to disagreement with flexibility and understanding

The final part of scoring the interaction concerns the physicians' response to disagreement by the patient. In our experience, such disagreements rarely occur. However, although rare, we consider the physician's response to such disagreement to be important in finding common ground.

Scoring

After the entire interview is coded, coders assign scores on the right side of the coding sheets and calculate the scores for components 1, 2 and 3. On the last coding sheet, an overall Patient-Centered Score (PCS) is calculated. Each of the three component scores can range theoretically from 0 to 100. The total PCS score is an average of the three component scores and it too can range theoretically from 0 (not at all patient-centered) to 100 (very patient-centered). A detailed description of the scoring procedure is provided in the MPCC manual (Brown *et al.*, 2001).

Descriptive results

Table 18.1 shows the means, ranges and standard deviations of the total MPCC and the three components as found in an observational cohort study of 39 family physicians and 315 of their patients (Stewart *et al.*, 2000).

Table 18.1   MPCC scores for a sample of family physicians ($n = 39$) and patient ($n = 315$) encounters

MPCC	Mean	Standard deviation	Actual range
Total score	50.77	17.86	8.13–92.52
Component 1	50.85	19.00	0.00–97.50
Component 2	39.70	42.76	0.00–100.00
Component 3	56.26	22.97	0.00–100.00

Source: Stewart *et al.*, 2000.

Conclusion

In this chapter, we have described the development, evolution and application of the MPCC. The most recent coding and scoring of the MPCC have been outlined in some detail.

19

Measuring patient perceptions of patient-centeredness

Moira Stewart and Leslie Meredith

Introduction

Measures of the patients' perception of patient-centered care have been developed which serve to supplement and complement the behavioral measure (MPCC) described in the previous chapter. What more patient-centered research approach could one imagine than asking patients to describe their experience of the visit with the doctor in a formal structured way? The measures, described in this chapter, have been used for research, as well as for education, by providing individual feedback to participating physicians on their patients' perceptions.

Patient perception measures are increasingly used to evaluate healthcare (Rosenthal and Shannon, 1997). Standard questionnaires to assess the patients' view of themselves or to assess their satisfaction with care (which includes implicit comparisons by patients between their perceptions of care and their expectations of care) are not the topic of this chapter. Rather, this chapter covers patients' reports of a recent experience of care. Other researchers have chosen such a focus to evaluate primary care generally (Haddad, 2000; Starfield, 1998). In general, such measures are: more sensitive to healthcare delivery changes than long-term health outcome measures; less expensive and more reliable than physician review methods; and focused on positive aspects of care (not mistakes), hence very suitable for quality improvement initiatives (Rosenthal and Shannon, 1997). These qualities make patient perception measures an important component of any healthcare research program.

Other researchers who have applied the patient perception approach to the study of patient-centered care include Little and colleagues (Little *et al.*, 2001a, b). They developed a 21-item questionnaire which they found to be reliable (Chronbach's alpha ranging from 0.96 to 0.84) and which factored into five factors very similar to the components of the patient-centered clinical method described in this book (Stewart, 2001). Little and colleagues' questionnaire was used before a visit to assess patient preferences (patients overwhelmingly preferred all facets of a patient-centered approach) and after the visit to assess patients' perceptions of their experience.

The current chapter presents the questionnaire measures of patients' perceptions of the patient-centered clinical method described in this book.

The measure of patient perception of patient-centeredness (PPPC)

Measure development and application

The 17 items developed by our colleagues Carol Buck and Martin Bass for a study of patient outcomes in family practice (Bass *et al.*, 1986), were adapted for a study of communication in family practice (Henbest and Stewart, 1990). The latter study served as a partial validation, in that the items on patients' perceptions of the doctors' ascertainment of the presenting problems were correlated with a patient-centered score of the audiotaped encounter (Spearman rank correlation coefficients ranging from 0.296 to 0.416, p values ranging from 0.006 to 0.001, $n = 73$, Henbest and Stewart, 1990). Revision of the 1990 version (eliminating four items for poor response or irrelevance to the concepts and adding one relevant item) led to the 14-item Patient Perception of Patient-Centeredness (PPPC) questionnaire which was used in two large studies: one of 39 randomly selected family physicians and 315 patients (Stewart *et al.*, 2000) and a version adapted for cancer care in a second study of 52 family physicians, oncologists and surgeons. The results of these two studies are described in Chapter 20.

In the late 1990s, pressure to create a shorter version for easy use in practice, especially for the purpose of continuous quality improvement, led to the selection of eight items which were found to associate significantly with either the MPCC (the audiotape measure) or a health outcome in the 2000 study, plus one new item thought to be necessary to reflect all the components of the patient-centered clinical method. This nine-item questionnaire has two versions, one for the patient to complete and one for the physician to complete. These were used in a national pilot project for specialists in Canada as part of the Royal College of Physicians and Surgeons maintenance of competence program. Similar programs with different questionnaires are being piloted in the USA by such organizations as the American Board of Internal Medicine for formative evaluation purposes.

Box 19.1 The 14-item Patient Perception of Patient-Centeredness

---

PATIENT PERCEPTION OF PATIENT-CENTEREDNESS

Please CIRCLE the response that best represents your opinion.

1. To what extent was your main problem(s) discussed today?

   Completely   Mostly   A little   Not at all

2. Would you say that your doctor knows that this was one of your reasons for coming in today?

   Yes   Probably   Unsure   No

3. To what extent did the doctor understand the importance of your reason for coming in today?

   Completely   Mostly   A little   Not at all

4. How well do you think your doctor understood you today?

   Very well   Well   Somewhat   Not at all

5. How satisfied were you with the discussion of your problem?

   Very satisfied   Satisfied   Somewhat satisfied   Not satisfied

6. To what extent did the doctor explain this problem to you?

   Completely   Mostly   A little   Not at all

7. To what extent did you agree with the doctor's opinion about the problem?

   Completely   Mostly   A little   Not at all

8. How much opportunity did you have to ask your questions?

   Very much   A fair amount   A little   Not at all

9. To what extent did the doctor ask about your goals for treatment?

   Completely   Mostly   A little   Not at all

10. To what extent did the doctor explain treatment?

    Very well   Well   Somewhat   Not at all

11. To what extent did the doctor explore how manageable this (treatment) would be for you? He/she explored this.

    Completely   Mostly   A little   Not at all

12. To what extent did you and the doctor discuss your respective roles? (Who is responsible for making decisions and who is responsible for what aspects of your care?)

    Completely   Mostly   A little   Not at all

13. To what extent did the doctor encourage you to take the role you wanted in your own care?

    Completely   Mostly   A little   Not at all

14. How much would you say that this doctor cares about you as a person?

    Very much   A fair amount   A little   Not at all

Box 19.2 Self-assessment and feedback on communication with patients – patient assessment

Please check (✓) the box that best represents your response.

1. To what extent was your main problem(s) discussed today?

    Completely ☐   Mostly ☐   A little ☐   Not at all ☐

2. How satisfied were you with the discussion of your problem?

    Very satisfied ☐   Satisfied ☐   Somewhat satisfied ☐   Not satisfied ☐

3. To what extent did the doctor listen to what you had to say?

    Completely ☐   Mostly ☐   A little ☐   Not at all ☐

4. To what extent did the doctor explain this problem to you?

    Completely ☐   Mostly ☐   A little ☐   Not at all ☐

5. To what extent did you and the doctor discuss your respective roles? (Who is responsible for making decisions and who is responsible for what aspects of your care?)

    Completely ☐   Mostly ☐   A little ☐   Not discussed ☐

6. To what extent did the doctor explain treatment?

    Very well ☐   Well ☐   Somewhat ☐   Not at all ☐

7. To what extent did the doctor explore how manageable this (treatment) would be for you? He/she explored this:

    Completely ☐   Mostly ☐   A little ☐   Not at all ☐

8. How well do you think your doctor understood you today?

    Very well ☐   Well ☐   Somewhat ☐   Not at all ☐

9. To what extent did the doctor discuss personal or family issues that might affect your health?

    Completely ☐   Mostly ☐   A little ☐   Not at all ☐

Reliability and validity of PPPC

While test–retest reliability has not been assessed, inter-item reliability has been found to be adequate for the 14-item PPPC (Chronbach's alpha = 0.71, $n = 315$).

Box 19.3 Self-assessment and feedback on communication with patients – specialist assessment

Please check (✓) the box that best represents your response.

1. To what extent was your patient's main problem(s) discussed today?

   Completely ☐   Mostly ☐   A little ☐   Not at all ☐

2. How satisfied were you with the discussion of your patient's problem?

   Very satisfied ☐   Satisfied ☐   Somewhat satisfied ☐   Not satisfied ☐

3. To what extent did you listen to what your patient had to say?

   Completely ☐   Mostly ☐   A little ☐   Not at all ☐

4. To what extent did you explain the problem to the patient?

   Completely ☐   Mostly ☐   A little ☐   Not at all ☐

5. To what extent did you and the patient discuss your respective roles? (Who is responsible for making decisions and who is responsible for what aspects of care?)

   Completely ☐   Mostly ☐   A little ☐   Not discussed ☐

6. To what extent did you explain treatment?

   Very well ☐   Well ☐   Somewhat ☐   Not at all ☐

7. To what extent did you and the patient explore how manageable this (treatment) would be for the patient? We explored this:

   Completely ☐   Mostly ☐   A little ☐   Not at all ☐

8. How well do you think you understood the patient today?

   Very well ☐   Well ☐   Somewhat ☐   Not at all ☐

9. Regarding today's problem, to what extent did you discuss personal or family issues that might be affecting your patient's health?

   Completely ☐   Mostly ☐   A little ☐   Not at all ☐

The validity of the 14-item PPPC was established through a significant correlation with the MPCC ($r = 0.16$, $p = 0.01$, $n = 315$); and significant correlations with patient health outcomes and with the efficiencies in the use of health services (Stewart *et al.*, 2000).

Chronbach's alpha reliability of the nine-item patient questionnaire is 0.80, $n = 85$. Similarly, Chronbach's alpha of the nine-item physician questionnaire is 0.79, $n = 117$.

Validity is based on the origin of the items. Eight items were significantly related to either the MPCC or a patient health outcome measure. The remaining item was added to enhance content validity.

The items

The 14-item PPPC is shown in Box 19.1. There are four items thought by the researchers to be relevant to component 1, 'Exploring both the disease and illness experience'; one item for component 2, 'Understanding the whole person'; and nine items for component 3, 'Finding common ground'.

Three scores can be created from PPPC. The 14-item measure was coded so that low scores meant positive perceptions in keeping with other patient outcomes where fewer problems/low scores means a better outcome. The total score is the sum of all responses divided by 14. The second score is for component 1 in which responses to items 1, 2, 3 and 4 are summed and divided by 4. (The reader will notice that there is only one item for component 2, item 14, so there is no computed score). The third score is for component 3 in which responses to items 5 through 13 are summed and divided by 9.

The nine-item questionnaire has two versions. The patient version is shown in Box 19.2. The physician version is shown in Box 19.3. A total score of the patient version is the sum of responses to all items divided by 9 and ranges from 1–4. The nine-item questionnaires were coded so that a high score meant positive perceptions in order to enhance the ease of interpretation of the feedback to doctors, with high scores intuitively meaning better performance. For formative feedback to the doctor, three displays were provided. First, scores on each item for all patients of one doctor were averaged, and compared to the average scores for other doctors in the dataset using the standard continuous quality improvement analysis method of the control chart (Berwick, 1991). Second, the proportion of patients of the doctor who responded with the most

Table 19.1   Descriptive results for PPPC – 14 items ($n = 315$)

Variables	Range	Mean (SD)
Patient perception of patient-centeredness total score	1–2.9	1.5 (0.37)
Patient perception that the illness experience has been explored	1–3.3	1.2 (0.29)
Patient perception that the patient and physician found common ground	1–3.3	1.7 (0.50)

Table 19.2   Control charts comparing six physicians' patient perceptions, with the explanation to the physician

Q5   *To what extent did the doctor discuss your respective roles?*
4   *Completely*   3   *Mostly*   2   *A little*   1   *Not at all*

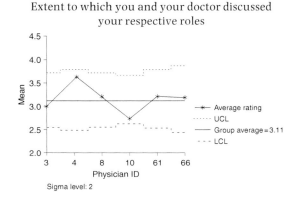

Extent to which you and your doctor discussed your respective roles

Sigma level: 2

As you can see from the chart, all physicians are within the control limits for this question. This indicates that the variation in ratings can be attributed to random fluctuations.

Your patients gave you an average rating of 3.00 indicating that the majority of patients felt you 'mostly' discussed your respective roles (i.e. who is responsible for making decisions and who is responsible for what aspects of your care). This is comparable to the overall average for the 5 physicians (3.11). You may notice that the range (2.6–3.7) is much wider and lower than previous questions.

Q6   *To what extent did the doctor explain treatment?*
4   *Very well*   3   *Well*   2   *Somewhat*   1   *Not at all*

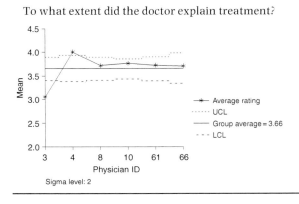

To what extent did the doctor explain treatment?

Sigma level: 2

As you can see, Physician 4 is above the upper control limit indicating a result attributable to performance and your rating puts you below the lower control limit. The group average level of explanation of treatment was 3.66. Your patients gave you an average rating of 3.00. This means that a majority of your patients felt you explained treatment 'well' to them. This may be an area that you could attend to more during visits.

positive rating was shown for each item in a bar graph, allowing each physician to see what aspect of patient-centered care he/she was better at or worse at. Third, the level of agreement between the patient and physician rating was shown for each item in a bar graph.

Descriptive results

Table 19.1 shows the means, standard deviations and ranges of the total 14-item PPPC and the two sub-scores for components 1 and 3 as found in the study of 39 family physicians and 315 patients (Stewart *et al.*, 2000).

Table 19.2 shows two control charts for a pilot study of six physicians each contributing between five and ten patients to the study. The written feedback was to doctor number 3.

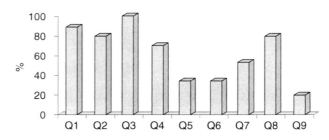

Q1   To what extent was your main problem(s) discussed today?
Q2   How satisfied were you with the discussion of your problem?
Q3   To what extent did the doctor listen to what you had to say?
Q4   To what extent did the doctor explain this problem to you?
Q5   To what extent did you and the doctor discuss your respective roles? (Who is responsible for making decisions and who is responsible for what aspects of your care?)
Q6   To what extent did the doctor explain treatment?
Q7   To what extent did the doctor explore how manageable this (treatment) would be for you?
Q8   How well do you think your doctor understood you today?
Q9   To what extent did the doctor discuss personal or family issues that might affect your health?

Summary
The vast majority of your patients were completely satisfied with the communication during the visit for Q1, Q2, Q4 and Q8. All eleven patients were completely satisfied regarding you listening to them during the visit – congratulations! For the remaining questions, a minority were completely satisfied. The lowest percentage occurs for question 9 (20%). Although there may be legitimate reasons for not discussing personal/family issues that may affect health, this is an area that was not covered completely. Less than half of your patients were not completely satisfied with the extent of the discussion regarding respective roles (Q5) and the extent you explained treatment (Q6). This may have been due to something you and the patient either could not cover or only had time to discuss superficially. Also, 46% of patients did not feel that a complete discussion occurred of how manageable treatment would be for them.

Figure 19.1   Proportion of one physician's patients who reported high ratings, with the explanation to the physician.

Figure 19. 1 shows the feedback on the proportion of patients giving the most positive rating for each item for one doctor. The physician can see for which aspects of patient-centered care their patients perceive them positively.

Figure 19.2 shows the level of agreement between one doctor and his/her patients along with the written feedback provided to that physician.

Conclusion

This chapter shows the versatility of the patient perception measures as both research and education tools. The chapter has presented an overview of two

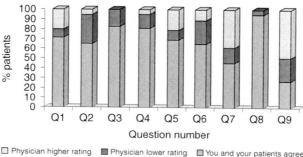

☐ Physician higher rating   ■ Physician lower rating   ■ You and your patients agree

The GRAY bar represents the percent of patients for which physician and patient rating agreed. On average, you agreed with 64% of your patients. In general your level of agreement is quite fairly inconsistent. The highest level of agreement, 92%, occurred on Q8 (How well do you think your doctor understood you today?) with Q3 (To what extent did the doctor listen to what you had to say?) a close second. The lowest level of agreement, 23% occurred on Q9 (To what extent did the doctor discuss personal/family issues that may affect your health?).

Now looking at the BLACK bar, on average, you rated your communication *lower* than 18% of your patients. The main source of disagreement occurred on Q2 (How satisfied were you with the discussion of your problem?), for which you rated yourself lower than 31% of your patients. There could be many reasons for this: you and your patients may have interpreted the question in different ways, you may have underestimated the impact of what you did discuss, and/or you are not as confident in yourself regarding this area of communication during patient visits. There were no other notable disagreements in this direction.

Now looking at the WHITE bar, on average, you rated your communication *higher* than 18% of your patients. Q7 (To what extent did the doctor explore how manageable this (treatment) would be for you?) and Q9 (To what extent did the doctor discuss personal or family issues that might affect your health?) both show fairly substantial disagreement in this direction (42% and 54% respectively).

*These percentages are based on the responses of 13 patients.

Figure 19.2   Level of agreement between the physician and that physician's patients, with the explanation to the physician.

questionnaire measures, showing their items, reliability and validity assessments, and their results. The two measures were:

1   the 14-item PPPC
2   the nine-item questionnaire which has a patient version and a physician version.

20

What these measures tell us about patient-centered care: interventions and outcomes

Moira Stewart and Judith Belle Brown

This chapter presents two recent studies using the Measure of Patient-Centered Communication and the Patient Perception of Patient-Centeredness question-naire. These two studies provide examples of rigorous epidemiologic methods and demonstrate that, while much has been learned, there is much left to be learned about the measurement and impact of patient-centered care.

The first study was called 'The impact of patient-centered care on patient outcomes in family practice' (Stewart *et al.*, 2000) and the second was 'Innovative training to improve physician communication with breast cancer patients, results of a randomized controlled trial'.

The study of impact

The hypothesis of this study (Stewart *et al.*, 2000) was that adult patients presenting a first episode of illness, who experienced a patient-centered visit, would more frequently demonstrate recovery from the discomfort of their symptom(s) and concerns two months after the encounter. They would also experience less subsequent medical care, that is, fewer patient-initiated visits, fewer diagnostic tests and fewer referrals in the two months after the visit.

This study used, first, the Measure of Patient-Centered Communication (MPCC) based on the audiotape of that initial visit, as described in Chapter 18. The second measure was of Patient Perception of Patient-Centeredness (PPPC) as described in Chapter 19. At the end of the audiotaped visit, the research assistant asked the 14 items of the PPPC questionnaire. A total score and two sub-scores were created: the patient perception sub-score that the illness experience had been fully explored; and the patient perception sub-score that the patient and doctor had found common ground. The health outcomes ascertained two months after the initial visit were: the patient's level of discomfort post-encounter compared to two months later (continuous variables measured on a visual analog scale based on pain studies, Klepac et al., 1981), and the patient's level of concern post-encounter compared to two months later (also a continuous variable). As well, patients were asked to complete the SF-36 (Stewart et al., 1988). There were sub-scores on physical health, mental health, perceptions of health, social health, pain (all continuous), and role function (a dichotomy). Finally, the study ascertained medical care outcomes (i.e. use of medical care resources) through a meticulous review of the patient's chart by three expert family physicians. The medical resources included: diagnostic tests over a two-month period (a dichotomous variable); number of referrals during the two months; and the number of visits during the two months after the study visit.

Step 1 of the analysis assessed confounding variables and identified two confounding variables to be included in later analyses: type of condition and marital status. Step 2 used multiple regressions for the continuous outcomes adjusted for the cluster sampling from the 39 practices using a statistical package on SAS called PROC-MIXED. For the two dichotomous outcomes we used a multiple logistic regression adjusting for the clustering of patients in practices, using the programs called PROC LOGISTIC and PROC IML.

A random sample of physicians was sought. There was a 52% refusal rate. The participants had the same year of graduation; location of practice within neighborhoods in the city of London, Ontario, Canada; and rural versus urban practice, as non-participants. But the participants were more likely to be a certificant of the College of Family Physicians of Canada. The 39 family physicians each contributed eight to ten patients (315 in total) and 28% of patients refused. The participants were the same age but more likely to be male than all eligible patients; 54% were female, the modal age category was 30–45 years old, 60% were married, and 42% had some post-secondary education.

Results in Table 20.1 show that the patient's perception of patient-centeredness (the PPPC) was significantly related to the patient's discomfort at the end of the two-month study period, controlling for baseline discomfort and the two confounding variables (type of presenting problem and marital status) and adjusting for clustering within practice. Significant findings with regard to the use of medical resources are shown in Table 20.2; when patients perceived that the visit was patient-centered, a lower proportion received diagnostic tests than if the patients perceived the visit was not patient-centered (14% versus 24%). Fewer patients were referred, as well (7% versus 16%).

In similar analyses, significant relationships were not found for the MPPC on the audiotape with patient health outcomes or use of medical resources.

Table 20.1 Multiple regression of patient perception of patient-centeredness (PPPC) total scores in relation to patients' post-encounter level of discomfort controlling for baseline discomfort (n = 297)*

Outcome: patients' level of discomfort

	Co-efficient	SE	Co-efficient/SE	p
Independent variables:				
PPPC total score	6.04	2.70	2.24	0.03
Baseline level of discomfort	0.84	0.04	22.50	0.0001
Patients' main presenting problem:				
• digestive	6.18	4.07	1.52	0.13
• musculoskeletal	2.42	3.39	0.71	0.48
• respiratory	6.56	3.25	2.02	0.04
• other	2.42	3.24	0.75	0.46
Patients' marital status	− 0.63	2.03	0.31	0.76

Mean level of discomfort by quartiles of the
PPPC total score

	Mean level of discomfort
First quartile – perception that the visit was patient-centered	42.5
Second quartile	45.0
Third quartile	45.2
Fourth quartile – perception that the visit was not patient-centered	48.8

* Adjusting for the clustering of patients within practices and controlling for two confounding variables (main presenting problem and marital status).

Figure 20.1 summarizes the pathway of relationships. The MPCC score based on the audiotape was significantly related to the total PPPC score, as well as the patient perception sub-score that the doctor and patient had found common ground. In addition, the PPPC was related to the patient health outcomes. However, the patient-centered behaviors (MPCC) although related to the patient perception were not directly related to the health outcomes. One conclusion is that only when the physician's patient-centeredness reaches a level that the patients notice will the outcomes be affected. One implication for teaching may

Table 20.2 Multiple logistic regression of patient perception of patient-centeredness (PPPC) total scores in relation to diagnostic tests ordered during the subsequent two months ($n = 297$)*

Outcome: diagnostic tests ordered (yes/no)

	Co-efficient	SE	Co-efficient/SE	p
Independent variables:				
PPPC total score	0.74	0.38	1.96	0.05
Patients' main presenting problem:				
• digestive	1.17	0.59	1.98	0.05
• musculoskeletal	0.27	0.53	0.52	0.61
• respiratory	0.05	0.40	0.11	0.91
• skin	−0.71	0.64	−1.11	0.26
Patients' marital status	0.64	0.31	2.06	0.04

Proportion of patients receiving diagnostic tests by
quartiles of the PPPC total score

	Proportion receiving diagnostic tests
First quartile – perception that visit was patient-centered	14.6%
Second quartile	17.0%
Third quartile	19.5%
Fourth quartile – perception that the visit was not patient-centered	24.3%

* Adjusting for the clustering of patients within practices and controlling for two confounding variables (main presenting problem and marital status).

be to incorporate patient perception as an important aspect in feedback to students about their patient-centeredness. These interesting findings are similar to findings of the next study.

The study of innovative training

The second study was titled 'Innovative training to improve physician communication with breast cancer patients, results of a randomized controlled trial' to

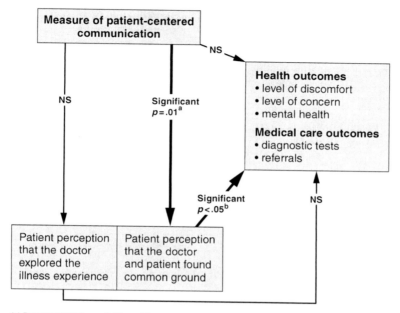

(a) Pearson correlation r = 0.16, p = .01
(b) Multiple regressions or multiple logistical regressions adjusted for clustering and
controlling for confounding variables

Figure 20.1   Diagram summarizing the relationships found among the measure of
patient-centered communication, patient perceptions of patient-centeredness and outcomes.
Reprinted with the permission of Dow Health Media Inc., from *The Journal of Family Practice*
49(9): 796–804.

address the question: does intensive training improve physician communication
with breast cancer patients? The purpose was to design a state-of-the-art educational program based on the real-life experiences of breast cancer survivors in the
hope of improving physicians' communication, and then formally evaluating this
program. This study was conducted in three phases: first, a qualitative study
exploring the real-life experiences of breast cancer survivors; second, a pretest of
the innovative CME program; and third, an evaluation of the CME program using
a randomized controlled trial.

In Phase I, the qualitative study revealed four important themes with regard
to breast cancer survivors' communication with healthcare providers around
the time of their diagnosis or recurrence of breast cancer (McWilliam *et al.*,
2000). Breast cancer survivors valued the ongoing, continuing relationship
with their healthcare providers, including trust and hope. The relationship-
building was intertwined with information-sharing. In other words, the vast
amount of information sharing with breast cancer patients must take place in

the context of a trusted relationship. The third theme was the experience of control. Patients recognized the importance of their attempts to regain control and to have some activities that they could do to participate in their healthcare. The fourth theme was mastering the whole person, i.e. the process of adjustment to the breast cancer as a chronic disease and as a part of the life of the patient, her family, her relationships, her sexual identity and her body image.

In Phase II a whole year was spent developing a state-of-the-art education intervention program based on the above four themes. The program contrasted with the control group program as illustrated in Table 20.3.

In Phase III, a randomized controlled trial evaluated the new intervention. We recruited 51 family physicians, surgeons and oncologists who were block randomized into two groups. Each physician started the study by seeing two announced standardized patients in their offices. One group received the six-hour state-of-the-art education intervention, and the other group received a two-hour education program (rather like a grand rounds with a video and a discussion). The small group six-hour continuing education interventions were led by a communication specialist and a clinician and included some important innovative educational components. After a short lecture on the relevant literature, we asked physicians to describe and discuss the barriers to good communication, followed by a discussion of solutions that they had tried. Then we turned to the patient's perception; a videotape was shown describing the findings of the qualitative study and we invited two breast cancer survivors into the small-group seminar to describe their experience of communication with health professionals around the time of diagnosis and to answer physicians' questions. The first segment of the CME concluded with two videotape demonstrations,

Table 20.3   Course outlines of the two continuing medical education programs

Course element	Intervention: state-of-the-art course	Control: traditional course
Length	6 hours	2 hours
Literature on the benefits of patient–physician communication	✓	✓
Physicians' perspective	✓	✕
Patients' perspective	✓	✕
Video demonstration and discussion	✓	✓
Two interviews with standardized patients followed by videotape review and feedback	✓	✕

a disease-centered and patient-centered communication between a doctor and a patient. After lunch the physicians participated in two standardized patient interviews. These were videotaped and participants received videotape feedback (following the rules of feedback in Chapter 13) from the group and from the group leaders, with a focus on the themes derived from the qualitative study.

After the intervention, both groups, once again, met two announced standardized patients in their offices. In addition, all of the surgeons and oncologists distributed questionnaires to ten real patients after the intervention. Family physicians did not hand out questionnaires because they rarely had more than three or four breast cancer patients in their practice at any one time. Therefore the list of outcome measures to assess the effectiveness of this state-of-the-art continuing education program was: the audiotapes of the standardized patients in the participant's office setting before compared to after the intervention and analyzed using a modified version of the MPCC; and the questionnaires administered to real patients including the PPPC and assessments of the patient's anxiety, satisfaction with information sharing, and perceived overall health.

The oncologists and surgeons who received the state-of-the-art education showed no difference in their actual behaviors on the modified MPCC as noted in the audiotaped analysis but the family physicians did. The six-hour education significantly improved the scores of family physicians by approximately 10 points on the 100 point scale of the modified MPPC whereas the control group remained the same.

In addition, the patients noticed differences between the state-of-the-art educated surgeons and oncologists, and the non-educated or the control group surgeons and oncologists in terms of their satisfaction with the doctor's information-giving and interpersonal skills. They also reported feeling better after the visit. The magnitude of these differences was large.

In conclusion the family physicians improved their communication behaviors. While the surgeons and oncologists did not improve their communication behaviors, their patients did notice a difference between the physicians who experienced the six-hour CME versus those who did not. There are at least two explanations for these contradictory results. First, there may be an educational reason. The surgeons and oncologists may have appreciated and responded to the patient's perspective, producing an attitude change. The two practice and feedback sessions may not have been successful for surgeons and oncologists because they perhaps did not believe that the standardized patients reflected real-life patient encounters. However, these sessions were successful for family physicians, perhaps because their residency training creates receptivity to learning from standardized patient visits. Second, there may be a measurement issue. Perhaps the modified MPCC, used to analyze the audiotapes, was not sensitive enough whereas the patient satisfaction measure and the self-related health measure were sensitive to the impact of the education.

Conclusion

Both of these studies indicate a need to look further to discern the physician behaviors that patients perceive. The patient-centered communication behaviors that we include in the MPCC do not, as a whole, correspond to what patients notice in either of the two studies. In the first study, an analytic study in family practice, the patient outcomes were not predicted by physician communication behaviors but were predicted by the patients' perceptions. In the second study, the education intervention affected the patients' views of the visits with the surgeons and oncologists but not the doctors' communication behaviors. Further research is therefore warranted to identify the sub-set of the patient-centered communication behaviors that matter to patients.

21

Conclusions

Moira Stewart

This book puts the patient at the center of medical care, education and research. It presents a clinical model and method relevant for all of medicine. No one medical specialty, and no particular type of patient problem, is better suited or less well suited to the approach outlined here. The patient-centered clinical method reveals the commonalities among medical disciplines rather than their distinctions. Indeed, it is a clinical method which shares much with other health professions as well. All practitioners can acknowledge the importance of the six components of the patient-centered clinical method: exploring both the disease and the illness experience; understanding the whole person; finding common ground; incorporating prevention and health promotion; enhancing the relationship; and being realistic.

One strength of the body of material contained in this book is that it represents two decades of work on four fronts simultaneously: conceptual/theoretical development; development of practical clinical approaches; educational development; and research. The first decade (1982–1992) saw great strides in the theoretical development of the patient-centered clinical method and patient-centered teaching. The second decade (1992–2002) saw the implementation of undergraduate medical education programs and residency programs based on patient-centered and learner-centered principles. As well, the second decade saw research programs come to fruition producing a harvest of new measures and provocative results.

Another strength of the patient-centered method is that it seeks to transcend some of the distinctions and limitations inherent in the conventional medical model, specifically the dichotomy between mind and body, art and science, feeling and thinking, subjective and objective, and tacit and explicit knowledge. Also, we challenge the notion that patient-centered medicine and evidence-based medicine are incompatible dichotomies; rather they are synergistic in creating improved clinical practice.

Medicine's attempts to embrace the whole rather than parts (i.e. both the mind and the body, both the subjective and the objective) is one aspect of a larger societal transformation toward a postmodern era. This turning point was allied with other recent changes such as the feminist movement, environmental action and community development. Nonetheless this broad embrace traces its origins not just to the postmodern trends of the twentieth century but to ancient Greece and the medical school of Kos.

One of the abiding strengths of this book and its predecessor is the presentation of the patient-centered framework in concise diagrams. Clinicians tell us that these pictures guide them even in the thick of an intense patient encounter. Educators have found them to be invaluable. However, these diagrams, even though helpful, are a double-edged sword; there are limitations. We have attempted to overcome the rather linear format of previous diagrams by locating component 3, 'Finding common ground' in its rightful place at the center of the process with the other components interacting around it. Still, none of these representations adequately depict the complex interactive process which circles around and around, always in motion. Although extremely helpful for clinical practice, for teaching and for clarity in research, diagrams can never fully capture the mysterious reality of a relationship between two people.

What does this book have to say to practicing clinicians? Putting the patient at the center of care is an important as well as somewhat daunting and long-term effort. It may be important, also, to say that aspiring to the practice of patient-centered medicine encompasses a change of heart as well as a change of mind. The change implies a new order, one in which the patient is a partner in care. There is, also, a change in the way physicians see themselves. Clinicians can be assured that patients are interested and will respond to being listened to, being respected and working in partnership with doctors.

What conclusions can be drawn from this book for medical educators? One message rings through loud and clear; putting the patient at the center is so much more than skills training. In order to assist students in the all-important change of heart, attention must be paid to their stage of development and to opportunities for enhancing their self-awareness. Another key point for educators is the parallel process between the patient-centered method of clinical care and the learner-centered method of education. In our view, continuing medical education must remain a priority to assist practicing clinicians in coping with the evolving demands of patients and the healthcare system. Finally and most importantly, the patient can be the center of education by being invited to teach, either directly in small or large group settings or indirectly by providing structured questionnaire feedback.

What key messages does this book have for researchers? Putting patients at the center of research has at least four meanings. The first is that research must embrace qualitative and quantitative approaches. Gaining insight into the illness experience and relationship through qualitative inquiry will assist a clinician's empathetic engagement. Data from quantitative studies are required to enhance analytic thinking about diagnosis and treatment. The second key message is that patients can be partners in the research enterprise, as advisors and co-leaders. Third, patients are the most appropriate evaluators of the degree to which the clinician is patient-centered. Finally, it is crucial that the striking research evidence about the effectiveness of the patient-centered clinical method be disseminated and acted upon, in order that the patient will remain at the center of practice.

Future directions

As the practice of medicine evolves, some internal and external pressures will facilitate the adoption of the patient-centered clinical method and others will impede it. Changes in healthcare in the past decade, and future changes, hold both threat and promise for patient-centered care, depending on the details of implementation. For example, some aspects of managed care disrupt continuity of care and intrude upon the patient–provider decision-making process regarding diagnostic tests and treatments. However, other aspects of managed care facilitate patient-centered care, such as the emphasis on patient satisfaction, malpractice risk reduction, and prevention and health promotion. Managed care should be scrutinized, with barriers to patient-centered practice being resisted and facilitators being promoted.

Similarly threat and promise exist with regard to the double-edged sword of information technology (IT). The opportunities that IT and the Internet provide for greater patient education and involvement should be encouraged. The problems arising in patient–physician encounters when the computer is the focus of attention, not the patient, need to be overcome through targeted policy and education.

In our view, each step in healthcare policy and planning should be scrutinized according to patient-centered criteria; if the innovation fails to support patient-centeredness, it should be returned to the drawing board for further analysis and revision. If this happens, then the important educational advances (in undergraduate, residency and continuing medical programs) aimed at enhancing the commitment of the clinician to be patient-centered will not be thwarted, but rather will be enhanced, by the clinical context.

An important next step in the development and evolution of the patient-centered clinical method, will be the application of the principles to a wide variety of problems hence evolving the concepts and making them tangibly relevant to concrete clinical situations. An exciting new series of books begins this task. They deal with: substance abuse (Floyd and Seale, 2002); chronic fatigue (Murdoch and Denz-Penhey, 2002); eating disorders (Berg *et al.*, 2002); and chronic myofascial pain (Malterud and Hunskaar, 2002).

This book identifies several important next steps for education of the patient-centered clinical method. Continued refinement of patient-centered curricula, for undergraduate medical education and for residency education, is necessary. An essential element for successful curriculum innovation is a well supported program of faculty development to provide opportunities to learn new teaching skills and to foster changes needed in the gestalt of the educational institutions. Also necessary is an energetic initiative for continuing medical education providing proven programs to a wider audience. Finally, including patients as partners in education can encourage the change of heart in the clinician so necessary for patient-centered relationships.

Two important next steps for research on the patient-centered clinical method have been highlighted in the book. First, research measures in the patient-centered domain, particularly measures based on review by a third party of a patient–doctor encounter, should be refined to ensure that they reflect dimensions which are important to patients. Second, the patient-centered interventions which researchers evaluate ought to be theory-based and should include the active participation of the patient.

Certain threads were woven throughout the chapters and the sections of this book: compassion, constancy, healing, caring and partnership. The book reveals parallels between clinical medicine advocating more emphasis on patient-centered clinical practice, education advocating learner-centered approaches and research seeking to understand meaning and experience as well as disease. One of these threads deserves special comment: *partnership*.

The changes we imagine in medical care, education and research are rooted in partnerships: between patients and doctors; between medical educators and medical students and residents; between continuing medical educators and practicing clinicians; among specialties within medicine; among the health professions; among researchers from a variety of backgrounds both quantitative and qualitative. Let us move medical care forward by first forging true and egalitarian partnerships in practice.

Appendix 1: Using review of videotaped interviews for learning and teaching

W Wayne Weston

It is difficult for doctors to change their interviewing methods. Byrne and Long (1984). Tuckett *et al.* (1985) and Verby *et al.* (1979) showed that older doctors' interviewing skills were no better than younger doctors', suggesting that they did not learn from experience. Walker (1988) evaluated the interviewing styles of part-time trainers in general practice before and after a one-year trainers' course. The course concentrated on attitudes and being more patient-centered. But after the course, the participants were actually more doctor-centered. One exception to this pessimistic review of the literature is the study by Verby *et al.* (1979). In this study, GPs provided peer review of their colleagues' videotaped interviews. A control group submitted videotapes that were not discussed. The peer learning group improved in a number of ways (compared with the control group) in that they:

- picked up more leads
- clarified more
- used more facilitation
- improved their questioning style
- ended the interview more smoothly.

Maguire and colleagues (1989) found similar results in a series of well-designed and controlled studies. Even four to six years later, the students who had received feedback on videotaped interviews were more likely to retain their skills than the control group.

The message is clear – review and feedback on videotaped interviews is a powerful teaching strategy; anything less may be ineffective in changing interviewing behavior.

Advantages of videotape review

- Provides an opportunity to see and hear yourself as others see and hear you – this is a remarkably powerful tool for enhancing self-awareness.

- Provides an opportunity to review the interview as it happened. So much is going on in a live interview that it is impossible to attend to everything important. Going over the interview again (or several times if necessary) reveals nuances of verbal and non-verbal behavior, sensitizing you to things you missed the first time so that you are more likely to see or hear them the next time.
- Because the tape can be reviewed at any time that suits the teacher's and learner's schedules, it is easier to arrange viewing and feedback than observation of live interviews.
- Provides an accurate record of what happened and does not rely on the frailties of memory thus avoiding arguments between student and teacher about what was said.
- Allows you to look at the interview with a colleague or supervisor to get more ideas about what was going on in the interaction and to consider ways to improve interviewing techniques or to consider new techniques.
- When the teacher and learner review the interview together it places the learner and teacher at the same level and facilitates a collaborative approach to teaching. Having the student review the tape first can enhance the student's role. This allows the student to select the segments of tape to watch with the teacher and to determine the agenda for the tape review. This places the learner in charge of his or her own learning. This is more effective than the traditional approach where the teacher has viewed a live interview as the expert and is expected to pronounce on the good and bad elements of the interview. From his or her detached and somewhat privileged position the teacher can always find things that the student could have done better. Because the student has been caught up in the interview and may need more time to think about it, he or she may feel in a 'one down' position, unable to be an equal participant in his or her own learning.
- When students know what to look for, they can review tapes on their own.
- Audiotapes are also very effective and cheaper and less complicated to set up than videotaping. Of course audiotapes do not pick up subtle non-verbal behavior. But audiotaping might be an effective way to get started with recording of interviews. Once the participants are comfortable with audiotaping, it is a small step to use videorecording.

Time and focus

One of the biggest reasons that videotape review is used so little is the misconception that it takes hours to do it properly. On the contrary, even brief review of a short segment of the videotape can be very effective. What takes time is setting everything up in the first place. But once the procedures are in place, taping can proceed without too much difficulty. Tape review should be goal oriented and can focus on components of the interview or on particular skills:

- The opening, e.g. 'How well am I introducing myself and my role on the team? Are there better or quicker ways to do this?'
- The closing, e.g. 'How well do I summarize the plans for treatment and follow-up?'
- Angry patients, e.g. 'How well do I respond to a patient's angry outburst? Are there other approaches I could use?'
- Management planning, e.g. 'How well do I find common ground with patients? Are there some other strategies I could use when the patient and I do not agree about the cause of the problem?'
- Screening for substance abuse, e.g. 'How well do I incorporate the CAGE questions into the interview?'
- Assessing a patient's stage of change, e.g. 'How well do I ask about a patient's readiness to consider changing a behavior?'
- Helping a patient in the maintenance stage of behavior change, e.g. 'How well do I work with patients, who are in the maintenance stage, to avoid relapse?'

The entire interview may be taped but only the relevant part needs to be reviewed with the teacher. Once the student knows what they are trying to accomplish, they can use tapes without supervision to continue to improve. A library of tapes made by teachers demonstrating each of the skills mentioned above would be a valuable resource for self-directed learning. This would save teacher time and would also give students a chance to see the teacher in action in situations that they might otherwise never see.

Guidelines for conducting videotape reviews

(Billings and Stoeckle, 1999; Butler and Englert, 2001; Carroll, 1981; Femino and Dube, 1995; Fuller and Manning, 1973; Paul *et al.*, 1998; Ram *et al.*, 1999)

1   The climate for the review should be psychologically safe. Remember – few people look good on videotape. Give participants time to get over the cosmetic effect – 'Good grief! Is that the way I look and sound!' Hargie and Saunders (1983) note that 'individuals viewing themselves for the first time are often preoccupied with the size, shape and general characteristics of their face and body, and ignore their actual behaviour' (1983: 159). But, with repeated exposure to video-feedback, they begin to focus on their performance and its consequences (Hargie and Morrow, 1986). They may need

to make a few tapes to watch on their own before being willing to show part of a tape to the teacher or to peers. But be careful – some students demand so much of themselves that they become excessively negative when they see minor imperfections on tape. Remind students that there is no such thing as a perfect interview – there is *always* something that could have been done better. This needs to be kept in mind whenever we are providing feedback – don't expect the impossible.

2   Keep the student's level of learning in mind – they are expected to have more to learn in the first and second years of medical school than in the third and fourth. Students in earlier years may be more interested in 'survival skills', e.g. how to deal with patients who seem to have limitless requests. Students who have little experience setting their own agenda for learning may need guidance about how to do this and some suggestions about what to focus on. The list included above in the section 'Time and focus' may help.

3   There should be prior agreement on the goals and behaviors to be focused on. Having clear objectives for these sessions is especially important; without goals you can easily lose your way. Also, without a focus, students tend to concentrate on their appearance rather than on their performance. When students are responsible for setting their own objectives for learning they are more engaged and motivated. Also, the process of goal-setting is itself highly educational. But be flexible – sometimes it is important to modify the agenda. Students may ignore an important issue on the tape because of a blind spot. But the teacher should avoid taking over and discarding the student's agenda – this may be embarrassing for the student and undermines the goal of helping learners be more self-directed. Clarify the roles of student and teacher before the tape review. Students welcome the opportunity to learn about their blind spots and will usually agree that one important role of the teacher is to point them out in a sensitive manner.

4   Optimum results are most likely with students who:

- are genuinely interested in participating
- have personal concerns or goals related to interviewing
- are open to change (at least at the stage of contemplation)
- have relatively good self-esteem
- can describe some deficiencies before the critique
- can identify discrepancies between observed and expected performance.

5   The feedback provided should:

- begin with the learner's observations first. Learning is more effective if it is self-initiated and self-critique generates less defensiveness than criticism from the teacher. Students tend to be more critical and demanding than the teacher and may be too hard on themselves. The teacher can

provide a more balanced perspective by pointing out the effective elements of the interview and reminding students that they are not expected to be perfect and that learning interviewing skills is a lifelong process
- include thanking students, if tape review is done in a group setting, for being willing to show their strengths and weaknesses so that all can learn
- focus on discrepancies that are moderate
- concentrate on two or three issues per session. Unless the review is focused on specific aspects of the interview, it is unlikely to effect any real change in behavior (Hargie and Morrow, 1986)
- be unambiguous, trustworthy, and informative
- be perceived by the student as accurate
- provide a balance between strengths and weaknesses. Too much negative criticism can overwhelm and discourage the student, whereas too little can create complacency and a lack of interest
- provide an opportunity to discuss feeling about the review process.

'Receiving feedback, whether negative or positive, always produces an emotional response ... Acknowledging that negative feedback is disappointing or embarrassing communicates understanding. The feelings of disappointment, frustration or embarrassment, although uncomfortable for both the giver and receiver, usually provide the motivation to make needed adjustments. Ignoring, minimizing or discounting the receiver's emotional response tends to distance the relationship' (Frankel, 1994a: 3).

There may also be strong feelings about the content of the interview or about the patient who was interviewed. This is common when the patient has problems with substance abuse. It is important to discuss these common reactions too.

6   The person(s) serving as facilitator(s) should:
- have previously been videotaped themselves
- communicate authenticity, positive regard and empathy
- collaborate with the learner regarding the goals of the feedback sessions
- confront the student with moderate discrepancies between observed and expected performance
- be non-judgmental toward the student.

7   Be watchful for 'parallel process' – issues present in the taped interview being replicated in the review process (also called 'isomorphism'). For example, if the student was having trouble finding common ground with the patient about the nature of the problem and the goals of management, the teacher may also have trouble reaching agreement with the student about his or her learning needs and the goals of the tape review. Drawing attention to these parallels may make the issue 'come alive' in the immediate experience of the student and teacher and may lead to better ideas about how to approach lack of agreement. Another example is a student who has trouble with time

management with patients because he feels it is impolite to negotiate with patients and to discuss how much time would be allotted for the visit. The teacher might ask if the student was offended when he had asked for the student's learning priorities because of time constraints. This parallel helps the student experience the issue from the patient's perspective and to realize that discussing time limitations with patients would not feel impolite to most patients (Frankel, 1994b: 4).

8   Discuss actions appropriate for establishing new behaviors, i.e. the student should leave the review with some *clear* ideas about how to perform at a higher level next time. It is helpful to ask the student to summarize what they are taking away from the feedback and discussion – their 'take home' message and planned learning activities. When there is a discrepancy between observed and expected behavior, consider two possible causes:

- a *skill* deficiency, i.e. the student has never learned the skill. In this case, plan opportunities for self-study and practice. Perhaps practice with role plays would be appropriate.
- a *performance* deficiency, i.e. the student is able to perform the skill but doesn't. This can be caused by several things:
  - The system makes it difficult to perform the task, e.g. too many patients to see in too short a time.
  - The performance is not rewarded, e.g. interviewing skills are often ignored.
  - Concentrating on interviewing skills may be punished because time taken from other tasks that are more highly valued, e.g. scut work.
  - The student is preoccupied with learning other things, e.g. management of serious organic disease, and has little time or energy for learning interviewing skills.
  - The student is 'burned out', depressed, preoccupied with a relationship problem or has a substance abuse problem.

The approach to these performance problems must obviously be tailored to the nature of the problem and speaks to the need for a broad view of student learning difficulties and the need for a program of assessment and support for all learners.

Common errors in using videotape review

(Frankel, 1994b)

1   Trying to do too much.
2   Confusing feedback and evaluation. Feedback is a gift – a chance to see yourself as others see you and provides an unparalleled opportunity to

learn; evaluation is always threatening and often provokes defensiveness thus reducing its educational value.

3   Applying gold standards to learners. Remember that medical education extends over the four years of medical school and the two to six more years of postgraduate education (and then forty years of practice). Don't expect students in second year, or even in clerkship, to have mastered all the intricacies of effective interviewing.

4   Deficit focus, i.e. concentrating on deficiencies rather than providing a balanced review of strengths and weaknesses.

5   Failure to take the learners' perspective into account.

6   Arguing about whether or not videotaping the interview created an artificial situation. The student may use this as an excuse for their inadequate performance and sometimes they are right. Performance anxiety may be increased so much by taping that they do not achieve their potential.

7   Being inflexible in a review agenda – be prepared to address unexpected issues if they are more important than the original agenda.

8   Failing to acknowledge the intensity of the experience and the vulnerability of the learner.

9   Ignoring the guidance, mentoring, nurturing and growth opportunities provided by these intense experiences.

10 Failing to solicit learner feedback on the session and the interaction. 'No feedback, no learning!' This applies to the teacher as well as the student. Feedback about the strengths and weaknesses of the review session will help make it better next time and provides a good model of the learning process.

11 Not respecting and/or protecting the participants' rights when showing tapes in settings outside the original tape review context. Always obtain informed consent if outside use of a tape is planned.

Consent for videotaping a patient

Most, if not all, medical schools and teaching hospitals have consent forms that the patient is asked to sign before taping is started. Patients need to have a clear explanation of the purpose of taping – to help the student learn more about interviewing – and assurance that no one except the student and teacher (and sometimes a small group of other students) will be viewing the tape and only for educational purposes. Some centers accept a verbal consent that is recorded at the start of the interview. Patient refusal to be videotaped is associated with younger age, being unemployed, female gender and psychological presentation (Howe, 1997).

Logistics

Videotape review is often not used because of misconceptions that it is too complicated, expensive or time-consuming. In fact, because it is so much more effective than any other method, it is probably a 'best buy' in terms of educational pay-off.

Modern videotape equipment is relatively inexpensive and the quality has improved dramatically in the past decade. There are two main methods to make recordings – using camcorders (either hand-held or on a tripod) and using wall-mounted cameras connected to a separate VCR.

Camcorders can be taken to patients' hospital rooms or to clinic examining rooms or even on house calls. Since many students have already had experience using camcorders for 'home movies', consider dividing the students into groups with each student taking turns recording the others. Tips can be provided on how to make a technically good recording.

The camera can be mounted on the wall of a clinic room and connected to a VCR and monitor in another room to permit recording as well as observation in real time. For wall-mounted cameras, you can use a camcorder or a remote camera that is simpler and cheaper – it is simply a camera without a microphone or cassette holder connected to a VCR. Remote microphones can be mounted in the ceiling and also connected to the VCR.

Sound quality leaves something to be desired with most camcorders although it has improved in recent years. Using external microphones will greatly improve the quality of sound recording. Small lapel microphones can be clipped onto the patient and physician to obtain excellent sound in an interview. Microphones can be suspended from the ceiling in clinic examining rooms. Note that when you use external microphones connected to a VCR you will need to use an amplifier to boost the audio signal.

Tips on making a technically good recording

- Mount the camera on a tripod if possible. This makes for a much steadier picture that is easier to watch than one in which the picture jumps around constantly. Electronic image stabilizers improve the quality of hand-held pictures but not as much as a tripod.
- Get the camera as close as possible to the subject in order to get the best possible sound quality. Note that the camera distorts the image so that people look fatter and farther apart than they really are. To get a 'natural looking' interview of two people requires them to be 'unnaturally close'.
- Avoid strong backlighting – the automatic iris will make the background look great but the foreground will be black, i.e. will look like shadows.

- Use remote microphones if available.
- Crop the picture by adjusting the zoom lens so that the subject fills as much of the screen as possible.
- Make sure the subject is in focus – use autofocus if available.
- If you pan or zoom during recording (to add variety), don't do too much – it is distracting.

Appendix 2: Learning the patient-centered clinical method: educational objectives

W Wayne Weston and Judith Belle Brown

This appendix to Chapter 15 describes each of the six interacting components of the patient-centered clinical method and outlines the knowledge, skills and attitudes needed by physicians practicing this approach. This list provides a quick synopsis of what we mean, in practical terms, by each component. In planning any learning experience, it is important for students to know where they are going (their objectives) otherwise they may end up somewhere else (Gronlund, 1999; Mager, 1968, 1997). Most lists of objectives are either so short and vague that they are unhelpful to the novice or they are so long and detailed that no one reads them. We have tried to avoid both extremes, to produce a usable list, by linking the educational objectives to the components of the medical interview. In this way, the curriculum is rooted in doctors' everyday interactions with their patients. But no list of objectives can stand alone. It is our hope that both students and teachers will use this list as a focus for joint discussion and for the development of learning plans. The list can also be utilized for evaluation by learners assessing their own learning needs and by teachers providing constructive feedback. This list is not intended to be exhaustive but rather to focus on what is most important. Objectives regarding the physician's conventional role are mentioned only briefly, not because they are less important, but because most readers will already be familiar with them.

Appendix 2 Learning the patient-centered clinical method: educational objectives

Objective	Knowledge	Skills	Attitudes
1 Exploring both the patient's disease and illness On the one hand, explores signs and symptoms of disease to develop a differential diagnosis; on the other hand, seeks to understand the patient's unique illness experience.	Detailed knowledge of common diseases – especially their presentations and natural history. General knowledge of treatable life-threatening, or disabling, conditions – even if rare – especially knowledge of early symptoms and signs. Understands why doctors and patients focus on organic manifestations of sickness and the limitations of this approach. Practical understanding of the distinction between disease and illness and the clinical relevance of this concept. Detailed knowledge of the common responses to sickness – their feelings, ideas, effects on function, and expectations. Working knowledge of illness behavior and the sick role: why people go to doctors when they do and the benefits and responsibilities of being sick.	Facilitates communication by balancing the use of open-ended and closed-ended techniques. Avoids behavior which 'cuts off' patients telling their own story of illness, e.g. ignoring important cues, interruptions, excessive focus on disease, jargon, premature reassurance, reading the chart, closed posture. Elicits patients' experience of illness by facilitating discussion of their feelings, ideas, effect of the illness on function, and their expectations of the physician. Pays attention to patients' feelings and responds appropriately to them. Searches for disease by zeroing in on cues to important disease processes. Conducts a reliable and efficient evaluation of patients' functional capacity – physical, emotional and social. Recognizes early cues to impending disaster.	Willingness to become involved in the full range of difficulties which patients bring to their doctors and not just their biomedical problems. Willingness to expend time, intellectual energy and emotional energy in working with patients.

Develops an efficient approach to the assessment of common presenting signs and symptoms.

Performs a reliable and efficient physical examination of all body systems, in patients of all ages in a manner which minimizes physical and emotional distress.

Avoids one-dimensional views of human sickness: skillfully weaves together the patient's story of illness with the physician's biomedical construct of the problem.

Critically analyzes data from any source – clinical evaluation. consultant's opinions or the medical literature.

Deals with uncertainty and ambiguity appropriately by focusing on the needs and welfare of the patient rather than the physician's desire for precision. Recognizes when it is necessary to make decisions on incomplete or conflicting data.

Appendix 2 Continued

Objective	Knowledge	Skills	Attitudes
2 Understanding the whole person	Deep knowledge of the human condition especially the nature of suffering and the responses of persons to sickness.	Able to explore patients' problems from multiple perspectives in an integrated fashion, e.g. molecules, tissues, organ systems, person, family and community.	Respect for the fundamental worth of all persons. Even when patients do not follow through with treatment or continue unhealthy lifestyles, physicians will demonstrate their belief in their value as persons.
Understands patients' diseases and their experiences of illness in relation to their life-setting, stage of personal and family development and broader context.	General understanding of the common effects of diseases on persons – physical, emotional, social and spiritual.	Defines patients' strengths.	
		Interviews more than one family member at a time to gather information about the patient and, also, about the influence of family interactions and relationships.	Shows respect for the values and beliefs of all cultural groups.
	Practical knowledge of the common developmental issues of each stage of human development.	Shows appropriate respect for patient confidentiality.	
	Deep knowledge of the effects of serious illness of one member of a family on the rest of the family.	Gathers information to construct a family genogram.	
	Understands the characteristics and hazards of the 'caretaker' role.	Uses housecalls to learn about the personal and family lives of patients.	
	Recognizes the impact of the family in ameliorating, aggravating, or even causing, illness in its members.	Takes an effective employment history to understand the role of work in causing, or alleviating, patients' problems.	
	Knowledge of the cultural beliefs and attitudes of patients which might influence their care.	Addresses patients' spiritual values and explores, when appropriate, how patients come to terms with their suffering.	
	Knowledge of the broader social, economic, political and environmental factors that influence patients' health.	Interviews patients within the context of their cultural background. Effectively interacts with patients using an interpreter.	

3 Finding common ground			
Reaches a mutual understanding and agreement on the problems, goals of treatment or management, and roles of doctor and patient.	Deep knowledge of the scientific treatment of diseases commonly seen in practice.	Expert use of conventional methods of treatment for common problems e.g. 'watchful expectancy', modification of lifestyle, medications, office procedures, hospitalization and referral. Also responds appropriately to emergencies and other serious problems, even if rare, for which early treatment makes a difference.	Willingness to collaborate with patients about management rather than needing always to 'take charge'.
	Understands the local folklore about common conditions seen.		Awareness of personal values and cultural differences and how these might interfere with providing unbiased assistance to patients with different values or points of view.
	Aware of the importance of patient autonomy.	Works with patients to manage, effectively, the full impact of disease and illness on themselves and their families.	
	Understands the issues that affect patient adherence.	Collaborates with patients to encourage and support them to take an active role in their own care.	
	Understands how medical decision making is fundamentally a moral enterprise.	Communicates information clearly to patients so that they are able to understand their problems, realize what may be done and what they can expect.	
	Working knowledge of clinical epidemiology especially regarding the predictive value of clinical and laboratory information and the critical appraisal of evidence.	Determines how much information, regarding their condition, patients want or are able to handle.	
	Understands the essential links between various components of the patient-centered clinical method and finding common ground.	Determines patients' ideas about their problems, their preferences about treatment and their concepts of the responsibilities of doctor and patient in management.	

Appendix 2 Continued

Objective	Knowledge	Skills	Attitudes
		Addresses differences of opinion with patients so that, together, they reach a conclusion that is both acceptable and safe for the patient.	
		Explicitly clarifies and summarizes the agreement with the patient.	
		Knows when to 'give in' gracefully to patients' urgent requests or demands and when, in the patients' best interests, it is essential to confront any differences of opinion.	

4 Incorporating prevention and health promotion			
Practices a systematic approach to prevention and health promotion that is congruent with patients' values.	Practical understanding of the importance of continuing comprehensive care and how this differs from episodic care.	Collaborates with the patient in developing a practical lifelong plan for health promotion and disease prevention.	Enthusiastic interest in all five stages of health promotion and prevention – health enhancement, risk avoidance, risk reduction, early detection, and complication reduction.
	General awareness of the characteristics of effective screening tests.	At appropriate intervals, monitors patients regarding already recognized problems and screens for unrecognized disease on the basis of an individualized assessment of each patient's risks.	Invests time and energy to incorporate screening, prevention and health promotion into day-to-day care of patients.
	Working knowledge of the evidence for or against the use of commonly recommended screening tests and the value of various preventive strategies, e.g. smoking counseling.	Uses the medical record system effectively as a reminder and also to document screening and prevention, e.g. problem lists, flow sheets, electronic records.	Accepts that some patients will not be interested, or ready to engage, in preventive or health promotion activities.
	Ability to define a protocol for screening all patients in the practice for those conditions for which screening has value.	Collaborates with the team to implement a program of screening and prevention in the practice.	
	Awareness of models of health promotion and their usefulness.	Enhances the patient's self-esteem and self-confidence in caring for themselves.	
		Effective use of motivational interviewing strategies.	
		Effectively finds common ground with patients regarding health promotion and prevention.	

Appendix 2 Continued

Objective	Knowledge	Skills	Attitudes
5 Enhancing the patient–doctor relationship At every visit, strives to build an effective long-term relationship with each patient as a foundation for their work together and to use the relationship for its healing power.	Understands the basic factors underlying an effective patient–doctor relationship – unconditional positive regard, empathy and genuineness. Understands the healing power and spiritual aspects of the patient–doctor relationship. Working knowledge of the placebo effect. Working knowledge of transference and counter-transference. Understands the potential for boundary violations and abuse of power. Self-awareness of personal strengths and weaknesses in working with patients. Awareness of emotional reactions to patients.	Communicates effectively both verbally and non-verbally to 'connect' with patients in meaningful and helpful ways. Creates a sense of safety and comfort, both by their interactions with patients and by their very presence. Uses personal qualities effectively – empathy, generating trust and confidence, providing support, encouragement and compassion. Uses physical contact with patients to allay fears, to establish therapeutic bonds and to provide comfort. Able to 'be with' patients in a healing relationship: attends fully to patients and their needs without always having to interpret or intervene. Uses repeated contacts to build up personal knowledge of patients and their families. Helps patients deal with termination of the patient–doctor relationship by preparing them in advance and providing opportunities to discuss their	Willingness to step into open-ended relationships with patients in which the expectations are often unknown in advance. Risks exposing areas of weakness and vulnerability. Risks being hurt. Willingness to make personal sacrifices when necessary for the well-being of patients. Exhibits long-term commitment to the well-being of patients. The relationship is a form of covenant: physicians promise to be faithful to their commitments even if patients do not follow through on theirs. Willingness to 'go to bat' for patients to protect them from the hazards of the healthcare system.

		feelings about the relationship and about their loss.	Self-awareness of limitations and personal responses to stress.
		Recognizes which patients require special approaches to interviewing and treatment e.g. ability to set appropriate limits.	Accepts that physicians cannot be all things to all people. Able to say no without guilt.
6 Being realistic about time and resources Manages resources, especially time and energy, to provide optimal care for each patient in the context of the whole practice and the community in which the physician works.	Aware of community resources.	Organizes time effectively and efficiently and, as much as possible, stays on schedule. Recognizes when a patient's situation requires extra time even if this disrupts the schedule.	Expends time and energy building personal relationships within his or her family.
	Understands the severe limitations of medicine to alter the natural course of disease.	Zeroes in on the heart of the problem: does not lose the forest for the trees.	Respects and values the roles and responsibilities of the other members of the healthcare team.
	Understands the task of medicine: 'To cure sometimes, to relieve often, to comfort always.'	Focuses on patients' prime needs and helps them to identify their central concerns.	Willingness to ask for help when needed.
	Understands the roles of the other members of the healthcare team.	Uses repeat visits effectively by not trying to do everything for every patient on each visit.	
	Understands how information technology can be incorporated into the practice of medicine, e.g. electronic medical records, e-mail, the Internet.	Works effectively as a member of a collaborative, interdisciplinary healthcare team.	
		Together with the patient, and other members of the team, sets reasonable goals and priorities.	

Appendix 2 Continued

Objective	Knowledge	Skills	Attitudes
		Wise stewardship of limited resources – balances needs of individual patients with the realities of the healthcare environment. Avoids being overextended by limiting responsibilities to what, realistically, can be accomplished.	

References

- Ablesohn A, Stieb D, Sanborn MD and Weir E (2002a) Identifying and managing adverse environmental health effects: 2. Outdoor air pollution. *CMAJ*. **166**(9): 1161–7.
- Ablesohn A, Gibson BL, Sanborn MD and Weir E (2002b) Identifying and managing adverse environmental health effects: 5. Persistent organic pollutants. *CMAJ*. **166**(12): 1549.
- Adjaye N (1981) Measles immunization. Some factors affecting non-acceptance of vaccine. *Public Health*. **95**(4): 185–8.
- Alonso A (1985) *The Quiet Profession – supervisors of psychotherapy*. Collier Macmillan, Canada, Toronto.
- Alonzo AA (2000) The experience of chronic illness and post-traumatic stress disorder: the consequences of cumulative adversity. *Soc Sci Med*. **50**(10): 1475–84.
- Anda RF, Croft JB, Felitti VJ, Nordenberg D, Giles WH, Williamson DF and Giovino GA (1999) Adverse childhood experiences and smoking during adolescence and adulthood. *JAMA*. **282**(17): 1652–8.
- Anderson ES, Winett RA, Wojcik JR, Winett SG and Bowden T (2001) A computerized social cognitive intervention for nutrition behavior: direct and mediated effects on fat, fiber, fruits, and vegetables, self-efficacy, and outcome expectations among food shoppers. *Ann Behav Med*. **23**(2): 88–100.
- Anderson JM, Anderson LJ and Felsenthal G (1993) Pastoral needs and support within an inpatient rehabilitation unit. *Arch Phys Med Rehabil*. **74**(6): 574–8.
- Anderson NR and West MA (1998) Measuring climate for work group innovation: development and validation of the team climate inventory. *J Organization Behav*. **19**: 235–58.
- Anderson RJ, Reed G and Kirk LM (1982) Compliance in elderly hypertensives. *Clinical Therapeutics*. **5**(Spec No.): 13–24.
- Andersson SO, Ferry S and Mattsson B (1993) Factors associated with consultation length and characteristics of short and long consultations. *Scand J Prim Health Care*. **11**: 61–7.
- Anspach RR (1988) Notes on the sociology of medical discourse: the language of case presentation. *J Health Social Behav*. **29**: 357–75.
- Arborelius E and Bremberg S (1992) What can doctors do to achieve a successful consultation? Videotaped interviews analysed by the 'consultation map' method. *Fam Pract*. **9**(1): 61–6.
- Armstrong D (1977) The structure of medical education. *Medical Education*. **11**: 244–8.
- Aronowitz RA (1998) *Making Sense of Illness: science, society, and disease*. Cambridge University Press, Cambridge.
- Audunsson GG (1986) *Preventive Infrastructure in Family Practice*. The Iceland Ministry of Health, Reykjavik, Iceland.
- Backett-Milburn K, Parry O and Mauthner N (2000) 'I'll worry about that when it comes along': osteoporosis, a meaningful issue for women at mid-life? *Health Educ Res*. **15**(2): 153–62.

- Baker SS (1985) *Information, Decision-making, and the Relationship Between Client and Health Care Professional in Published Personal Narratives.* University Microfilms International, Ann Arbor, MI.
- Baldwin DC, Jr, Daugherty SR and Eckenfels EJ (1991) Student perceptions of mistreatment and harrassment during medical school – a survey of ten United States schools. *West J Med.* **155**: 140–5.
- Bales RF (1950) *Interactive Process Analysis: a method for the study of small groups.* Addison-Wesley, Reading, MA.
- Balint E, Courtenay AE, Hull S and Julian P (1993) *The Doctor, the Patient, and the Group.* Routledge, London.
- Balint M (1957) *The Doctor, His Patient, and the Illness.* International Universities Press, New York.
- Balint M (1964) *The Doctor, His Patient, and the Illness* (2e). International Universities Press, New York.
- Balint M, Hunt J, Joyce D, Marinker M and Woodcock J (1970) *Treatment or Diagnosis: a study of repeat prescriptions in general practice.* JB Lippincott, Philadelphia, PA.
- Bandura A (1986) *Social Foundations of Thought and Action: a social cognitive theory.* Prentice-Hall, Englewood Cliffs, NJ.
- Barbee RA and Feldman SE (1970) A three year longitudinal study of the medical interview and its relationship to student performance in clinical medicine. *J Med Educ.* **45**(10): 770–6.
- Barry CA, Bradley CP, Britten N, Stevenson FA and Barber N (2000) Patients' unvoiced agendas in general practice consultations: qualitative study. *BMJ.* **320**: 1246–50.
- Barry CA, Stevenson FA, Britten N, Barber N and Bradley CP (2001) Giving voice to the lifeworld. More humane, more effective medical care? A qualitative study of doctor–patient communication in general practice. *Soc Sci Med.* **53**: 487–505.
- Bartz R (1993) *Interpretive Dialogue: a multi-method qualitative approach for studying doctor–patient interactions.* Paper presented at the Annual Meeting of the North American Primary Care Research Group, San Diego, CA.
- Bartz R (1999) Beyond the biopsychosocial model: new approaches to doctor–patient interactions. *J Fam Pract.* **48**(8): 601–7.
- Baskett HK and Marsick VJ (1992) Professionals' ways of knowing: new findings on how to improve professional education. In: HK Baskett and VJ Marsick (eds) *New Directions for Adult and Continuing Education,* 55. Jossey-Bass, San Francisco, CA.
- Bass MJ, Buck C, Turner L, Dickie G, Pratt G and Campbell Robinson CH (1986) The physician's actions and the outcome of illness in family practice. *J Fam Pract.* **23**: 43–7.
- Battista RN and Lawrence RS (eds) (1988) Implementing preventive services. *Am J Prev Med.* **4**(Supp 8).
- Battle CU (1975) Symposium on behavioral pediatrics. Chronic physical disease. Behavioral aspects. *Pediatr Clin North Am.* **22**(3): 525–31.
- Baur C (2000) Limiting factors on the transformative powers of e-mail in patient–physician relationships: a critical analysis. *Health Commun.* **12**(3): 239–59.
- Beaudoin C, Maheux B, Cote L, Des Marchais JE, Jean P and Berkson L (1998) Clinical teachers as humanistic caregivers and educators: perceptions of senior clerks and second-year residents. *CMAJ.* **159**: 765–9.
- Becker MH and Janz NK (1990) Practicing health promotion: the doctor's dilemma. *Ann Int Med.* **113**(6): 419–22.
- Beckman HB and Frankel RM (1984) The effect of physician behavior on the collection of data. *Ann Int Med.* **101**(5): 692–6.

- Beckman HB, Markakis KM, Suchman AL and Frankel RM (1994) The doctor–patient relationship and malpractice: lessons from plaintiff depositions. *Arch Int Med.* **154**: 1365–70.
- Beeker C, Kraft JM, Southwell BG and Jorgensen CM (2000) Colorectal cancer screening in older men and women: qualitative research findings and implications for intervention. *J Community Health.* **25**(3): 263–78.
- Belenky MF, Clinchy BM, Goldberger NR and Tarule JM (1986) *Women's Ways of Knowing: the development of self, voice, and mind.* Basic Books, New York.
- Berger AS (2002) Arrogance among physicians. *Academic Medicine.* **77**(2): 145–7.
- Berger J and Mohr J (1967) *A Fortunate Man: the story of a country doctor.* Pantheon Books, New York.
- Berkman LF and Syme SL (1979) Social networks, host resistance, and mortality: a nine-year follow-up of Alameda County residents. *Am J Epidemiol.* **109**: 186–204.
- Berwick DM (1991) Controlling variation in health care: a consultation from Walter Shewhart. *Med Care.* **29**(12): 1212–25.
- Berzoff J, Flanagan LM and Hertz P (1996) *Inside Out and Outside In. Psychodynamic clinical theory and practice in contemporary multicultural contexts.* Jason Aronson Inc., North Vale, NJ.
- Bevis O and Watson J (2000) *Toward a Caring Curriculum: a new pedagogy for nursing.* Jones and Bartlett Publishers, Sudbury, MA.
- Biegel DE, Npparstek AJ and Khan MM (1980) Determinants of social support systems. In: RR Stough and A Wandersman (eds) *Optimizing Environments: research, practice and policy.* Environmental Design Research Association, Washington, DC.
- Billings JA and Stoeckle JD (1999) *The Clinical Encounter – a guide to the medical interview and case presentation* (2e). Mosby, St Louis, MO.
- Bird J and Cohen-Cole SA (1990) The three function model of the medical interview: an educational device. In: MS Hale (ed.) *Methods in Teaching Consultation-liaison Psychiatry.* Karger, Basel.
- Blacklock SM (1977) Symptom of chest pain in family practice. *J Fam Pract.* **4**: 429–33.
- Blackwell B (1996) From compliance to alliance. A quarter century of research. *Netherlands J Med.* **48**: 140–9.
- Blane D, Hart CL, Smith GD, Gillis C, Hole DJ and Hawthorne VJ (1997) Association of cardiovascular disease risk factors with socioeconomic position during childhood and during adulthood. *BMJ.* **313**: 1434–8.
- Blumenthal D, Causino N, Chang YC, Culpepper L, Marder W, Saglam D, Stafford R and Starfield B (1999) The duration of ambulatory visits to physicians. *J Fam Pract.* **48**(4): 264–71.
- Boaden N and Leaviss J (2000) Putting teamwork in context. *Med Educ.* **34**(11): 921–7.
- Boon H, Brown JB, Gavin A, Kennard MA and Stewart M (1999) Breast cancer survivors' perceptions of complementary/alternative medicine (CAM): making the decision to use or not to use. *Qual Health Res.* **9**(5): 639–53.
- Borkan J, Reis S, Steinmetz D and Medalie JH (1999) *Patients and Doctors. Life-changing stories from primary care.* The University of Wisconsin Press, Madison, WI.
- Borkan JM (1999) Examining American family medicine in the new world order: a study of 5 practices. *J Fam Pract.* **48**(8): 620–7.
- Bosma H, Schrijvers C and Mackenbach JP (1999) Socioeconomic inequalities in mortality and importance of perceived control: cohort study. *BMJ.* **319**: 1469–70.
- Botelho R (2002) *Beyond Advice: becoming a motivational practitioner.* Motivative Healthy Habits Press, Rochester, NY.

- Bowen M (1976) Theory in the practice of psychotherapy. In: PJ Guerin (ed.) *Family Therapy: theory and practice*. Gardner Press, New York.
- Bowen M (1978) Toward the differentiation of self in one's family of origin. In: M Bowen (ed.) *Family Therapy in Clinical Practice*. Jason Aronson, New York.
- Boyer EL (1990) *Scholarship Reconsidered: priorities of the professoriate*. The Carnegie Foundation for the Advancement of Teaching, Princeton, NJ.
- Braddock CH, Edwards KA, Hasenberg NM and Levinson W (1999) Informed decision making in outpatient practice: time to get back to basics. *JAMA*. **282**(24): 2313–20.
- Brent DA (1981) The residency as a developmental process. *J Med Educ*. **56**(5): 417–22.
- Brett AS (1999) Views of managed care. *NEJM*. **341**(8): 616–18.
- Britten N, Stevenson FA, Barry CA, Barber N and Bradley CP (2000) Misunderstandings in prescribing decisions in general practice: qualitative study. *BMJ*. **320**: 484–8.
- Brody H (1992) *The Healer's Power*. Yale University Press, New Haven, CT.
- Brody H (1999) The biopsychosocial model, patient-centered care, and culturally sensitive practice. *J Fam Pract*. **48**(8): 585–7.
- Brookfield SB (1985) Self-directed learning: from theory to practice. In: *New Directions for Adult and Continuing Education, 25*. Jossey-Bass, San Francisco, CA.
- Brookfield SB (1986) *Understanding and Facilitating Adult Learning: a comprehensive analysis of principles and effective practices*. Jossey-Bass, San Francisco, CA.
- Broom B (1997) *Somatic Illness and the Patient's Other Story. A practical integrative mind/body approach to disease for doctors and psychotherapists*. Free Association Books Ltd, New York.
- Broom BC (2000) Medicine and story: a novel clinical panorama arising from a unitary mind/body approach to physical illness. *Adv Mind Body Med*. **16**(3): 161–77.
- Brown JB, Stewart M and Ryan B (forthcoming) Outcomes of patient–provider interaction. In: T Thompson *et al.* (eds) *Handbook of Health Communication*. Lawrence Erlbaum, Mahwah, NJ.
- Brown JB, Stewart MA, McCracken EC, McWhinney IR and Levenstein JH (1986) Patient-centered clinical method II. Definition and application. *Fam Pract*. **3**(2): 75–9.
- Brown JB, Weston WW and Stewart MA (1989) Patient-centered interviewing Part II: Finding common ground. *Canadian Family Physician*. **35**: 153–7.
- Brown JB, Stewart MA and Tessier S (1995) Assessing communication between patients and doctors: a manual for scoring patient-centered communication. *CSFM Working Paper Series*. **95**(2). Centre for Studies in Family Medicine, The University of Western Ontario, London, Ontario.
- Brown JB, Handfield-Jones R, Rainsberry P and Brailovsky CA (1996) The Certification Examination of the College of Family Physicians of Canada: IV: Simulated Office Orals. *Canadian Family Physician*. **42**: 1539–48.
- Brown JB, McWilliam C and Mai V (1997a) Barriers and facilitators to seniors' independence: perceptions of seniors, caregivers and health care providers. *Canadian Family Physician*. **43**: 469–79.
- Brown JB, Dickie I, Brown L and Biehn J (1997b) Long-term attendance at a family practice teaching unit. *Canadian Family Physician*. **43**: 901–6.
- Brown JB, Sangster M and Swift J (1998) Factors influencing palliative care. Qualitative study of family physicians' practices. *Canadian Family Physician*. **44**: 1028–34.
- Brown JB, Stewart M and Ryan B (2001) Assessing communication between patients and physicians: the measure of patient-centered communication (MPCC) (2e). *Working Paper Series*. **95**(2). UWO, London, Ontario.
- Brown JB, Sangster LM, Ostbye T, Barnsley JM, Mathews M and Ogilvie G (2002a) Walk-in clinics: patient expectations and family physician availability. *Fam Pract*. **19**(2): 202–6.

- Brown JB, Lent B, Stirling A, Takhar J and Bishop J (2002b) Caring for seriously mentally ill patients: qualitative study of family physicians' experiences. *Canadian Family Physician.* **48**: 915–20.
- Brown JB, Sangster LM, Ostbye T, Barnsley J, Mathews M and Ogilvie G (2002c) Walk-in clinics in Ontario: an atmosphere of tension. *Canadian Family Physician.* **48**: 531–6.
- Brown JB, Stewart M and Weston WW (2002d) *Challenges and Solutions in Patient-centered Care: a case book.* Radcliffe Medical Press, Oxford.
- Brown JB, Harris SB, Webster-Bogaert S, Wetmore S, Faulds C and Stewart M (2002e) The role of patient, physician and systemic factors in the management of type 2 diabetes mellitus. *Fam Pract.* **19**(4): 344–9.
- Brown JB, Carroll J, Boon H and Marmoreo J (2002f) Women's decision-making about their health care: views over the life cycle. *Patient Educ Couns.* **48**(3): 225–31.
- Broyard A (1992) *Intoxicated By My Illness. And other writings on life and death.* Clarkson Potter Publishers, New York.
- Bruce N and Burnett S (1991) Prevention of lifestyle-related disease: general practitioners' views about their role, effectiveness, and resources. *Fam Pract.* **8**(4): 373–7.
- Burke V, Giangiulio N, Gillam HF, Beilin LJ, Houghton S and Milligan RA (1999) Health promotion in couples adapting to a shared lifestyle. *Health Educ Res.* **14**(2): 269–88.
- Burtt EA (1954) *The Metaphysical Foundations of Modern Science* (2e). Doubleday, Garden City, NY.
- Butler DJ and Englert L (2001) On the rise and fall of videotaping programs. *Fam Med.* **33**(2): 89–90.
- Byrne PS and Long BEL (1984) *Doctors Talking to Patients.* HMSO, London.
- Calnan M (1988) Examining the general practitioner's role in health education: a critical review. *Fam Pract.* **5**(3): 217–23.
- Campbell TL, McDaniel SH and Seaburn DB (1998) Principles of collaborative family healthcare. In: AL Suchman, RJ Botelho and P Hinton-Walker (eds) *Partnerships in Health Care: transforming relational process.* University of Rochester Press, Rochester, NY.
- Canadian Task Force on the Periodic Health Examination (1994) *The Canadian Guide to Clinical Preventive Health Care.* Health Canada, Ottawa.
- Candib LM (1987) What doctors tell about themselves to patients: implications for intimacy and reciprocity in the relationship. *Fam Med.* **19**(1): 23–30.
- Candib LM (1988) Ways of knowing in family medicine: contributions from a feminist perspective. *Fam Med.* **20**(2): 133–6.
- Candib LM (1995) *Medicine and the Family. A feminist perspective.* Basic Books, New York.
- Candy PC (1991) *Self-direction for Lifelong Learning – a comprehensive guide to theory and practice.* Jossey-Bass, San Francisco, CA.
- CanMEDS 2000 (2000) Extract from the CanMEDS 2000 project societal needs working group report. *Medical Teacher.* **22**(6): 549–54.
- Cannon WB (1990) The case method of teaching systematic medicine. *Boston Medical Surgery Journal.* **142**: 31–6.
- Carroll J, Brown JB, Blaine S, Glendon G, Pugh P and Medved W (2003) Genetic susceptibility to cancer: family physicians' concerns and needs. *Canadian Family Physician.* **49**: 45–52.
- Carroll JC, Brown JB, Reid AJ and Pugh P (2000) Women's experience of maternal serum screening. *Canadian Family Physician.* **46**: 614–20.
- Carroll JG (1981) Faculty evaluation. In: *Handbook of Teacher Evaluation.* Sage Publications, Beverly Hills, CA.
- Carson R (1962) *Silent Spring.* Fawcett Publications, Greenwich, CT.

- Carter AH (1989) Metaphors in the physician–patient relationship. *Soundings.* **72**(1): 153–64.
- Carter B and McGoldrick M (eds) (1989) *The Changing Family Life Cycle: a framework for family therapy.* Allyn and Bacon, Boston, MA.
- Carter H and Jones I (1985) Measles immunization: results of a local programme to increase vaccine uptake. *BMJ.* **290**:1717–19.
- Carter WB, Belcher DW and Inui TS (1981) Implementing preventive care in clinical practice II. Problems for managers, clinicians and patients. *Med Care Rev.* **38**(4): 195–216.
- Casbergue J (1978) The role of faculty development in clinical education. In: MK Morgan and DM Irby (eds) *Evaluating Clinical Competence in the Health Professions.* CV Mosby, St Louis, MO.
- Cassell EJ (1985a) *Talking with Patients II. Clinical technique.* The MIT Press, Cambridge, MA.
- Cassell EJ (1985b) *The Healer's Art.* The MIT Press, Cambridge, MA.
- Cassell EJ (1991) *The Nature of Suffering and the Goals of Medicine.* Oxford University Press, New York.
- Charon R (1986) To render the lives of patients. *Lit Med.* **5**: 58–74.
- Charon R (1989) Doctor–patient/reader–writer: learning to find the text. *Soundings.* **72**(1): 137–52.
- Charon R (2001) The patient–physician relationship. Narrative medicine: a model for empathy, reflection, profession, and trust. *JAMA.* **286**(15): 1897–1902.
- Cheren M (1983) Helping learners achieve greater self-direction. In: RM Smith (ed.) *Helping Adults Learn How to Learn.* Jossey-Bass, San Francisco, CA.
- Cherry JD (1984) The epidemiology of pertussis and pertussis immunization in the United Kingdom and the United States: a comparative study. *Curr Probl Pediatr.* **14**(2): 1–78.
- Chickering AW (1981) *The Modern American College.* Jossey-Bass, San Francisco, CA.
- Chovanec DM (1998) Self-directed learning: highlighting the contradictions. In: SM Scott, B Spencer and AM Thomas (eds) *Learning for Life – Canadian readings in adult education.* Thompson Educational Publishing, Toronto.
- Christie-Seeley J (1984) *Working with the Family in Primary Care.* Praeger, New York.
- Churchill LR (1997) 'Damaged humanity': the call for a patient-centered medical ethic in the managed care era. *Theor Med.* **18**(12): 113–26.
- Coe RM, Prendergast CG and Psathas G (1984) Strategies for obtaining compliance with medications regimens. *JAMA.* **32**: 589–94.
- Cohen SJ (1985) An educational psychologist goes to medical school. In: EW Eisner (ed.) *The Educational Imagination: on the design and evaluation of school programs* (2e). Macmillan, New York.
- Coombs RH (1998) *Surviving Medical School.* Sage Publications, Thousand Oaks, CA.
- Cooper AF (1998) Whose illness is it anyway? Why patient perceptions matter. *Int J Clin Pract.* **52**(8): 551–6.
- Corin E (1994) The social and cultural matrix of health and disease. In: A De Gruyter (ed.) *Why Are Some People Healthy and Others Not? The determinants of health of populations.* Hawthorne, New York.
- Cortese L, Malla AK, McLean T and Diaz JF (1999) Exploring the longitudinal course of psychotic illness: a case study approach. *Can J Psychiatr.* **44**(9): 881–6.
- Cousins N (1979) *Anatomy of an Illness as Perceived by the Patient.* Norton, New York.
- Craigie FC, Jr and Hobbs RF, III (1999) Spiritual perspectives and practices of family physicians with an expressed interest in spirituality. *Fam Med.* **31**(8): 578–85.

- Crookshank FG (1926) The theory of diagnosis. *Lancet.* **2**: 934–42; 995–9.
- Curry L (2002) Individual differences in cognitive style, learning style and instructional preference in medical education. In: GR Norman, CPM van der Vleuten and DI Newble (eds) *Handbook of Research in Medical Education*, Kluwer Academic, Dordrecht.
- Cushing H (1925) *The Life of Sir William Osler*. Clarendon Press, Oxford.
- D'Eon M, Overgaards V and Harding SR (2000) Teaching as a social practice: implication for faculty development. *Adv Health Sciences Educ.* **5**: 151–62.
- Daloz LA (1999) Mentor: guiding the journey of adult learners. In: *Effective Teaching and Mentoring* (2e). Jossey-Bass, San Francisco, CA.
- Daniels N, Kennedy B and Kawachi I (2000) *Is Inequality Bad for Our Health?* Beacon Press, Boston, MA.
- David DS (1999) Views of managed care. *NEJM.* **341**(8): 617–18.
- de Bourdeaudhuij I and Van Oost P (1998) Family members' influence on decision making about food: differences in perception and relationship with healthy eating. *Am J Health Promotion.* **13**(2): 73–81.
- de Leeuw E (1989) Concepts in health promotion: the notion of relativism. *Soc Sci Med.* **29**(11): 1281–8.
- Dietrich AJ and Marton KI (1982) Does continuous care from a physician make a difference? *J Fam Pract.* **15**: 929–37.
- Doherty WJ and Baird MA (1986) Developmental levels in family-centered medical care. *Fam Med.* **18**(3): 153–6.
- Doherty WJ and Baird MA (1987) *Family-centered Medical Care: a clinical casebook*. Guilford Press, New York.
- Donnelly WJ (1986) Medical language as symptom: doctor talk in teaching hospitals. *Perspect Biol Med.* **30**(1): 81–94.
- Donnelly WJ (1989) Righting the medical record: transforming chronicle into story. *Soundings.* **72**(1): 127–36.
- Dowell J and Hudson H (1997) A qualitative study of medication-taking behaviour in primary care. *Fam Pract.* **14**(5): 369–75.
- Dowell J, Jones A and Snadden D (2002) Exploring medication use to seek concordance with 'non-adherent' patients: a qualitative study. *Br J Gen Pract.* **52**(474): 24–32.
- Dowell JS, Snadden D and Dunbar JA (1996) Rapid prescribing change, how do patients respond? *Soc Sci Med.* **43**(11): 1543–9.
- Doxiadis S (ed.) (1987) *Ethical Dilemmas in Health Promotion*. John Wiley and Sons, New York.
- Drinka TJK and Clark PG (2000) Health care teamwork. In: *Interdisciplinary Practice and Teaching*. Greenwood, Westport, CT.
- Dubos R (1980) *Man Adapting*. Yale University Press, New Haven, CT.
- Dubovsky SL (1981) *Psychotherapeutics in Primary Care*. Grune and Stratton, New York.
- Dudley RA and Luft HS (2001) Managed care in transition. *NEJM.* **344**(14): 1087–92.
- Eagle MN (1984) *Recent Developments in Psychoanalysis: a critical evaluation*. McGraw-Hill, New York.
- Eberhart-Phillips J, Hall D, Herbison GP, Jenkins S, Lambert J, Ng R, Nicholson M and Rankin L (2000) Internet use amongst New Zealand general practitioners. *New Zealand Medical Journal.* **113**: 135–7.
- Egbert LD, Battit GE, Welch CE and Bartlett MK (1964) Reduction of post-operative pain by encouragement and instruction of patients. A study of doctor–patient rapport. *NEJM.* **270**: 825–7.

- Ehman JW, Ott BB, Short TH, Ciampa RC and Hansen-Flaschen J (1999) Do patients want physicians to inquire about their spiritual or religious beliefs if they become gravely ill? *Arch Int Med.* **159**(15): 1803–6.
- Eichna L (1980) Medical-school education, 1975–1979: a student's perspective. *NEJM.* **303**(13): 727–34.
- Eisner EW (1985) *The Educational Imagination: on the design and evaluation of school programs* (2e). Macmillan, New York.
- Ellis MR, Vinson DC and Ewigman B (1999) Addressing spiritual concerns of patients: family physicians' attitudes and practices. *J Fam Pract.* **48**(2): 105–9.
- Ellis MR, Campbell JD, Detwiler-Breidenbach A and Hubbard DK (2002) What do family physicians think about spirituality in clinical practice? *J Fam Pract.* **51**(3): 249–54.
- Elwyn G and Smail J (1999) *Integrated Teams in Primary Care.* Radcliffe Medical Press, Oxford.
- Elwyn G, Edwards A, Kinnersley P and Grol R (2000) Shared decision making and the concept of equipoise: the competences of involving patients in healthcare choices. *Br J Gen Pract.* **50**: 892–7.
- Elwyn G and Charles C (2001) Shared decision making: the principles and the competences. In: GEA Edwards (ed.) *Evidence-based Patient Choice. Inevitable or impossible?* Oxford University Press, New York.
- Emanuel EJ and Dubler NN (1995) Preserving the physician–patient relationship in the era of managed care. *JAMA.* **273**(4): 323–9.
- Engel GL (1977) The need for a new medical model: a challenge for biomedicine. *Science.* **196**(4286): 129–36.
- Engel GL (1980) The clinical application of the biopsychosocial model. *Am J Psychiatry.* **137**(5): 535–44.
- Entralgo PL (1961) *The Therapy of the Word in Classical Antiquity.* Yale University Press, New Haven, CT.
- Entralgo PL (1956) *Mind and Body.* PJ Kennedy, New York.
- Epp J (1986) *Achieving Health for All: a framework for health promotion.* Health and Welfare Canada, Ottawa.
- Epstein PR (1995) Emerging diseases and ecosystem instability: new threats to public health. *Am J Public Health.* **Feb**: 168–72.
- Epstein RM, Campbell TL, Cohen-Cole SA, McWhinney IR and Smilkstein G (1993) Perspectives on patient–doctor communication. *J Fam Pract.* **37**(4): 377–88.
- Epstein RM (1999) Mindful practice. *JAMA.* **282**(9): 833–9.
- Erikson EH (1950) *Childhood and Society.* Norton, New York.
- Erikson EH (1982) *The Life Cycle Completed: a review.* Norton, New York.
- Ettner SL (1999) The relationship between continuity of care and the health behaviors of patients: does having a usual physician make a difference? *Med Care.* **37**(6): 547–55.
- Evans BJ, Kiellerup FD, Stanley RO, Burrows GD and Sweet B (1987) A communication skills programme for increasing patients' satisfaction with general practice consultations. *Br J Med Psychology.* **60**: 373–8.
- Evans JM, Newton RW, Ruta DA, MacDonald TM and Morris AD (2000) Socio-economic status, obesity and prevalence of Type 1 and Type 2 diabetes mellitus. *Diabetic Medicine.* **17**(6): 478–80.
- Faber K (1923) *Nosography in Modern Internal Medicine* (trans. Jean Martin). Paul B Hoeber, New York.
- Feinstein J (1993) The relationship between socioeconomic status and health: a review of the literature. *Milbank Quarterly.* **71**(2): 279–322.

- Feldman RH, Damron D, Anliker J, Ballesteros RD, Langenberg P, DiClemente C and Havas S (2000) The effect of the Maryland WIC-5-A-Day promotion program on participants' stages of change for fruit and vegetable consumption. *Health Educ Behav.* **27**(5): 649–63.

- Femino J and Dube C (1995) Instructional use of audio and video recording. In: M Lipkin Jr, SM Putnam and A Lazare (eds) *The Medical Interview: clinical care, education and research.* Springer, New York.

- Ferris TG (1998) Today's primary care doctors offer more time and counseling to children but also prescribe more medications. *AHCPR.* **217**: 8–9.

- Festinger L (1957) A theory of cognitive dissonance. Quoted in: LA Daloz (1999) *Mentor: guiding the journey of adult learners* (2e of *Effective Teaching and Mentoring.* Jossey-Bass, San Francisco, CA). University Press, Stanford, CA.

- Fields HJ (1990) About men: a whole new ballgame. *New York Times Magazine.*

- Fleck L (1979) *The Genesis and Development of a Scientific Fact.* University of Chicago Press, Chicago.

- Flexner A (1910) *Medical Education in the United States and Canada.* The Carnegie Foundation for the Advancement of Teaching.

- Ford-Gilboe M (1997) Family strengths, motivation, and resources as predictors of health promotion behavior in single-parent and two-parent families. *Res Nurs Health.* **20**(3): 205–17.

- Forrest CB and Starfield B (1998) Entry into primary care and continuity: the effects of access. *Am J Public Health.* **88**(9): 1330–6.

- Forsyth DR and McMillan JH (1991) Practical proposals for motivating students. In: RJ Menges and MD Svinicki (eds) *College Teaching: from theory to practice* (New Directions for Teaching and Learning Series, 45). Jossey-Bass, San Francisco, CA.

- Foss L (2002) *The End of Modern Medicine: biomedical science under a microscope.* State University of New York, Albany, NY.

- Fowler JW (1981) *Stages of Faith: the psychology of human development and the quest for meaning.* Harper and Row, San Francisco, CA.

- Fraiberg S, Adelson E and Shapiro V (1975) Ghosts in the nursery. A psychoanalytic approach to the problems of impaired infant–mother relationships. *J Am Acad Child Psychiatry.* **14**(3): 387–421.

- Frank A (1991) *At the Will of the Body: reflections on illness.* Houghton Mifflin, Boston, MA.

- Frankel R (1994a) *Giving Effective Feedback.* Unpublished manuscript presented to Miles Research Forum, Tucson, AZ.

- Frankel R (1994b) *Coaching Learners to Improve Communication Skills Using Audio and Videotape.* Unpublished manuscript presented to the Miles Research Forum, Tucson, AZ.

- Frankel RM (2001) Cracking the code: theory and method in clinical communication analysis. *Health Commun.* **13**(1): 101–10.

- Freeman R (1998) *Mentoring in General Practice.* Butterworth Heinemann, Oxford.

- Freer CB (1980) Self-care: a health diary study. *Med Care.* **18**(8): 853–61.

- Friedewald VE, Jr (2000) The Internet's influence on the doctor–patient relationship. *Health Manag Technol.* **21**(11): 80, 79.

- Fries JF, Bloch DA, Harrington H, Richardson N and Beck R (1993) Two-year results of a randomized controlled trial of a health promotion program in a retiree population: the Bank of America Study. *Am J Med.* **94**(5): 455–62.

- Fugelli P (2001) Trust – in general practice. *Br J Gen Pract.* **51**: 575–9.

- Fuller FF and Manning BA (1973) Self-confrontation reviewed: a conceptualization for video playback in teacher education. *Rev Educ Res.* **43**: 469–528.

- Gagne RM, Briggs LJ and Wager WW (1992) *Principles of Instructional Design* (4e). Holt, Rinehart and Winston, New York.
- Gagne RM and Medsker KL (1996) *The Conditions of Learning*. Training Applications, Belmont, CA.
- Galazka SS and Eckert JK (1986) Clinically applied anthropology: concepts for the family physician. *J Fam Pract.* **22**: 159–65.
- Garrett L (1994) *The Coming Plague: newly emerging diseases in a world out of balance*. Penguin Books, New York.
- Garrity TF (1981) Medical compliance and the clinician–patient relationship: a review. *Social Science and Medicine – Part E: Medical Psychology*. **15**: 215–22.
- Garrity TF and Leaviss J (1989) Patient–physician communication as a determinant of medication misuse in older, minority women. *J Drug Issues*. **19**: 245–59.
- Gerhardt U (1990) Qualitative research on chronic illness: the issue and the story. *Soc Sci Med*. **30**(11): 1149–59.
- Gieger JH (1993) Community oriented primary care: the legacy of Sidney Kark. *Am J Public Health*. **83**(7): 946–7.
- Gilligan C (1982) *In a Different Voice: psychological theory and women's development*. Harvard University Press, Cambridge, MA.
- Gilligan C and Pollack S (1988) The vulnerable and invulnerable physician. In: C Gilligan *et al.* (eds) *Mapping the Moral Domain – A Contribution of Women's Thinking to Psychological Theory and Education*. Harvard University Press, Cambridge, MA.
- Gillis AJ (1993) Determinants of a health-promoting lifestyle: an integrative review. *J Adv Nurs*. **18**(3): 345–53.
- Gilman S (1988) *Disease and Representation: images of illness from madness to AIDS*. Cornell University Press, Ithaca, NY and London.
- Glass TA, de Leon CM, Marottoli RA and Berkman LF (1999) Population based study of social and productive activities as predictors of survival among elderly Americans. *BMJ*. **319**: 478–83.
- Glasser M and Pelto GH (1980) *The Medical Merry-go-round: a plea for reasonable medicine*. Redgrave, Pleasantville, NY.
- Glassick CE, Huber MT and Maeroff GI (1997) *Scholarship Assessed – evaluation of the professoriate* (The Ernest L Boyer Project of the Carnegie Foundation for the Advancement of Teaching). Jossey-Bass, San Francisco, CA.
- Glick TH and Moore GT (2001) Time to learn: the outlook for renewal of patient-centred education in the digital age. *Med Educ*. **35**(5): 505–9.
- Godkin MA and Catlin RJO (1984) Office design. In: RE Rakel (ed.) *Textbook of Family Practice* (3e). WB Saunders, Philadelphia, PA.
- Godolphin W, Towle A and McKendry R (2001) Challenges in family practice related to informed and shared decision-making: a survey of preceptors of medical students. *JAMA*. **165**(4): 434–5.
- Goldberg PE (2000) The physician–patient relationship: three psychodynamic concepts that can be applied to primary care. *Arch Fam Med*. **9**(10): 116–48.
- Golin CE, DiMatteo MR and Gelberg L (1996) The role of patient participation in the doctor visit. Implications for adherence to diabetes care. *Diabetes Care*. **19**(10): 1153–64.
- Good BJ and Good M (1981) Meaning of symptoms: a cultural-hermeneutic model for clinical practice. In: L Eisenberg and A Kleinman (eds) *Relevance of Social Science for Medicine*. D Reidel, Boston, MA.

- Good BJ, Herrera H, Delvecchio-Good M and Cooper J (1985) Reflexivity, countertransference, and clinical ethnography: A case from a psychiatric cultural consultation clinic. In: RA Hahn and AD Gaines (eds) *Physicians of Western Medicine*. D Reidel, Boston, MA.
- Goodyear-Smith F and Buetow S (2001) Power issues in the doctor–patient relationship. *Health Care Analysis*. 9: 449–62.
- Goold SD and Lipkin M, Jr (1999) The doctor–patient relationship. Challenges, opportunities, and strategies. *J Gen Intern Med*. 14(1): S26–S33.
- Gordon GH, Baker L and Levinson W (1995) Physician–patient communication in managed care. *West J Med*. 163(6): 527–31.
- Green AR, Carrillo JE and Betancourt JR (2002) Why the disease-based model of medicine fails our patients. *West J Med*. 176(2): 141–3.
- Greenfield S, Kaplan S and Ware JE, Jr (1985) Expanding patient involvement in care. Effects on patient outcomes. *Ann Int Med*. 102(4): 520–8.
- Greenfield S, Kaplan SH and Ware JE, Jr (1988) Patients' participation in medical care: effects on blood sugar and quality of life in diabetes. *J Gen Intern Med*. 3: 448–57.
- Greenhalgh T and Hurwitz B (1998) *Narrative Based Medicine. Dialogue and discourse in clinical practice*. BMJ Books, London.
- Grol R (2001) Improving the quality of medical care: building bridges among professional pride, payer profit, and patient satisfaction. *JAMA*. 286(20): 2578–85.
- Gronlund NE (1999) *How to Write and Use Educational Objectives* (6e). Prentice-Hall, Englewood Cliffs, NJ.
- Gross DA, Zyzanski SJ, Borawski EA, Cebul RD and Stange KC (1998) Patient satisfaction with time spent with their physician. *J Fam Pract*. 47: 133–7.
- Grow GO (1991) Teaching learners to be self-directed. *Adult Education Quarterly*. 41(3) 125–49.
- Grumbach K, Selby JV, Damberg C, Bindman AB, Quesenberry C, Jr, Truman A and Uratsu C (1999) Resolving the gatekeeper conundrum: what patients value in primary care and referrals to specialists. *JAMA*. 282(3): 261–6.
- Guy K (1997) *Our Promise to Children*. Canadian Institute of Child Health, Ottawa, ON.
- Haddad S, Potvin L, Roberge D, Pineault R and Remondin M (2000) Patient perception of quality following a visit to a doctor in a primary care unit. *Fam Pract*. 17(1): 21–9.
- Hafferty FW (1998) Beyond curriculum reform: confronting medicine's hidden curriculum. *Academic Medicine*. 73(4): 403–7.
- Hajek P, Najberg E and Cushing A (2000) Medical students' concerns about communicating with patients. *Med Educ*. 34(8): 656–8.
- Hall JA and Dornan MC (1988a) Meta-analysis of satisfaction with medical care: description of research domain and analysis of overall satisfaction levels. *Soc Sci Med*. 27: 637–44.
- Hall JA and Dornan MC (1988b) What patients like about their medical care and how often they are asked: a meta-analysis of the satisfaction literature *Soc Sci Med*. 27: 935–9.
- Hamilton E and Cairns H (1961) *The Collected Dialogues of Plato, inc. letters*. Bollingen Foundation, New York.
- Hammond M and Collins R (1991) *Self-directed Learning: a critical practice*. Kogan Page, London.
- Hanckel FS (1984) The problem of induction in clinical decision making. *Medical Decision Making*. 4(1): 59–68.
- Haney AC (1971) Psychosocial factors involved in medical decision-making. In: RH Coombs and CE Vincent (eds) *Psychosocial Aspects of Medical Training*. Charles C Thomas, Springfield, IL.

- Hansen PA and Roberts KB (1992) Putting teaching back at the centre. *Teach Learning Medicine.* **4**(3): 136–9.
- Hargie O and Saunders C (1983) Individual differences and social skills training. In: R Ellis and D Whittington (eds) *New Directions in Social Skills Training.* Croom Helm, Beckenham.
- Hargie OD and Morrow NC (1986) Using videotape in communication skills training: a critical evaluation of the process of self-viewing. *Med Teach.* **8**(4): 359–65.
- Hartman A and Laird J (1983) *Family-centred Social Work Practice.* Free Press, New York.
- Haug M and Lavin B (1983) *Consumerism in Medicine: challenging physician authority.* Sage, Beverly Hills, CA.
- Havelock P and Schofield T (1999) Making change happen: developing primary healthcare teams. In: P Moreton (ed.) *The Very Stuff of General Practice.* Radcliffe Medical Press, Oxford.
- Hawk J and Scott CD (1986) A case of family medicine: sources of stress in residents and physicians in practice. In: CD Scott and J Hawk (eds) *Heal Thyself – the health of health care professionals.* Brunner/Mazel, New York.
- Hawkins AH (1986) AR Luria and the art of clinical biography. *Lit Med.* **5**: 1–15.
- Hawkins AH (1993) *Reconstructing Illness: studies in pathology.* Purdue University Press, West Lafayette, IN.
- Haynes RB, Devereaux PJ and Guyatt GH (2002) Physicians' and patients' choices in evidence based practice. *BMJ.* **324**: 1350.
- Headache Study Group of The University of Western Ontario (1986) Predictors of outcome in headache patients presenting to family physicians – a one year prospective study. *Headache.* **26**: 285–94.
- Helfer RE (1970) An objective comparison of the pediatric interviewing skills of freshman and senior medical students. *Pediatrics.* **45**(4): 623–7.
- Helsing KJ and Szklo M (1981) Mortality after bereavement. *Am J Epidemiol.* **114**: 41–52.
- Henbest RJ and Stewart M (1990) Patient-centredness in the consultation 2: Does it really make a difference? *Fam Pract.* **7**(1): 28–33.
- Henbest RJ and Fehrsen GS (1992) Patient-centredness: is it applicable outside the West? Its measurement and effect on outcomes. *Fam Pract.* **9**(3) 311–17.
- Hendley B (1978) Martin Buber on the teacher–student relationship: a critical appraisal. *J Philosophy Educ.* **12**: 144.
- Hepworth DH and Larsen J (1990) *Direct Social Work Practice: theory and skills* (3e). Wadsworth, Belmont, CA.
- Herwaldt LA (2001) Treating the patient, not the disease. In: *The Stories. Experiences of relationship-centered care.* Fetzer Institute, Kalamazoo, MI
- Hickson GB, Clayton EW, Githens PB and Sloan FA (1992) Factors that prompted families to file medical malpractice claims following perinatal injuries. *JAMA.* **267**: 1359–63.
- Hickson GB, Clayton EW, Entman SS, Miller CS, Githens PB, Whetten-Goldstein K and Sloan FA (1994) Obstetricians' prior malpractice experience and patients' satisfaction with care. *JAMA.* **272**(20): 158–37.
- Hinds PS, Chaves DE and Cypress SM (1992) Context as a source of meaning and understanding. In: JM Morse (ed.) *Qualitative Health Research.* Sage, Newbury Park, CA.
- Hippocrates (1982) *The Aphorisms of Hippocrates.* The Classics of Medicine Library, Gryphon Editions, Birmingham, AL.
- Hippocrates (1986) *Airs, Waters, Places: an essay on the influence of climate, water supply and situation on health.* Penguin Books, Harmondsworth.
- Hjortdahl P and Borchgrevink CF (1991) Continuity of care: influence of general practitioners' knowledge about their patients on use of resources in consultations. *BMJ.* **303**: 1181–4.

- Hoffmaster B (1992) Values: the hidden agenda in preventive medicine. *Canadian Family Physician.* **38**: 321–7.
- Hornberger J, Thorn D and MaCurdy T (1997) Effects of a self-administered previsit questionnaire to enhance awareness of patients' concerns in primary care. *J Gen Intern Med.* **12**: 597–606.
- House JS, Landis KR and Umberson D (1988) Social relationships and health. *Science.* **241**: 540–5.
- Howe A (1997) Refusal of videorecording: what factors may influence patient consent? *Fam Pract.* **14**(3): 233–7.
- Howie JG, Porter AM, Heaney DJ *et al.* (1991) Long to short consultation ratio: a proxy measure of quality of care for general practice. *Br J Gen Pract.* **41**: 48–54.
- HSC (1998) *The New NHS: modern, dependable.* Department of Health, London.
- Hull FM and Hull FS (1984) Time and the general practitioner: the patient's view. *J Royal Coll General Pract.* **34**: 71–5.
- Hunter KM (1991) *Doctors' Stories: the narrative structure of medical knowledge.* Princeton University Press, Princeton, NY.
- Hurowitz JC (1993) Toward a social policy for health. *NEJM.* **329**(2): 130–3.
- Ingelfinger FJ (1980) On arrogance. *NEJM.* **33**(206): 507–11.
- Irby DM (1978) Clinical teacher effectiveness in medicine. *J Med Educ.* **53**(10): 808–15.
- Jacobson LD, Wilkinson C and Owen PA (1994) Is the potential of teenage consultations being missed? A study of consultation times in primary care. *Family Practice.* **11**: 296–9.
- Jadad AR (1999) Promoting partnerships: challenges for the internet age. *BMJ.* **319**: 761–4.
- Jaen CR, McIlvain H, Pol L, Phillips RL, Jr, Flocke S and Crabtree BF (2001) Tailoring tobacco counseling to the competing demands in the clinical encounter. *J Fam Pract.* **50**(10): 859–63.
- James W (1958) *The Varieties of Religious Experience: a study in human nature.* The New American Library, New York.
- Jerritt WA (1981) Lethargy in general practice. *Practitioner.* **225**: 731–7.
- Johnson JE, Nail LM, Lauver D, King KB and Keys H (1988) Reducing the negative impact of radiation therapy on functional status. *Cancer.* **61**(1): 46–51.
- Jonas S (1978) *Medical Mystery: the training of doctors in the United States.* WW Norton, New York.
- Jones I and Morrell D (1995) General practitioners' background knowledge of their patients. *Fam Pract.* **12**(1): 49–53.
- Jordan JV, Kaplan AG, Miller JB, Stiver IP and Surrey JL (1991) *Women's Growth in Connection: writings from the Stone Center.* The Guilford Press, New York.
- Kaplan GA and Neil JE (1993) Socioeconomic factors and cardiovascular disease: a review of the literature. *Circulation.* **88**(4, Part 1): 1973–98.
- Kaplan SH, Greenfield S and Ware JE (1989a) Impact of the doctor–patient relationship on outcomes of chronic disease. In: M Stewart and D Roter (eds) *Communicating with Medical Patients.* Sage, Beverly Hills, CA.
- Kaplan SH, Greenfield S and Ware JE, Jr (1989b) Assessing the effects of physician–patient interactions on the outcomes of chronic disease. *Med Care.* **27**(3): S110–27.
- Kaprio J, Koskenvou M and Rita H (1987) Mortality after bereavement: a prospective study of 95,647 widowed persons. *Am J Public Health.* **77**: 283–7.
- Kassirer JP (2000) Patients, physicians, and the internet. *Health Affairs.* **19**(6): 115–23.
- Katon W and Kleinman A (1981) Doctor–patient negotiation and other social science strategies in patient care. In: L Eisenberg and A Kleinman (eds) *Relevance of Social Science for Medicine.* D Reidel, Boston, MA.

- Kawachi I, Kennedy BP and Wilkinson RG (1999a) Crime: social disorganization and relative deprivation. *Soc Sci Med.* **43**(6): 719–31.
- Kawachi I, Kennedy BP and Wilkinson RG (1999b) *The Society and Population Health Reader: income inequality and health.* The New Press, New York.
- Kearley KE, Freeman GK and Heath A (2001) An exploration of the value of the personal doctor–patient relationship in general practice. *Br J Gen Pract.* **51**: 712–18.
- Kelly L and Brown JB (2002) Listening to native patients. *Canadian Family Physician.* **48**: 1645–52.
- Kelman EG and Straker KC (2000) *Study without Stress – mastering medical sciences.* Sage, Thousand Oaks, CA.
- Kern DE, Thomas PA, Howard DM and Bass EB (1998) *Curriculum Development for Medical Education. A six-step approach.* The Johns Hopkins University Press, Baltimore.
- Kern DE, Wright SM, Carrese JA, Lipkin M, Jr, Simmons JM, Novack DH, Kalet A and Frankel R (2001) Personal growth in medical faculty: a qualitative study. *West J Med.* **175**(2): 92–8.
- Kernick D and Scott A (2002) Economic approaches to doctor/nurse skill mix: problems, pitfalls, and partial solutions. *Br J Gen Pract.* **52**: 42–6.
- Kestenbaum V (1982) *Humanity of the Ill: phenomenological perspectives.* University of Tennessee Press, Knoxville, TN.
- King DE and Bushwick B (1994) Beliefs and attitudes of hospital inpatients about faith healing and prayer. *J Fam Pract.* **39**(4): 349–52.
- Kinnersley P, Stott N, Peters TJ and Harvey I (1999) The patient-centredness of consultations and outcome in primary care. *Br J Gen Pract.* **49**: 771–6.
- Kinra S, Nelder RP and Lewendon GJ (2000) Deprivation and childhood obesity: a cross sectional study of 20,973 children in Plymouth, UK. *J Epidemiol Community Health.* **54**(6): 456–60.
- Kitagawa EM and Hauser PM (1973) *Differential Mortality in the United States: a study in socio-economic epidemiology.* Harvard University Press, Cambridge, MA.
- Kjellgren KI, Ahlner J and Saljo R (1995) Taking antihypertensive medication – controlling or co-operating with patients? *Int J Cardiology.* **47**: 257–8.
- Klass P (1987) *A Not Entirely Benign Procedure: four years as a medical student.* GP Putman, New York.
- Klass P (1992) *Baby Doctor.* Random House, New York.
- Klaus MH and Kennell JH (1976) *Maternal–Infant Bonding.* CV Mosby, St Louis, MO.
- Kleinman A (1988) *The Illness Narratives. Suffering, healing and the human condition.* Basic Books, New York.
- Kleinman A (1999) Prologue. In: J Borkan *et al.* (eds) *Patients and Doctors. Life-changing stories for primary care.* University of Wisconsin Press, Madison, WI.
- Kleinman AM, Eisenberg L and Good B (1978) Culture, illness, and care: clinical lessons from anthropologic and cross-cultural research. *Ann Int Med.* **88**(2): 251–8.
- Klepac RK, Dowling J, Rokke P, Dodge L and Schafer L (1981) Interview vs. paper-and-pencil administration of the McGill Pain Questionnaire. *Pain.* **11**(2): 241–6.
- Klitzman R (1989) *A Year-long Night.* Penguin Books, New York.
- Knowles MS (1984) *Andragogy in Action: applying modern principles of adult learning.* Jossey-Bass, San Francisco, CA.
- Knowles MS (1986) *Using Learning Contracts.* Jossey-Bass, San Francisco, CA.
- Knowles MS (1989) *The Making of an Adult Educator – an autobiographical journey.* Jossey-Bass, San Francisco, CA.

- Knowles MS, Holton EF, III and Swanson RA (1998) *The Adult Learner – the definitive classic in adult education and human resource development* (5e). Gulf Publishing, Houston, TX.
- Kohut H (1971) *The Analysis of the Self*. International Universities Press, New York.
- Kohut H (1977) *The Restoration of the Self*. International Universities Press, New York.
- Konner M (1987) *Becoming a Doctor: a journey of initiation in medical school*. Viking-Penguin, New York.
- Korzybski A (1958) *Science and Sanity: an introduction to non-Aristotelian systems and general semantics* (4e). International Non-Aristotelian Library, Lake Bille, CT.
- Kumar P and Basu D (2000) Substance abuse by medical students and doctors. *J Indian Med Assoc*. **98**(8): 447–52.
- Laitakari J and Asikainen TM (1998) How to promote physical activity through individual counseling – a proposal for a practical model of counseling on health-related physical activity. *Patient Educ Couns*. **33**(1): S13–24.
- Lang F, Floyd MR and Beine KL (2000) Clues to patients' explanations and concerns about their illnesses. A call for active listening. *Arch Fam Med*. **9**(3): 222–7.
- Lang F, Marvel K, Sanders D, Waxman D, Beine KL, Pfaffly C and McCord E (2002) Interviewing when family members are present. *Am Fam Physician*. **65**(7) 1351–4.
- Lantz PM, House JS, Lepkowski JM, Williams DR, Miller JB and Chen J (1998) Socioeconomic factors, health behaviors, and mortality: results from a nationally representative prospective study of US adults. *JAMA*. **279**(21): 1703–8.
- LeBaron C (1981) *Gentle Vengeance*. Richard Marek, New York.
- Leder D (1990) Clinical interpretation: the hermeneutics of medicine. *Theor Med*. **11**(1): 9–24.
- Lee JM (1993) Screening and informed consent. *NEJM*. **328**(6): 438–40.
- Leichtman F (1975) Social and psychological development of adolescents and the relationship to chronic illness. *Medical Clin North Am*. **59**: 13–15.
- Leigh JP, Richardson N, Beck R, Kerr C, Harrington H, Parcell CL and Fries JF (1992) Randomized controlled study of a retiree health promotion program: The Bank of America Study. *Arch Int Med*. **152**: 1201–6.
- Lester GW and Smith SG (1993) Listening and talking to patients. A remedy for malpractice suits? *West J Med*. **158**: 268–72.
- Levenstein JH, McCracken EC, McWhinney IR, Stewart MA and Brown JB (1986) The patient-centred clinical method 1. A model for the doctor–patient interaction in family medicine. *Fam Pract*. **3**(1): 24–30.
- Levinson DJ (1978) *Seasons of a Man's Life*. Knopf, New York.
- Levinson W, Roter DL, Mullooly JP, Dull VT and Frankel RM (1997) Physician–patient communication. The relationship with malpractice claims among primary care physicians and surgeons. *JAMA*. **277**(7) 553–9.
- Levinson W, Gorawara-Bhat R and Lamb J (2000) A study of patient clues and physician responses in primary care and surgical settings. *JAMA*. **284**(8): 1021–7.
- Ley P (1982) Satisfaction, compliance and communication. *Br J Clin Psychology*. **21**(4): 241–54.
- Lilley R with Davies G and Cain B (1999) *The PCG Team Builder. Creating and maintaining effective team working. A workbook for the health service and primary care team*. Radcliffe Medical Press, Oxford.
- Linn MW, Linn BS and Stein SR (1982) Satisfaction with ambulatory care and compliance in older patients. *Med Care*. **20**(6): 606–14.
- Little M and Midtling JEE (1989) *Becoming a Family Physician*. Springer-Verlag, New York.

- Little P, Everitt H, Williamson I, Warner G, Moore M, Gould C, Ferrier K and Payne S (2001a) Preferences of patients for patient centred approach to consultation in primary care: observational study. *BMJ*. **322**: 468–72.
- Little P, Everitt H, Williamson I, Warner G, Moore M, Gould C, Ferrier K and Payne S (2001b) Observational study of effect of patient centredness and positive approach on outcomes of general practice consultations. *BMJ*. **323**: 908–11.
- Lockhart-Wood K (2000) Collaboration between nurses and doctors in clinical practice. *Br J Nurs*. **9**(5): 276–80.
- Longhurst JF and Grant HF (1989) Images of illness: blindness. *Canadian Family Physician*. **35**: 1623–6.
- Longhurst MF (1989) Physician self-awareness: the neglected insight. In: M Stewart and D Roter (eds) *Communicating with Medical Patients*. Sage, Newbury Park, CA.
- Lowenstein J (2002) Excerpt from: Can you teach compassion? In: R Coles and R Testa (eds) *A Life in Medicine – a literary anthology*. The New Press, New York.
- Loxterkamp D (1991) Being there: on the place of the family physician. *J Am Board Fam Pract*. **4**(5): 354–60.
- Loxterkamp D (2001) A vow of connectedness: views from the road to Beaver's farm. *Fam Med*. **33**(4): 244–7.
- Lucas AF (1990) Using psychological models to understand student motivation. *New Directions Teaching Learning*. **42**: 103–14.
- Lynch JW, Kaplan GA and Salonen JT (1997) Why do poor people behave poorly? Variation in adult health behaviours and psychosocial characteristics by stages of socio-economic lifecourse. *Soc Sci Med*. **44**(6): 809–19.
- MacLeod A (1992) *Vision*. McClelland and Stewart New Canadian Library, Toronto.
- Mager RF (1968) *Developing Attitude Toward Learning*. Fearon, Palo Alto, CA.
- Mager RF (1997) *Preparing Instructional Objectives: a critical tool in the development of effective instruction* (3e). The Center for Effective Performance, Atlanta, GA.
- Maguire P, Fairbairn S and Fletcher C (1989) Consultation skills of young doctors: benefits of undergraduate feedback training in interviewing. In: M Stewart and D Roter (eds) *Communicating with Medical Patients*. Sage, Thousand Oaks, CA.
- Mailick M (1979) The impact of severe illness on the individual and family: an overview. *Soc Work Health Care*. **5**(2): 117–28.
- Main DS, Holcomb S, Dickinson P and Crabtree BF (2001) The effect of families on the process of outpatient visits in family practice. *J Fam Pract*. **50**(10): 888.
- Main DS, Tressler C, Staudenmaier A, Nearing KA, Westfall JM and Silverstein M (2002) Patient perspectives on the doctor of the future. *Fam Med*. **34**(4): 251–7.
- Malterud K (1994) Key questions – a strategy for modifying clinical communication. Transforming tacit skills into a clinical method. *Scand J Prim Health Care*. **12**(2): 121–7.
- Malterud K (1998) Understanding women in pain. New pathways suggested by Umea researchers: qualitative research and feminist perspectives. *Scand J Prim Health Care*. **16**(4): 195–8.
- Marmoreo J, Brown JB, Batty HR, Cummings S and Powell M (1998) Hormone replacement therapy: determinants of women's decisions. *Patient Educ Couns*. **33**(3): 289–98.
- Marmot MG, Kogevinas M and Elston MA (1987) Social/economic status and disease. *Ann Rev Public Health*. **8**: 111–35.
- Marshall L, Weir E, Ablesohn A and Sanborn MD (2002) Identifying and managing adverse environmental health effects: 1. Taking an exposure history. *CMAJ*. **166**(8): 1041–3.
- Marteau TM (1990) Reducing the psychological costs. *BMJ*. **301**: 26–8.

- Martin CM, Banwell CL, Broom DH and Nisa M (1999) Consultation length and chronic illness care in general practice: a qualitative study. *Med J Australia.* **171**: 77–81.
- Martinelli AM (1999) An explanatory model of variables influencing health promotion behaviors in smoking and nonsmoking college students. *BMJ.* **319**: 263–9.
- Marvel K, Major G, Jones K and Pfaffly C (2000) Dialogues in the exam room: medical interviewing by resident family physicians. *Fam Med.* **32**(9): 628–32.
- Marvel MK (1993) Involvement with the psychosocial concerns of patients. Observations of practising family physicians on a university faculty. *Arch Fam Med.* **2**(6): 629–33.
- Marvel MK, Doherty WJ and Weiner E (1998) Medical interviewing by exemplary family physicians. *J Fam Pract.* **47**: 343–8.
- Marvel MK, Epstein RM, Flowers K and Beckman HB (1999) Soliciting the patient's agenda: have we improved? *JAMA.* **281**(3): 283–7.
- Matthews DA, McCullough ME, Larson DB, Koenig HG, Swyers JP and Milano MG (1998) Religious commitment and health status. A review of the research and implications for family medicine. *Arch Fam Med.* **7**(2): 118–24.
- Mattingly C and Fleming MH (1994) *Clinical Reasoning – forms of inquiry in a therapeutic practice.* FA Davis, Philadelphia, PA.
- Maudsley RF, Wilson DR, Neufeld VR, Hennen BK, DeVillaer MR, Wakefield J, MacFadyen J, Turnbull JM, Weston WW, Brown MG, Frank JR and Richardson D (2000) Educating future physicians for Ontario: Phase II. *Academic Medicine.* **75**(2): 113–26.
- May WF (1991) *The Patient's Ordeal.* Indiana University Press, Bloomington, IN.
- Mayer JD (1984) Medical geography. *JAMA.* **251**: 2680–3.
- Mayeroff M (1972) *On Caring.* Harper and Row, New York.
- McBride JL, Arthur G, Brooks R and Pilkington L (1998) The relationship between a patient's spirituality and health experiences. *Fam Med.* **30**(2): 122–6.
- McCullough LB (1989) The abstract character and transforming power of medical language. *Soundings.* **72**(1): 111–25.
- McDaniel S, Campbell TL and Seaburn DB (1990) *Family-oriented Primary Care: a manual for medical providers.* Springer-Verlag, New York.
- McEwen BS (1999) Stress, adaptation and disease: allostasis and allostatic load. *Ann NY Acad Sci.* **840**: 33–44.
- McEwen BS (2000) Allostatis and allostatic load: implication for neuropharmacology. *Neuropharmacology.* **22**(2): 108–24.
- McGinnis JM and Hamburg MA (1988) Opportunities for health promotion and disease prevention in the clinical setting. *West J Med.* **149**: 468–74.
- McKeachie WJ (1978) *Teaching Tips – a guidebook for the beginning college teacher* (7e). DC Heath, Lexington, MA.
- McLane CG, Zyzanski, SJ and Flocke SA (1995) Factors associated with medication noncompliance in rural elderly hypertensive patients. *Am J Hypertens.* **8**: 206–9.
- McLeod ME (1998) Doctor–patient relationship: perspectives, needs, and communication. *Am J Gastroenterology.* **93**(5) 676–80.
- McMichael C, Kirk M, Manderson L, Hoban E and Potts H (2000) Indigenous women's perceptions of breast cancer diagnosis and treatment in Queensland. *Australian New Zealand J Public Health.* **24**(5): 515–19.
- McMurray C and Smith R (2001) *Diseases of Globalization: socioeconomic transitions and health.* Earthscan Publications, London and Sterling, VA.
- McNeilis KS (2001) Analyzing communication competence in medical consultations. *Health Commun.* **13**(1): 5–18.

- McPhee SJ, Richard RJ and Solkowit SN (1986) Performance of cancer screening in a university internal medicine practice. *J Gen Intern Med.* **1**: 275–8.
- McPhee SJ and Schroeder SA (1987) Promoting preventive care: changing reimbursement is not enough. *Am J Public Health.* **77**(7): 780–1.
- McWhinney IR (1972) Beyond diagnosis. An approach to the integration of behavioural science and clinical medicine. *NEJM.* **287**: 384–7.
- McWhinney IR (1988) *Through Clinical Method to a More Humane Medicine in the Task of Medicine: dialogue at Wickenberg.* The Henry J Kaiser Family Foundation, Menlo Park, CA.
- McWhinney IR (1989a) *An Acquaintance with Particulars.* The Curtis Hames Lecture. Society of Teachers of Family Medicine, Annual Spring Conference, Denver, CO.
- McWhinney IR (1989b) The need for a transformed clinical method. In: M Stewart and D Roter (eds) *Communicating with Medical Patients.* Sage, Newbury Park, CA.
- McWhinney IR (1997) *A Textbook of Family Medicine* (2e). Oxford University Press, New York.
- McWhinney IR, Epstein RM and Freeman TR (1997) Rethinking somatization. *Ann Int Med.* **126**(9): 747–50.
- McWhinney IR (2001) The value of case studies. *Eur J Gen Pract.* **7**: 88–9.
- McWilliam CL (1993) Health promotion: strategies for family physicians. *Canadian Family Physician.* **39**: 1079–85.
- McWilliam CL, Stewart M, Brown JB, Desai K and Coderre P (1996) Creating health with chronic illness. *Adv Nurs Sci.* **18**(3): 1–15.
- McWilliam CL, Stewart M, Brown JB, McNair S, Desai K, Patterson ML, Del Maestro N and Pittman BJ (1997) Creating empowering meaning: an interactive process of promoting health with chronically ill older Canadians. *Health Promotion International.* **12**(2): 111–23.
- McWilliam CL, Stewart M, Brown JB, McNair S, Donner A, Desai K, Coderre P and Galajda J (1999) A randomized controlled trial of a critical reflection approach to home-based health promotion for chronically ill older persons. *Health Promotion International.* **14**(1): 27–41.
- McWilliam CL, Brown JB and Stewart M (2000) Breast cancer patients' experiences of patient–doctor communication: a working relationship. *Patient Educ Couns.* **39**(2–3): 191–204.
- Mead N and Bower P (2000) Patient-centredness: a conceptual framework and review of the empirical literature. *Soc Sci Med.* **51**: 1087–110.
- Meade MS (1986) Geographic analysis of disease and care. *Annu Rev Public Health.* **7**: 313–35.
- Mechanic D and Meyer S (2000) Concepts of trust among patients with serious illness. *Soc Sci Med.* **51**: 657–68.
- Mechanic D (2001) How should hamsters run? Some observations about sufficient patient time in primary care. *BMJ.* **323**: 266–8.
- Mechanic D, McAlpine DD and Rosenthal M (2001) Are patients' office visits with physicians getting shorter? *NEJM.* **344**(3): 198–204.
- Medalie JH and Cole-Kelly K (2002) The clinical importance of defining family. *Am Fam Physician.* **65**(7): 1277–9.
- Meredith L, Stewart M and Brown JB (2001) Patient-centered communication scoring method report on nine coded interviews. *Health Commun.* **13**(1): 19–31.
- Merriam SB (1993) *An Update on Adult Learning Theory. New directions for adult and continuing education.* Jossey-Bass, San Francisco, CA.
- Merriam SB and Caffarella RS (1999) *Learning in Adulthood – a comprehensive guide* (2e). Jossey-Bass, San Francisco, CA.

- Mezirow J *et al.* (2000) *Learning as Transformation – critical perspectives on a theory in progress.* Jossey-Bass, San Francisco, CA.
- Michels R (1999) Views of managed care. *NEJM.* **341**: 8.
- Miller GE, Abrahamson S, Cohen IS, Grasin HP, Harnack RS and Land A (1961) *Teaching and Learning in Medical School.* Harvard University Press, Cambridge, MA.
- Miller WL (1992) Routine, ceremony, or drama: an exploratory field study of the primary care clinical encounter. *J Fam Pract.* **34**(3): 289–96.
- Mishler EG (1984) *Discourse of Medicine: dialectics of medical interviews.* Ablex, Norwood, NJ.
- Mishne JM (1993) *The Evolution and Application of Clinical Theory. Perspectives from four psychologies.* The Free Press, New York.
- Montgomery CL (1993) *Healing Through Communication: the practice of caring.* Sage, Newbury Park, CA.
- Moore PJ, Adler NE and Robertson PA (2000) Medical malpractice: the effect of doctor–patient relations on medical patient perceptions and malpractice intentions. *West J Med.* **173**(4): 244–50.
- Morgan M, Lakhani AD, Morris RW and Vaile MS (1987) Parents' attitudes to measles immunization. *J Royal Coll General Pract.* **37**: 25–7.
- Morris A (1998) *Illness and Culture in the Postmodern Age.* University of California Press, Berkeley, CA.
- Morris BAP (1991) Case reports: boon or bane? In: PG Norton *et al.* (eds) *Primary Care Research: traditional and innovative approaches.* Sage, Newbury Park, CA.
- Mukand J (1990) *Vital Lines: contemporary fiction about medicine.* St Martin's Press, New York.
- Mundy GR (1991) Presidential address of the SSCI – Can the triple threat survive biotech? *Am J Med Sci.* **302**(1): 38–41.
- Murphy J, Chang H, Montgomery JE, Rogers WH and Safran DG (2001) The quality of physician–patient relationships. Patients' experiences 1996–1999. *J Fam Pract.* **50**(2): 123–9.
- Murray M (2001) *Beyond the Myths and Magic of Mentoring – how to facilitate an effective mentoring process.* Jossey-Bass, San Francisco, CA.
- Myers MF (2000) *Intimate Relationships in Medical School – how to make them work.* Sage, Thousand Oaks, CA.
- National Health Assessment Group for the US Global Change Research Program (2001) *Climate Change and Human Health: the potential consequences of climate variability and change.* A Report of the National Health Assessment Group for the US Global Change Research Program.
- National Research Council, CoRPaC (1989) *Improving Risk Communication.* National Academy Press, Washington, DC.
- Neufeld V, Maudsley R, Turnbull J, Weston W, Pickering R and Brown M (1998) Educating future physicians for Ontario. *Academic Medicine.* **73**(11): 1133–48.
- Newman B and Young RJ (1972) A model for teaching the total person approach to patient problems. *Nursing Research.* **21**: 264–9.
- Norman GK and Scherger JE (1999) Views of managed care. *NEJM.* **341**(8): 616–18.
- Northrup DE, Moore-West M, Skipper B and Teaf SR (1983) Characteristics of clinical information searching: investigation using critical incident technique. *J Med Educ.* **58**: 873–81.
- Novack DH, Suchman AL, Clark W, Epstein RM, Najberg E and Kaplan C (1997) Calibrating the physician. Personal awareness and effective patient care. *JAMA.* **278**(6): 502–9.

- Novack DH, Epstein RM and Paulsen RH (1999) Toward creating physician-healers: fostering medical students' self-awareness, personal growth, and well-being. *Academic Medicine.* **74**(5): 516–20.
- Nutting PA (ed.) (1990) *Community-oriented Primary Care: from principle to practice.* University of New Mexico Press, Albuquerque, NM.
- Odegaard CE (1986) *Dear Doctor – a personal letter to a physician.* The Henry J Kaiser Family Foundation, Menlo Park, CA.
- Olesen J (1994) Understanding the biologic basis of migraine. *NEJM.* **331**(25): 1713–14.
- Opie A (2000) *Knowledge-based Teamwork. Thinking teams/thinking clients.* Columbia University Press, New York.
- Ottawa Charter for Health Promotion (1986) *Ottawa Charter for Health Promotion.*
- Oxford Textbook of Medicine (2002) *The Maladies of Modernization: sickness in the system itself.* Edited by DJ Weatherall, JGG Ledingham and DA Worrell. Oxford University Press, Oxford.
- Palmer P (1998) *The Courage to Teach – exploring the inner landscape of a teacher's life.* Jossey-Bass, San Francisco, CA.
- Pappas G, Queen S, Hadden W and Fisher G (1993) The increasing disparity in mortality between socioeconomic groups in the United States, 1960 and 1986. *NEJM.* **329:** 103–9.
- Parchman M, Ferrer R and Blanchard S (2002) Geography and geographic information systems in family medicine research. *Family Medicine.* **34**(2): 132–7.
- Participants in the Bayer-Fetzer Conference on Physician–Patient Communication in Medical Education (2001) Essential elements of communication in medical encounters: the Kalamazoo consensus statement. *Academic Medicine.* **76**(4) 390–3.
- Patterson F (1979) *Photography and the Art of Seeing.* Van Nostrand Reinhold, Toronto.
- Patz JA, Epstein PR, Burke TA and Balbus JM (1996) Global climate change and emerging infectious diseases. *JAMA.* **275**(3): 217–23.
- Paul S, Dawson KP, Lanphear JH and Cheema MY (1998) Video recording feedback: a feasible and effective approach to teaching history-taking and physical examination skills in undergraduate paediatric medicine. *Med Educ.* **32**(3): 332–6.
- Pavis S, Cunningham-Burley S and Amos A (1998) Health related behavioural change in context: young people in transition. *Soc Sci Med.* **47**(10): 1407–18.
- Payer L (1988) *Medicine and Culture.* Penguin Books, New York.
- Payne M (2000) *Teamwork in Multiprofessional Care.* Lyceum Books, Chicago, IL.
- Pearlman DN, Rakowski W, Clark MA, Ehrich B, Rimer BK, Goldstein MG, Woolverton H, III and Dube CE (1997) Why do women's attitudes toward mammography change over time? Implications for physician–patient communication. *Cancer Epidemiol Biomarkers Prevention.* **6**(6): 451–7.
- Penchansky R and Macnee C (1994) Initiation of medical malpractice suits: a conceptualization and test. *Medical Care.* **32:** 813–31.
- Pendleton D, Schofield T, Tate P and Havelock P (1984) *The Consultation: an approach to learning and teaching.* Oxford University Press, Oxford.
- Peremans L, Hermann I, Avonts D, Van Royen P and Denekens J (2000) Contraceptive knowledge and expectations by adolescents: an explanation by focus groups. *Patient Educ Couns.* **40**(2): 133–41.
- Perry WG, Jr (1970) *Forms of Intellectual and Ethical Development in the College Years.* Holt, Rinehart and Winston, New York.
- Piaget J (1950) *The Psychology of Intelligence.* Harcourt Brace, New York.

- Piazza J, Conrad K and Wilbur J (2001) Exercise behavior among female occupational health nurses. Influence of self efficacy, perceived health control, and age. *AAOHN Journal*. **49**(2): 79–86.
- Plsek PE and Greenhalgh T (2001) Complexity science: the challenge of complexity in health care. *BMJ*. **324**: 625–8.
- Pommerenke FA and Dietrich A (1992) Improving and maintaining preventive services. Part 1: Applying the patient model. *Family Practice*. **34**(1): 86–91.
- Post SG, Puchalski CM and Larson DB (2000) Physicians and patient spirituality: professional boundaries, competency, and ethics. *Ann Int Med*. **132**(7): 578–83.
- Poulton BC and West MA (1999) The determinants of effectiveness in primary health care teams. *J Interprofessional Care*. **13**(1): 7–18.
- Power C, Li L and Manor O (2000) A prospective study of limiting longstanding illness in early adulthood. *Int J Epidemiol*. **29**(1): 131–9.
- Preven DW, Kachur EK, Kupfer RB and Waters JA (1986) Interviewing skills of first-year medical students. *J Med Educ*. **61**(10): 842–4.
- Prochaska JO, DiClemente CC and Norcross JC (1992) In search of how people change: applications to addictive behaviors. *American Psychologist*. **47**(9): 1102–14.
- Quill TE (1989) Recognizing and adjusting to barriers in doctor–patient communication. *Ann Int Med*. **111**(1): 51–7.
- Quill TE and Brody H (1996) Physician recommendations and patient autonomy: finding a balance between physician power and patient choice. *Ann Int Med*. **125**(9): 763–9.
- Ram P, Grol R, Rethans JJ, Schouten B, Van DC and Kester A (1999) Assessment of general practitioners by video observation of communicative and medical performance in daily practice: issues of validity, reliability and feasibility. *Med Educ*. **33**(6): 447–54.
- Redelmeier DA, Molin JP and Tibshirani RJ (1995) A randomised trial of compassionate care for the homeless in an emergency department. *Lancet*. **345**: 1131–4.
- Reifman A, Barnes GM, Dintcheff BA, Uhteg L and Farrell MP (2001) Health values buffer social-environmental risks for adolescent alcohol misuse. *Psychol Addictive Behav*. **15**(3): 249–51.
- Reilly P (1987) *To Do No Harm – a journey through medical school*. Auburn House, Dover, MA.
- Reiser D and Schroder AK (1980) *Patient Interviewing: the human dimension*. Williams and Wilkins, Baltimore.
- Rhoades DR, McFarland KF, Finch WH and Johnson AO (2001) Speaking and interruptions during primary care office visits. *Fam Med*. **33**(7): 528–32.
- Richlin L (1993) *New Directions for Teaching and Learning. Preparing faculty for the new conceptions of scholarship* (summer ed.). Jossey-Bass, San Francisco, CA.
- Ridsdale L, Morgan M and Morris R (1992) Doctors' interviewing technique and its response to different booking time. *Fam Pract*. **9**: 57–60.
- Rimal RN (2000) Closing the knowledge–behavior gap in health promotion: the mediating role of self-efficacy. *Health Commun*. **12**(3): 219–37.
- Rimal RN (2001) Analyzing the physician–patient interaction: an overview of six methods and future research directions. *Health Commun*. **13**(1): 89–99.
- Roberts LW, Warner TD, Lyketsos C, Frank E, Ganzini L and Carter D (2001) Perceptions of academic vulnerability associated with personal illness: a study of 1,027 students at nine medical schools. Collaborative Research Group on Medical Student Health. *Compr Psychiatry*. **42**(1): 1–15.

- Robinson WD, Priest LA, Susman JL, Rouse J and Crabtree BF (2001) Technician, friend, detective, and healer: family physicians' responses to emotional distress. *J Fam Pract.* **50**(10): 864–70.
- Roff S and McAleer S (2001) What is educational climate? *Medical Teacher.* **23**(4): 333–4.
- Rogers C (1951) *Client-centered Therapy – its current practice implications and theory.* Riverside Press, Cambridge, MA.
- Rogers C (1961) Significant learning. In: C Rogers (ed.) *On Becoming a Person.* Houghton Mifflin, Boston, MA.
- Roland MO, Bartholomew J, Courtenay MJ, Morris RW and Morrell DC (1986) The 'five minute' consultation: effect of time constraint on verbal communication. *BMJ (Clinical Research ed.).* **292**: 874–6.
- Rolland J (1989) Chronic illness and the family life cycle. In: B Carter and M McGoldrick (eds) *The Changing Family Life Cycle: a framework for family therapy.* Allyn and Bacon, Boston, MA.
- Rollnick S, Mason P and Butler C (1999) *Health Behavior Change: a guide for practitioners.* Churchill Livingstone, Edinburgh.
- Rose G (1981) Strategy of prevention: lessons from cardiovascular disease. *BMJ.* **282**: 1847.
- Rosenthal GE and Shannon SE (1997) The use of patient perceptions in the evaluation of health-care delivery systems. *Med Care.* **35**(11): NS58–68.
- Roter D (1989) Which facets of communication have strong effects on outcome – a meta-analysis. In: M Stewart and D Roter (eds) *Communication with Medical Patients.* Sage, Newbury Park, CA.
- Roter D and Hall J (1992) *Improving Psychosocial Problem Address in Primary Care: is it possible and what difference does it make?* The International Consensus Conference on Doctor–Patient Communication, Toronto.
- Roter DL (1977) Patient participation in the patient–provider interaction: the effects of patient question-asking on the quality of interaction, satisfaction and compliance. *Health Educ Monogr.* **5**(4): 281–315.
- Roter DL, Cole KA, Kern DE, Barker LR and Grayson M (1990) An evaluation of residency training in interviewing skills and the psychosocial domain of medical practice. *J Gen Intern Med.* **28**: 375–88.
- Roter DL, Stewart M, Putnam SM, Lipkin M, Jr, Stiles W and Inui TS (1997) Communication patterns of primary care physicians. *JAMA.* **277**(4): 350–6.
- Roter DL and Larson S (2001) The relationship between residents' and attending physicians' communication during primary care visits: an illustrative use of the Roter Interaction Analysis System. *Health Commun.* **13**(1): 33–48.
- Royal College of General Practitioners (2001) *Quality Team Development. Standards and criteria.* RCGP, London.
- Rudebeck CE (1992) General practice and the dialogue of clinical practice. *Scand J Prim Health Care.* Supp **1**: 1–94.
- Rudebeck CE (2002) Imagination and empathy in the consultation. *Br J Gen Pract.* **52**: 450–3.
- Sackett DL, Straus SE, Richardson WS, Rosenberg W and Haynes RB (2000) *Evidence-based Medicine. How to practise and teach EBM* (2e). Churchill Livingstone, New York.
- Sacks O (1982) *Awakenings.* Pan Books, London.
- Sacks O (1984) *One Leg to Stand On.* Gerald Duckworth, London.
- Sacks O (1986) Clinical tales. *Lit Med.* **5**: 16–23.
- Sacks O (1989) *Seeing Voices: a journey into the world of the deaf.* University of California Press, Berkeley, CA.

- Saltz CC and Schaefer T (1996) Interdisciplinary teams in health care: integration of family caregivers. *Soc Work Health Care.* **22**(3): 59–70.
- Salzman C (1995) Medication compliance in the elderly. *J Clin Psychiatry.* **56**(Supp 1): 18–22.
- Sanson-Fisher R and Maguire P (1980) Should skills in communicating with patients be taught in medical schools? *Lancet.* **2**: 523–6.
- Sanson-Fisher RW, Campbell EM, Redman S and Hennrikus DJ (1995) Patient–provider interactions and patient outcomes. *Diabetes Educator.* **15**: 134–8.
- Savage R and Armstrong D (1990) Effect of a general practitioner's consulting style on patients' satisfaction: a controlled study. *BMJ.* **301**: 968–70.
- Sawa RJ (1992) *Family Health Care.* Sage, Newbury Park, CA.
- Sbarbaro JA (1990) The patient–physician relationship: compliance revisited. *Ann Allergy.* **64**: 325–31.
- Scarf M (1995) *Intimate Worlds: life inside the family.* Random House, New York.
- Schamess G (1996) Ego psychology. In: J Berzoff, L Melano Flanagan and P Hertz (eds) *Inside Out and Outside In. Psychodynamic clinical theory and practice in contemporary multicultural contexts.* Jason Aronson, London.
- Scherger JE (1996) Does the personal physician continue in managed care? *J Am Board Fam Pract.* **9**(1): 67–8.
- Schlesinger EG (1985) *Health Care Social Work Practice. Concepts and strategies.* Times Mirror/Mosby College Publishing, St Louis, MO.
- Schoenbach VJ, Wagner EH and Karon JM (1983) The use of epidemiologic data for personal risk assessment in health hazard/health risk appraisal programs. *J Chronic Dis.* **36**(9): 625–38.
- Schön DA (1983) *The Reflective Practitioner: how professionals think in action.* Basic Books, New York.
- Schön DA (1987) *Educating the Reflective Practitioner.* Jossey-Bass, San Francisco, CA.
- Schwartz MA and Wiggins O (1985) Science, humanism, and the nature of medical practice: a phenomenological view. *Perspect Biol Med.* **28**(3): 331–66.
- Schwenk TL and Whitman NA (1987) *The Physician as Teacher.* William and Wilkins, Baltimore.
- Scott JG, Cohen D, DiCicco-Bloom B, Orzano AJ, Jaen CR and Crabtree BF (2001) Antibiotic use in acute respiratory infections and the ways patients pressure physicians for a prescription. *J Fam Pract.* **50**(10): 853–8.
- Seeman TE (1996) Social ties and health: the benefits of social integration. *Ann Epidemiol.* **6**(5): 442–51.
- Seifert MH, Jr (1992) Qualitative designs for assessing interventions in primary care: examples from medical practice. In: F Tudiver, MJ Bass and EV Dunn (eds) *Assessing Interventions: traditional and innovative methods.* Sage, Newbury Park, CA.
- Shaikh A, Knobloch LM and Stiles WB (2001) The use of a verbal response mode coding system in determining patient and physician roles in medical interviews. *Health Commun.* **13**(1): 49–60.
- Shanafelt TD, Bradley KA, Wipf JE and Back AL (2002) Burnout and self-reported patient care in an internal medicine residency program. *Ann Int Med.* **136**(5): 358–67.
- Shannon J, Kirkley B, Ammerman A, Keyserling T, Kelsey K, DeVellis R and Simpson RJ, Jr (1997) Self-efficacy as a predictor of dietary change in a low-socioeconomic-status southern adult population. *Health Educ Behav.* **24**(3): 357–68.
- Shapiro RS, Simpson DE, Lawrence SL, Talsky AM, Sobocinski KA and Schiedermayer DL (1989) A survey of sued and nonsued physicians and suing patients. *Arch Int Med.* **149**: 2109–96.

- Sherwood NE and Jeffery RW (2000) The behavioral determinants of exercise: implications for physical activity interventions. *Annu Rev Nutr*. **20**: 21–44.
- Silver HK and Glicken AD (1990) Medical student abuse – incidence, severity, and significance. *JAMA*. **263**(4): 527–32.
- Simon SR, Pan RJ, Sullivan AM, Clark-Chiarelli N, Connelly MT, Peters AS, Singer JD, Inui TS and Block SD (1999a) Views of managed care – a survey of students, residents, faculty, and deans at medical schools in the United States. *NEJM*. **340**(12): 928–36.
- Simon SR, Pan RJD and Block SD (1999b) Views of managed care. *NEJM*. **341**(8).
- Skeff KM and Mutha S (1998) Role models – guiding the future of medicine. *NEJM*. **339**: 2015–17.
- Skelton JR, Wearn AM and Hobbs FDR (2002) A concordance-based study of metaphoric expressions used by general practitioners and patients in consultation. *Br J Gen Pract*. **52**: 114–18.
- Smith GD, Hart C, Blane D, Gillis C and Hawthorne V (1997) Lifetime socioeconomic position and mortality: prospective observational study. *BMJ*. **314**: 547–52.
- Smucker DR, Zink T, Susman JL and Crabtree BF (2001) A framework for understanding visits by frequent attenders in family practice. *J Fam Pract*. **50**(10): 847–52.
- Sobel DS (2000) MSJAMA: mind matters, money matters: the cost-effectiveness of mind/body medicine. *JAMA*. **284**(13): 1705.
- Sotile WM and Sotile MO (2002) *The Resilient Physician – effective emotional management for doctors and their medical organizations*. American Medical Association, Chicago, IL.
- Sox CM, Swartz K, Burstin HR and Brennan TA (1998) Insurance or a regular physician: which is the most powerful predictor of health care? *Am J Public Health*. **88**(3): 364–70.
- Speidel J (2000) Environment and health: 1. Population consumption and human health. *CMAJ*. **163**(5): 551–6.
- Spiegel DA (1981) Motivating the student in the psychiatry clerkship. *J Med Educ*. **56**(7): 593–600.
- Squier RW (1990) A model of emphatic understanding and adherence to treatment regimens in practitioner–patient relationships. *Soc Sci Med*. **30**: 325–39.
- Stachtchenko S and Jenicek M (1990) Conceptual differences between prevention and health promotion: research implications for community health programs. *Canadian J Public Health*. **81**(1): 53–9.
- Stafford RS, Saglam D, Causino N, Starfield B, Culpepper L, Marder WD and Blumenthal D (1999) Trends in adult visits to primary care physicians in the United States. *Arch Fam Med*. **8**(1): 26–32.
- Stange KC, Zyzanski SJ, Jaen CR *et al*. (1998) Illuminating the 'black box': a description of 4454 patient visits to 138 family physicians. *J Fam Pract*. **46**: 377–89.
- Stapleton SR (1998) Team building. Making collaborative practice work. *J Nurse Midwifery*. **43**(1): 12–18.
- Starfield B, Wray C, Hess K, Gross R, Birk PS and D'Lugoff BC (1981) The influence of patient–practitioner agreement on outcome of care. *Am J Public Health*. **71**(2): 127–31.
- Starfield B (1998) *Primary Care. Balancing health needs, services, and technology*. Oxford University Press, New York.
- Starfield B (2001) New paradigms for quality in primary care. *Br J Gen Pract*. **April**: 303–9.
- Stein HF (1985a) What is therapeutic in clinical relationships? *Fam Med*. **17**(5): 188–94.
- Stein HF (1985b) *The Psycho-dynamics of Medical Practice. Unconscious factors in patient care*. University of California Press, Berkeley, CA.

- Stenhouse L (2001) Introduction to curricular research and development. In: JM Genn (ed.) *AMEE Medical Education Guide 23 (Part 1): curriculum, environment, climate, quality and change in medical education – a unifying perspective.* AMEE.
- Stensland P and Malterud K (1999) Approaching the locked dialogues of the body. Communicating symptoms through illness diaries. *Scand J Prim Health Care.* 17(2): 75–80.
- Stensland P and Malterud K (2001) Unravelling empowering internal voices – a case study on the interactive use of illness diaries. *Fam Pract.* 18(4): 425–9.
- Stephens GG (1982) *The Intellectual Basis of Family Practice.* Winter Publishing, Tucson, AZ.
- Stephens GG (1993) Patients on patienthood: new voices from the high-tech area. *J Am Board Fam Pract.* 6(2): 224–6.
- Stephenson S (2002) A memorable patient. No other medicine but only hope. *BMJ.* 324: 713.
- Stetten D, Jr (1981) Coping with blindness. *NEJM.* 305: 458.
- Stevens J (1974) Brief encounter. *J Royal Coll General Pract.* 24: 5–22.
- Stevenson FA, Barry CA, Britten N, Barber N and Bradley CP (2000) Doctor–patient communication about drugs: the evidence for shared decision making. *Soc Sci Med.* 50: 829–40.
- Stewart AL, Hays RD and Ware JE, Jr (1988) The MOS short-form general health survey. Reliability and validity in a patient population. *Med Care.* 26(7): 724–35.
- Stewart M and Roter D (1989) *Communicating with Medical Patients.* Sage, Newbury Park, CA.
- Stewart M, Brown JB and Weston WW (1989) Patient-centred interviewing III: five provocative questions. *Canadian Family Physician.* 35: 159–61.
- Stewart M, Brown JB, Weston WW, McWhinney IR, McWilliam CL and Freeman TR (1995) *Patient-Centered Medicine: transforming the clinical method.* Sage Publications, Thousand Oaks, CA.
- Stewart M (1995) Effective physician–patient communication and health outcomes: a review. *CMAJ.* 152(9): 1423–33.
- Stewart M, Brown JB, Boon H, Galajda J, Meredith L and Sangster M (1999) Evidence on patient–doctor communication. *Cancer Prev Control.* 3(1): 25–30.
- Stewart M, Brown JB, Donner A, McWhinney IR, Oates J, Weston WW and Jordan J (2000) The impact of patient-centred care on outcomes. *J Fam Pract.* 49(9): 796–804.
- Stewart M (2001) Towards a global definition of patient-centred care. *BMJ.* 322: 444–5.
- Stewart MA, McWhinney IR and Buck CW (1975) How illness presents: a study of patient behavior. *J Fam Pract.* 2(6): 411–14.
- Stewart MA and Buck CW (1977) Physicians' knowledge of and response to patients' problems. *Med Care.* 15(7): 578–85.
- Stewart MA, McWhinney IR and Buck CW (1979) The doctor/patient relationship and its effect upon outcome. *J Royal Coll General Pract.* 29: 77–81.
- Stewart MA (1984) What is a successful doctor–patient interview? A study of interactions and outcomes. *Soc Sci Med.* 19: 167–75.
- Stewart MA, Brown JB, Levenstein JH, McCracken EC and McWhinney IR (1986) The patient-centred clinical method III. Changes in residents' performance over two months of training. *Family Practice – An International Journal.* 3: 164–7.
- Stichler JF (1995) Professional interdependence: the art of collaboration. *Adv Pract Nurs Q.* 1(1): 53–61.
- Strasser T, Jeanneret O and Raymond L (1987) Ethical aspects of prevention trials. In: S Doxiadis (ed.) *Ethical Dilemmas in Health Promotion.* John Wiley and Sons, Toronto.

- Street RL, Jr and Millay B (2001) Analyzing patient participation in medical encounters. *Health Commun.* **13**(1): 61–73.
- Stuifbergen AK, Seraphine A and Roberts G (2000) An explanatory model of health promotion and quality of life in chronic disabling conditions. *Nurs Res.* **49**(3): 122–9.
- Styron W (1990) *Darkness visible.* Random House, New York.
- Suchman AL and Matthews DA (1988) What makes the patient–doctor relationship therapeutic? Exploring the connexional dimension of medical care. *Ann Int Med.* **108**(1): 125–30.
- Suchman AL, Botelho RJ and Hinton-Walker P (eds) (1998) *Partnerships in Healthcare: transforming relational process.* University of Rochester Press, Rochester, NY.
- Suchman AL (1998) Control and relation: two foundational values and their consequences. In: AL Suchman, RJ Botelho and P Hinton-Walker (eds) *Partnerships in healthcare: transforming relational process.* University of Rochester Press, Rochester, NY.
- Susser M (1993) A South Africa odyssey in community health: a memoir of the impact of the teachings of Sidney Kark. *Am J Public Health.* **83**(7): 1039.
- Svarstad BL (1985) The relationship between patient communication and compliance. In: DD Breimer and P Speiser (eds) *Topics in Pharmaceutical Science.* Elsevier, Amsterdam.
- Szasz TS and Hollender MH (1956) The basic model of the doctor–patient relationship. *Arch Int Med.* **97**: 585.
- Tait I (1979) *The history and function of clinical records.* Unpublished MD dissertation, University of Cambridge, Cambridge.
- Tarlow B (1996) Caring: a negotiated process that varies. In: S Gordon, P Benner and N Noddings (eds) *Caregiving. Readings in knowledge, practice, ethics, and politics.* University of Pennsylvania Press, Philadelphia, PA.
- Tate P, Foulkes J, Neighbour R, Campion P and Field S (1999) Assessing physicians' interpersonal skills via videotaped encounters: a new approach for the Royal College of General Practitioners Membership examination. *J Health Commun.* **4**(2): 143–52.
- Thom DH and Campbell B (1997) Patient–physician trust: an exploratory study. *J Fam Pract.* **44**(2): 169–76.
- Thomas KB (1978) The consultation and the therapeutic illusion. *BMJ.* **1**: 1327–8.
- Thomas KB (1987) General practice consultations: is there any point in being positive? *BMJ.* **294**: 1200–2.
- Thompson SC, Nanni C and Schwankovsky L (1990) Patient-oriented interventions to improve communication in a medical office visit. *Health Psychology.* **9**: 390–404.
- Thorsen H, Witt K, Hollnagel H and Malterud K (2001) The purpose of the general practice consultation from the patient's perspective – theoretical aspects. *Fam Pract.* **18**(6): 638–43.
- Tiberius RG (1986) Metaphors underlying the improvement of teaching and learning. *Br J Educ Technol.* **2**(17): 144–56.
- Tiberius RG, Sinai J and Flak E (2002) The role of teacher–learner relationships in medical education. In: GR Norman, CPM van der Vleuten and DI Newble (eds) *International Handbook of Research in Medical Education.* Kluwer Academic, Dordrecht.
- Toombs K (1992) *The Meaning of Illness: a phenomenological account of the different perspectives of physician and patient.* Kluwer Academic, Norwell, MA.
- Tough A (1979) *The Adult's Learning Projects: a fresh approach to theory and practice in adult learning* (2e). Ontario Institute for Studies in Education, Toronto.
- Toulmin S (1991) *Return to Reason.* Harvard University Press, Cambridge, MA.
- Toulmin S (1992) *Cosmopolis: the hidden agenda of modernity.* University of Chicago Press, Chicago.

- Towle A and Godolphin W (1999) Framework for teaching and learning informed shared decision making. *BMJ.* **319**: 766–71.
- Tresolini CP (1994) *Health Professions: education and relationship-centered care.* Fetzer Institute and the Pew Health Professions Commission, San Francisco, CA.
- Tuckett D, Boulton M, Olson C and Williams A (1985) *Meetings Between Experts: an approach to sharing ideas in medical consultations.* Tavistock, New York.
- Tudiver F, Brown JB, Medved W *et al.* (2001) Making decisions about cancer screening when the guidelines are unclear or conflicting. *J Fam Pract.* **50**(8): 682–7.
- Urquhart J (2001) The vision of Alistair MacLeod. In: I Guildford (ed.) *Alistair MacLeod – essays on his works.* Guernica, Toronto.
- US Preventive Services Task Force (1989) *Guide to Clinical Preventive Services: an assessment of the effectiveness of the 169 interventions.* Williams and Wilkins, Baltimore.
- Veatch R (1972) Models for ethical medicine in a revolutionary age. *Hastings Center Report.* **2**: 5.
- Verby JE, Holden P and Davis RH (1979) Peer review of consultations in primary care: the use of audiovisual recordings. *BMJ.* **1**: 1686–8.
- Vincent C, Young M and Phillips A (1994) Why do people sue doctors? A study of patients and relatives taking legal action. *Lancet.* **343**: 1609–13.
- Virshup BB, Oppenberg AA and Coleman MM (1999) Strategic risk management: reducing malpractice claims through more effective patient–doctor communication. *Am J Medical Quality.* **14**(4): 153–9.
- von Friederichs-Fitzwater MM and Gilgun J (2001) Relational control in physician–patient encounters. *Health Commun (Coding Provider–Patient Interaction).* **13**(1): 75–88.
- Waitzkin H (1984) The micropolitics of medicine. *Int J Health Sci.* **14**(3): 339–80.
- Wald PS and Brody MR (1999) Views of managed care. *NEJM.* **341**(8): 616–17.
- Walker EA, Gelfand A, Katon WJ, Koss MP, Von Korff M, Bernstein D and Russo J (1999) Adult health status of women with histories of childhood abuse and neglect. *Am J Med.* **107**(4): 332–9.
- Walker M (1988) Training the trainers: socialization and change in general practice. *Sociol Health Illness.* **10**: 282–302.
- Wanek V, Born J, Novak P and Reime B (1999) [Attitudes and health status as determinants of participation in individually oriented health promotion]. *Gesundheitswesen.* **61**(7): 346–52.
- Wasson JH, Sox HC and Sox CH (1981) Diagnosis of abdominal pain in ambulatory male patients. *Medical Decision Making.* **1**: 215–24.
- Wasylenki DA, Cohen CA and McRobb BR (1997) Creating community agency placements for undergraduate medical education: a program description. *CMAJ.* **156**(3): 379–83.
- Watson J (1984) *Health – a need for new direction. A task force on the allocation of health care resources.* Canadian Medical Association, Ottawa.
- Watson J (1985) *Nursing: human science and human care.* Appleton-Century-Crofts, New York.
- Watson WH and McDaniel SH (2000) Relational therapy in medical settings: working with somatizing patients and their families. *Psychother Pract.* **56**(8): 1065–82.
- Way D, Jones L, Baskerville B and Busing N (2001) Primary health care services provided by nurse practitioners and family physicians in shared practice. *CMAJ.* **165**(9): 1210–14.
- Ways P, Engel JD and Finkelstein P (2000) *Clinical Clerkships – the heart of professional development.* Sage, Thousand Oaks, CA.

- Webb E, Ashton CH, Kelly P and Kamah F (1998) An update on British medical students' lifestyles. *Med Educ*. **32**(3): 325–31.
- Weed LL (1969) *Medical Records, Medical Education and Patient Care*. Year Book Medical Publishers, Chicago.
- Weimer M (2002) *Learner-centered Teaching – five key changes to practice*. Jossey-Bass, San Francisco, CA.
- Westcott R (1977) The length of consultations in general practice. *J Royal Coll General Pract*. **27**: 552–5.
- Weston WW, Brown JB and Stewart MA (1989) Patient-centred interviewing. Part I: Understanding patients' experiences. *Canadian Family Physician*. **35**: 147–51.
- White KL (1988) *The Task of Medicine: dialogue at Wickenburg*. The Henry J Kaiser Family Foundation, Menlo Park, CA.
- Whitehead AN (1975) *Science and the Modern World*. Collins Fontana, San Francisco, CA.
- Whyte A and Burton I (1982) Perception of risks in Canada. In: I Burton and R McCullough (eds) *Living with risk*. Institute for Environmental Studies, University of Toronto, Toronto.
- Wiggers JH and Sanson-Fisher R (1997) Duration of general practice consultations: association with patient occupational and educational status. *Soc Sci Med*. **44**(7): 925–34.
- Williams M and Neal RD (1998) Time for a change? The process of lengthening booking intervals in general practice. *Br J Gen Pract*. **48**: 1783–6.
- Wilson A (1991) Consultation length in general practice: a review. *Br J Gen Pract*. **41**: 119–122.
- Wilson BM (1995) Promoting compliance: the patient–provider partnership. *Adv Renal Replacement Therapy*. **2**(3): 199–206.
- Wolfish MG and McLean JA (1974) Chronic illness in adolescents. *Pediatr Clin North Am*. **21**(4): 1043–9.
- Wood ML (1991) Naming the illness: the power of words. *Fam Med*. **23**(7): 534–8.
- Woods ME and Hollis F (1990) *Casework: a psychosocial therapy*. McGraw-Hill, New York.
- World Health Organization (1986a) Health promotion: a discussion document on the concept and principles, ICP/HSR 602. *Health Promotion*, WHO Reg Off Eur (reprinted). **1**: 736.
- World Health Organization (1986b) *Health Promotion: concept and principles in action – a policy framework*. WHO, London.
- Wright HJ and MacAdam DB (1979) *Clinical Thinking and Practice: diagnosis and decision in patient care*. Churchill Livingstone, Edinburgh.
- Wright SM, Kern DE, Kolodner K, Howard DM and Brancati FL (1998) Attributes of excellent attending-physician role models. *NEJM*. **339**: 1986–93.
- Wulff HR, Pedersen SA and Rosenberg R (1986) *Philosophy of Medicine: an introduction*. Blackwell Scientific Publications, Oxford.
- Yaffe MJ, Dulka IM and Kosberg JI (2001) Interdisciplinary health-care teams. What should doctors be aware of? *Canadian Journal CME*. **May**: 153–60.
- Yates FE (1993) Self-organizing systems. In: DNCAR Boyd (ed.) *The Logic of Life: the challenge of integrative physiology*. Oxford University Press, New York.
- Zwarenstein M and Bryant W (2001) *Interventions to Promote Collaboration between Nurses and Doctors* (Cochrane Review). Update Software, Oxford.
- Zyzanski SJ, McWhinney IR, Blake R, Crabtree B and Miller W (1992) Qualitative research: perspectives on the future. In: B Crabtree and W Miller (eds) *Doing Qualitative Research: research methods for primary care, vol. 3*. Sage, Newbury Park, CA.
- Zyzanski SJ, Stange KC, Langa D and Flocke SA (1998) Trade-offs in high-volume primary care practice. *J Fam Pract*. **46**: 397–402.

Index

psychomotor skills, patient-centered
 curriculum 233–4

realism, patient-centered clinical method
 component 5–7
realistic, being 131–48, 259–60
 case examples 144–5, 146–8
 learner-centered method of medical
  education 168, 181–3
 resources, accessing 142–5
 teamwork and teambuilding
  135–42
 time and timing 132–5
reflection on action 173
relationship, patient–doctor see
  patient–doctor relationship
religious issues 60–2
reorganization, illness stage 39–40
resources
 accessing 142–5
 case example 144–5
 and communication 143–5
 stewardship 142–5
return, MPCC 280
role models, teachers as 195–7
role play, teaching 213–14

self-awareness
 case examples 190–1
 need for 188–91
 patient–doctor relationship 125–6
smoking, case example 187–8
social support, proximal context
  factor 74–5
socio-historical circumstances, distal
  context factor 79
specific context 72–3
spiritual issues 60–2
Stephenson, S 126
stewardship, accessing resources
  142–5
substance abuse, medical students
  174–5
supervision, clinical, tips on 211–14
supervisory skills 177
support, mentoring 161
swallowing, case example 129–30
Sydenham, Thomas 19–20

teachers
 competing demands 194
 guidelines 165
 inexperience 193–4
 issues 199–200
 over-protectiveness 195
 as role models 195–7
 roles in teaching 207–10
teaching
 conceptual framework 212
 feedback 201, 204–7
 metaphors 154–6
 methods 177–8, 202–4
 patient-centered clinical method
  153–66, 185–97
 role play 213–14
 roles 207–10
 strategies 207, 208–11
 teacher roles 178
 videotape review 213
 see also learner-centered method of
  medical education
teamwork and teambuilding 135–42,
  181–3
 interdisciplinary teams 137–8
 interdisciplinary teamwork challenges
  139–42
 multidisciplinary teams 137–8
 team composition 138
 teams, defined 137–8
 transdisciplinary teams 137–8
technical competence, dealing with
  disease 156
time, patient-centered consultations
  132–3, 264–5
timing, patient-centered
  consultations 133–5
transdisciplinary teams 137–8
transference, patient–doctor relationship
  127–9
transformational journey, learning as
  158–9
transmission metaphor, teaching 154
treatment, goals 278
trust 120
 patient–doctor relationship 129–30

understanding the patient's world
  103–8